SPORTS
& EXERCISE
INJURIES

SPORTS & EXERCISE INJURIES

Conventional, Homeopathic & Alternative Treatments

Steven Subotnick

North Atlantic Books
Homeopathic Educational Services
Berkeley, California

Sports & Exercise Injuries:
Conventional, Homeopathic and Alternative Treatments

Copyright © 1991 by Steven Subotnick
ISBN 1–55643–114-7
All rights reserved

Published by
North Atlantic Books
P.O. Box 12327
Berkeley, California 94701
and
Homeopathic Educational Services
2124 Kittredge Street
Berkeley, California 94704

The illustrations on pages 297, 299, and 300 are excerpted from *Stretching,* © 1980 by Bob and Jean Anderson. $9.95, Shelter Publications, Inc., P.O. Box 279, Bolinas, California 94924. Distributed in bookstores by Random House. Reprinted by permission.

Cover photograph by Richard Blair
Cover and book design by Paula Morrison
Printed in the United States of America

Sports & Exercise Injuries: Conventional, Homeopathic and Alternative Treatments is sponsored by the Society for the Study of Native Arts and Sciences, a nonprofit educational corporation whose goals are to develop an educational and crosscultural perspective linking various scientific, social, and artistic fields; to nurture a holistic view of arts, sciences, humanities, and healing; and to publish and distribute literature on the relationship of mind, body, and nature.

Library of Congress Cataloging-in-Publication Data

Subotnick, Steven I.
    Sports and exercise injuries : conventional, homeopathic, and
alternative treatments / by Steven Subotnik.
      p.   cm.
    Includes index.
    ISBN 1-55643-114-7 : $18.95
    1. Sports medicine. 2. Sports—accidents and injuries—Alternative
treatment. 3. Sports—accidents and injuries—Homeopathic treatment.
I. Title.
    [DNLM: 1. Alternative Medicine. 2. Athletic Injuries—therapy.
3. Exercise. 4. Homeopathy. 5. Sports Medicine.   QT 260 S941s]
RC1210.S83 1991
617.1'027—dc20
DLNM/DLC
for Library of Congress   91-20892
                                                 CIP

To my wife, Janice and to my children, Mark, Ali and Kari for the love and happiness that they have brought into my life.

Acknowledgments

The impeccable faculty at the Hahnemann College of Homeopathy in Berkeley, California: Peggy Chipkin, Nancy Herrick, Bill Gray, Vicky Menear, Roger Morrison, Michael Quinn, and Jonathan Shore, have been invaluable in teaching me the spirit and practice of homeopathy. My colleague Dana Ullman, Director of Homeopathic Educational Services, inspired and encouraged me greatly in this project of bringing together an integrated approach to healing. His editorial comments were a core contribution. Carol Adrienne created the form of the book by organizing and writing the text and producing all the artwork including the original drawings at the beginning of each chapter. Lindy Hough brought her publishing knowledge of homeopathy and alternative therapies to bear in her meticulous editing. Barbara Howard was an early support in the process by typing the original notes for the work. And finally, my teacher and dear friend, Lazaris, gave the spark of inspiration that continues to light my way.

Contents

Chapter 1. The First Key to Health: Balance

Chapter 2. Biomechanics: You, Your Body, and Running

Chapter 3. Training For Runners, Walkers, and Sportspeople

Chapter 12. Knee Injuries

Chapter 13. Hip, Pelvis, and Groin Injuries

Chapter 14. Lower Back Injuries

Chapter 17. Arthritis and Sports

Chapter 18. Sports Injuries in Childhood and Adolescence

Chapter 19. The Aging Athlete

List of Illustrations

Chapter 3. Training for Runners, Walkers, and Sportspeople
Fig.

Chapter 6. Alternative Treatments
Fig.

Chapter 7. Basic First Aid
Fig.

Chapter 8. Foot Injuries
Fig.

Chapter 9. Heel Injuries
Fig.

Chapter 10. Ankle Injuries
Fig.

Chapter 11. Lower Leg Injuries
Fig.

Chapter 12. Knee Injuries
Fig.

Chapter 13. Hip, Pelvis, and Groin Injuries
Fig.

Chapter 14 Lower Back Injuries
Fig.

Chapter 15. Exercises
Fig.

Chapter 18. Sports Injuries in Childhood and Adolescence
Fig.

FOREWORD

I have known Dr. Steven Subotnick for over twenty years, and during that time I have been amazed at his many different fields of interest. He is truly a polymath: a person with a wide range of knowledge. This is unusual in medical professionals, who often become narrow specialists.

Dr. Subotnick has achieved widespread recognition in the field of podiatric medicine as a foot surgeon and an innovator in conservative management of foot diseases. He has also developed an integrative approach to foot health and sports medicine by using the various alternative modalities mentioned in this book—chiefly homeopathy—in combination with the most sophisticated developments from conventional medicine.

During my own forty year medical practice I have explored many techniques of alternative medicine, or as they say in England, "complementary medicine." As one of the first physicians to use acupuncture in the United States, I came in contact with holistic practitioners who not only opened my awareness to the importance of Chinese medicine but also to various other therapies as well.

Prior to 1900 15 percent of American physicians practicing in the United States used homeopathy. Twenty-two homeopathic colleges included some of the finest medical schools in the country—among them Boston University, the University of Michigan, and Hahnemann Medical College.

With the ascendancy of the pharmaceutical industry, homeopathy was literally driven from the American health scene for many decades — not because it was an invalid medicine for many ailments, but because it was an inexpensive system that prevented lucrative commercial markets from growing for the new "wonder" drugs. In the nineteen fifties Americans became interested in the very rapid "cure" of their ills which various conventional drugs promised. The side effects of chemically produced substances were not widely known. The pharmaceutical industry began to make much greater profits in producing medicines that we use today than they ever could have made in the manufacturing of homeopathic remedies, and medical researchers became occupied with developing commercial products rather than testing inexpensive and often commonly found remedies to "cure" common ailments. Patenting, licensing and selling new drugs, including vaccinations, became very lucrative. A look at the American stock market will show that drug industry stocks are at the top of the American market today, and have been since World War II.

The general public, however, is becoming more aware of the dangers of dependence on antibiotics, pain killers, tranquilizers, and various other drugs. They are currently joined by a growing number of practitioners who are exploring natural remedies which have few side effects. My own experience with acupuncture and homeopathy is perhaps typical of a type of physician who is looking beyond pharmaceutical samples and highly advertised products.

As a scientist trained to question any form of therapy which could not be explained in scientific terms, I was initially skeptical about the potential of acupuncture to provide any valid relief for my patients. As I worked with it, I began to have a great deal of success treating my patients with acupuncture, and have confirmed my results with double-blind research.

Much to my surprise, I have discovered that numerous other alternative therapies are also effective in treating acute and chronic health problems. Because these therapies are considerably safer than conventional medical treatments, I have been surprised and distressed that few of my fellow American medical collegues are seriously investigating these valuable alternatives.

Dr. Subotnick's enthusiasm for homeopathic medicines is the result of his spectacular successes in using it with patients, but he has also been affected, as we all have, by the growing body of research in Europe and England confirming the value of these natural medicines.

My own experience using the various alternative modalities covered by Dr. Subotnick has proven to me that combining various forms of therapy frequently brings about significant alleviation of a patient's health problem ... and changes the patient's attitude towards taking responsibility for the health care of his or her own body. This kind of work demands more patient involvement. The more you and your family know about the various treatment alternatives available, the more you can make decisions and become truly educated about different ways to treat sickness and injury.

Although this book deals primarily with injuries to the foot and lower extremities, the lessons to be learned from reading about the various homeopathic remedies and physical therapies available are a model that can be applied to the whole body. The comprehensive nature of this book and the pragmatic discussions it engages in certainly lead me to commend it for a general readership.

Ronald M. Lawrence, M.D.
President, American Medical Athletic Association;
Assistant Clinical Professor, Neuropsychiatric Institute,
UCLA School of Medicine.
July, 1991

PROLOGUE

A wise man should consider that health is the greatest of human
blessings, and learn how by his own thought to derive benefit from his
illnesses.

—Hippocrates 460–400 B.C.

There seems to be a purpose in even the most frustrating of experiences. I don't believe this book would have been written if it were
not for my son's serious illness about six years ago. It was because of
his seemingly miraculous recovery that I was introduced to homeopathy.

At that time Mark was fourteen and was battling recurring bouts
of serious bronchitis; three times it had progressed to pneumonia. As
a doctor and a parent, I felt doubly helpless when he did not seem to
get better after our family doctor prescribed the usual antibiotics.
There seemed to be nothing we could do.

My wife, Jan, however, had always been interested in less conventional methods of healing. She had started giving our family "health
foods" in the seventies, and had been interested in acupuncture and
hypnosis. She investigated homeopathy after a friend had been cured
of a chronic ear problem with homeopathic remedies when conventional medicine failed. I had to admit that I didn't like the idea of repeatedly using antibiotics on Mark since they can sometimes depress
the body's immune system, and after awhile the body builds up a resistance to them.

So Jan decided to take Mark to a homeopath. She took him to
see Dr. William Gray at the Hahnemann Clinic in Berkeley, California.
I thought, "Well, it can't hurt."

However, when she came home and said that the doctor had given
Mark a super-dilute dose of mercury, I really panicked. Mercury is a
poison. It causes diseases like Minamata disease, an illness resembling
multiple sclerosis. Since he'd already taken the remedy, there was
nothing I could do but wait.

During the first day Mark got much sicker. He went to bed and
slept. I worried about him all night. But, he woke up in the morning
much better. I was amazed. I'd never seen a recovery like that.

Over the following year, he had two more bouts of bronchitis. Both times he took the homeopathic mercury, and each time the infection cleared up overnight. Since then, he has not had another attack of bronchitis.

During that first year, I happened to have a few patients with chronic medical conditions who had also found improvement with homeopathy after conventional medicine had not worked. Obviously, in light of my own observations of Mark, I was beginning to be intrigued about this type of medicine. Soon thereafter, I met Dana Ullman, director of Homeopathic Educational Services in Berkeley, California. He asked me if I would be willing to participate in a clinical trial using homeopathic medicines for my patients with various sports injuries. I read a considerable amount of literature on homeopathy and came to the conclusion that it might just be a fantastic adjunct to my conventional medical procedures.

What appealed to me about this system (described in more detail in Chapter 5) is that it's safe, the remedies are inexpensive, and they often have positive and lasting effects on the immune system. Homeopathic medicines do not have side effects. How such a small dose of a substance can do anything at all involves the mystery of "potentizing" a remedy. Suffice to say that homeopathy has been used for generations in Europe, England, Australia and this country, and preceeded pharmaceutical drugs. The history of homeopathy and its relation to American medicine is ably described in Harris Coulter's *Divided Legacy: The Conflict Between Homeopathy and the American Medical Association* (North Atlantic Books).

I first used the remedies for conditions such as Achilles tendinitis, heel spur syndrome, plantar fasciitis, shin splint, painful runner's knee, overuse exhaustion with aching muscles, and generalized stiffness. The results were surprisingly good. These homeopathic remedies improved the overall condition of my patients and helped their specific symptoms. I remember two cases that were quite interesting.

The first was June, the wife of a patient of mine. She was a good runner, quite active in sports and a great tennis player. She came to me with a painful knee. When I asked about her medical history, she said she had been using cortisone for ten years for Crohn's disease, an inflammatory bowel disease.

Her knee was quite swollen, and her characteristics fit the homeopathic remedy *Ruta Grav.* I gave her this remedy for the knee problem plus temporary orthotics for her running shoes and tennis shoes.

The next time I saw June, about two weeks later, she told me that her Crohn's disease had gone away. She no longer needed the cortisone, and her knee eventually healed up. Needless to say, I was very excited. When I studied some more about *Ruta Grav*, I found that it is also beneficial for inflammation—which explains why it worked on her inflamed bowel as well as her swollen knee. This really hit home to me about treating the whole person.

The second example was a gentleman about sixty-five who came in complaining of a very sore heel. He had heel spur syndrome and bursitis at the back of the heel. I made him some orthotics, and gave him *Ruta Grav* for the heel problem. As it happened he also had prostatitis (inflammation of the prostate.) He called not long after I gave him the remedy to tell me that his prostatitis had gone away along with the bursitis in the heel!

These two examples got me to thinking that a homeopathic remedy can take care of a lot more than just the symptom in the leg, knee, or foot. These experiences with my son and my patients convinced me that homeopathy has a useful place in our current medical system for both prevention and treatment.

Modern, orthodox medicine is often extolled for its ability to diagnose disease, to correct surgically, to treat trauma, to ease pain, and to give relief. Indeed, we would all be at a great loss without the strides the medical profession has made. Modern medicine has the capacity to add days, if not years to life. With the wizardry of technical advancements, it can also add quality to life, as well as length.

Unfortunately, the very things that give modern medicine its power—quick-acting drugs, pain-suppressing medicine, specialized disciplines—also can interfere with true healing. Modern medicine has responded beautifully to our—the consumer/patient's—demand for a "quick-fix." Pain-killers eradicate the pain sometimes instantly. Western medicine excels in the science of diagnosis. We applaud the expertise of the specialist who, after examining and testing a millimeter of your tissue, locates and names the "problem." Thanks to ever-advancing diagnostic and surgical techniques such as magnetic resonance imaging and arthroscopy, to name only two, we can travel micro-scopically throughout your body. Science has forever influenced how we attend to ourselves in illness.

Yet we have all experienced the typical scenario of a five or ten-minute visit with an orthodox medical doctor, which most often results in a prescription for a pill. We go away with a drug—a drug that often merely exchanges one disease for another, one problem for another. The drug may be as invasive and possibly as harmful as the virus or illness that has overtaken our defense system. The drug is not designed to truly heal, although it may take care of the symptoms. It is designed to suppress symptoms.

In the average conventional treatment, you, the patient, are never known as a person with a life history that speaks through your medical history. Your specialist, or team of specialists, has looked at a piece of you but never looked into your eyes or held your hand or talked with you about how your life is really going. Your original complaint becomes something to be suppressed, gotten rid of, with no real understanding of what its message is for you at this time in your life. The doctor goes on to the next patient, the next prescription, with the limited, albeit admirable, goal of adding days to your life.

But what of adding life to your days? Isn't that the real goal? Wouldn't you rather have days filled with joy and aliveness instead of merely more days devoid of the vitality of true health? What is true health? I have given this a lot of thought, both as a doctor and as a man, a father, a husband, and even as a runner.

True health, as I see it, encompasses more than just the absence of disease in the physical body. True health is living with the magic of desire, the expectation of realizing dreams, and the miracle of self-creation. Indira Gandhi once said,

> Wellness is not the absence of illness but a glowing vitality, a feeling of wholeness with a capacity for continuous intellectual and spiritual growth.

Homeopathy, naturopathic medicine, and alternative therapies, when properly chosen, can add life to days. Why is this? For one thing, these systems of natural remedies are oriented around health—being healthy and staying healthy—not disease. For example, homeopathy and naturopathy emphasize prevention, and treat you according to the type of person you are—not for a specific disease symptom—so that your immune system is as strong as possible to do its job of protecting the whole of you. Natural remedies enhance the healing power you were born with. They help you stay tuned to the unparalleled inner guidance that is always present if you choose to pay attention.

Secondly, homeopathy and alternative treatments assist you to come into balance—your balance. Each of us is an individual, and no two people will heal in exactly the same way. Natural medicines boost your ability to deal with not just your present symptoms, but your whole constitution—including physical, mental, emotional, and spiritual dimensions. Good natural health practitioners are as interested in your level of joy and spiritual connection as in the level of your cholesterol. I like what George Leonard said in *The Silent Pulse:*

> At the heart of each of us, whatever our imperfections, there exists a silent pulse and a perfect rhythm, a complex wave of forms and resonances, which is absolutely individual and unique, and connects us to everything in the universe.

Thirdly, natural remedies are safe and non-toxic. They can be used by you and your family for self-medication with no harmful side-effects. As a matter of fact, the side effect you might experience is increased self-esteem and personal power as a result of your higher level of participation in your health and the health of those you love.

By using alternative medicines or therapies either in combination with orthodox medicine or instead of orthodox medicine, you are not simply replacing prescription drugs for natural remedies. The real benefit is the opportunity to learn more about the care and keeping of body, mind, and soul.

Our way of life in the West has demanded that we accept and adjust to increased demands on our time. We forego rest and nurturing mealtimes, for example, in favor of rushing to meetings and duties. We tend to see ourselves at the effect of the outer world, demanding, therefore, medicine that fixes the outer symptoms . . . quickly. The scientific focus on cures for specific diseases has led us to believe that someone else with specialized knowledge will assume responsibility for our health. Instead of paying attention to the level of suitability, harmony and satisfaction in our worklife and homelife, we focus on how good a health insurance plan we have—assuming, then, that we have taken care of our future health.

Changing your reference point from a "victim of the times" mentality to one of personal responsibility means that you will have to recognize that you are ill or healthy by your own choice. The true teaching of illness brings you to the realization that, at some level, you are responsible for what you have created. At that point, you add life to your days, and, in so doing, truly heal yourself, not just suppress your suffering.

Symptoms all have a message as well as a cause. Symptoms manifested are a call for healing—a blinking red light to "stop, and look both ways," perhaps to change directions, perhaps to continue along your way. A symptom may indicate that it's time to forgive yourself for something, heal and go on with your life. The truth is, you either allow or create your illness or injury more than you realize.

Many of my patients are dedicated runners, and many are determined to follow a healthy walking program. When they do get an injury, they arc often very hard on themselves, sometimes angry or depressed because they were, they thought, doing the "healthy thing." I try to explain to them that it does no good to beat yourself up or to belittle yourself for having an injury or illness. All illness, even your running injury, is a lesson. The lesson may be to slow down, or stop being so compulsive—not only with your running, but perhaps in other areas, too.

One of my favorite stories about how insights or perceptions can be revealed through our sport comes from *Golf In The Kingdom*, by Michael Murphy. The narrator, a golf pro, was haunted by a recurring thought:

> "You're not lined up straight." It kept creeping into my thoughts as I was playing. "You're not lined up straight." I tried to adjust my swing and stance, but the thought persisted week after week. Slowly, inexorably, the meaning came clear; indeed I was not lined up straight, in my work, with my friends, during most of the day. I was sleeping in my office then, rising to telephone calls . . . doing business over every meal. I was as disorganized as I had ever been and my unconscious knew it . . . only during a round of golf did I slow down enough for the word to get through.

Use your running as a way to enjoy life, not to cover up or avoid what's really going wrong—a relationship that's not working, a career that you hate. You can escape the world by running, and sometimes that's healthy because running is an excellent way to deal with stress. But when you deny feelings and problems in your life, focusing only on running or any sport as a way to achieve a goal or avoid relationships, eventually the blinking red light of illness or injury goes on.

Let your walks or runs, your bike rides or swims, be quiet times; get to know yourself. Tune in to what I call "the whispers." The whispers tell you what's really going on—if you're on-course or if you're off-course. If you don't listen to the whispers—those initial aches and pains—or, if you don't attend to your anxiety or repressed anger, you will hear shouts, loud warnings like a foghorn in the night. These are the more serious injuries and illnesses: perhaps a badly sprained ankle, a consistently aching hip or high blood-pressure. If you continue to ignore the foghorns, then don't be surprised at a broken bone, an ulcerated colon, cancer, or a heart attack while running. Even these illnesses allow you the opportunity to change—to forgive yourself, heal and move on. Your health and well-being are a manifestion of your consciousness, level of development, and insight.

The fact that you are reading this page is an indication that you are willing to learn more about yourself, and participate in your own health. I realized a few years ago, that patients usually came to a doctor when they had *already* made a decision to get well. Basically, you give yourself permission to get well. A doctor can't do that for you. In the past, the doctor functioned as rabbi, priest, counselor or shaman to provide the setting and the stage for healing to occur. There is no healing without a change of awareness. The doctor agrees that yes, it's time to get well, and, in essence, gives his or her permission to the patient to begin the healing process. As doctors, we try to suspend the disease long enough for the body to reprogram its beliefs and attitudes and get well.

Interestingly enough, when you empower your health practitioner (by giving him or her your confidence and attention), you should be taking back your own power to begin healing. Once you have made that decision to heal, almost any kind of treatment will be successful because *the power is within you to heal.* I think of myself (as the doctor) as providing the *context* while you, the patient provides the *content* of healing energy. Don't fret endlessly over whether you have made the right decision in a doctor, whether or not traditional medicine is better or worse than alternative treatments. Trust that your body will tell you what is working, what is right. Get all the information you can, then use your intuition.

Another important point about the healing interaction between doctor and patient is that it works both ways. As a doctor, I am very aware that my patients, those particular people who have chosen to work with *me*, are my teachers and mirrors for issues that need work within myself. When I treat people, I am essentially treating myself. What I see as fears in my patients, I recognize as fears within myself. I have learned to pay attention to how I feel with each person, because in becoming "at one" with them, my intuition usually leads me not only to the right treatment for them, but also to my own self-discovery. Many health practitioners, such as psychotherapists, have learned that our feelings and emotions during the treatment interaction give us incredibly rich and relevant information.

There is no such thing as an observer. You're either an active participant or a passive participant. If you're active, you are "responding" (being responsible). If you're passive, you're asking other people to be responsible. So many times, people give their power away in the conventional medical setting. "You're the doctor, tell me what to do."

Healing is a dynamic, ongoing process. It's not static. You are continually renewing your committment to wholeness and wellness by the choices you make every day regarding your diet, exercise, friendships, pastimes, and the means by which you choose to educate yourself.

My goal in this book is to help you pick and choose among the many healing approaches, to guide you as much as I can towards what may best suit you and your injury. Together we will explore the modalities, the therapies, the remedies or prescriptions. I want to help you add life to your days—and may your days be many!

Steve Subotnick
Doctor of Podiatric Medicine, M.S.

HOW TO USE THIS BOOK

This book is designed for people who want to take a more active and informed role in treating and planning their fitness program to prevent injuries.

The first three chapters provide an overview of fitness principles and biomechanics of sensible training for beginning and advanced runners, walkers, and other sportspeople. Chapters 4 and 5 describe conventional and homeopathic treatment of sports injuries. The major questions people have when they begin to use homeopathy are answered in Chapter 5. Further descriptions of homeopathy are available through the resource list in Chapter 20. Treatment modalities which are useful in healing sports injuries and bringing the body to relaxed health are described in Chapter 6. Chapters 8 to 14 deal specifically with foot, heel, ankle, lower leg, knee, pelvis, and back injuries, showing how alternative and conventional treatments can be combined. First aid—what to do at the moment of injury—is treated in Chapter 7.

Some treatment in this book is appropriate for self-care. In other instances, you will need to see a practitioner, whether a podiatrist, a homeopath, a sports medicine medical professional like myself who uses and recommends a wide range of alternative treatments as well as orthodox medicine. My intention is to give you an over-view of the possibilities for integrating conventional treatment with homeopathic remedies and body work therapies, internal martial arts, physical therapies and age-old arts like T'ai Chi, Chi Gong and yoga.

Chapter 1

THE FIRST KEY TO HEALTH: BALANCE

I live in light's extreme; I stretch in all directions; sometimes I think I'm several.

—Theodore Roethke

"I just didn't want to 'give-in' to that pain I kept feeling in my knee—with the race only two days away," admitted Patrick, my patient whose leg had given out four minutes into the San Francisco Bay-to-Breakers marathon after six months of progressive training. What he said made me smile, a bit ruefully, because I, too, have had those exact feelings of wanting to push through to my goal no matter what.

As he was speaking, I saw myself training for that same race several years ago—training, sometimes straining, gasping like a snorting draught-horse, a far-off checkered goal in my mind. I can still smell those days, all those days of running, running through drizzle and downpour in my rain jacket, hood pulled up and breath steaming in the dark when I ran before work. Listening to Patrick, I knew that the thought of missing the race, of having to wait another year, had kept him running in spite of his pain. I knew, too, that he didn't want to admit defeat to Matt, his friend and training buddy; he didn't have to tell me that. I knew the feeling. I knew all about the feeling of invulnerability, pride, expectation of a new personal record, not to mention the camaraderie. Half the fun of the race was goofing around with my pals, Rob and Joe, at the picnic our wives always made after the big run. Not to run? Not to participate? Unthinkable. Patrick was the same intense kind of runner I used to be.

How do you talk about balance to a lover? Runners are lovers. We love it all—well, let's be honest. Anybody who says he loves to exercise is lying. Nobody who runs likes getting ready to run, or the initial fifteen to thirty minutes into it, when they're stiff and just warming

1

up. Sometimes it takes a *lot* of strength just to open the door on a dark morning when the wind is raging. Thoughts of turning back or of taking just a short run almost always come up for me as I'm starting to lope down the driveway with the sun coming up behind the houses in my neighborhood.

Another patient of mine, Tom Robinson, who helped promote Dr. George Sheehan's new book on running, made the comment, "George, you must love to run and exercise." Dr. Sheehan replied, "No. I hate to run!" Now, George Sheehan, cardiologist, author, speaker, and runner is a man who has built a philosophy and a career around running. His reply stunned Tom; in fact, he said, it changed his life because he thought everybody who ran, loved it, and since he didn't love it, he decided there was no reason to do it. "From that time on," Tom told me, "I started to run, and the more I ran the more I loved it, and, at the same time, the more I hated it."

I can well understand what George and Tom mean. I start loving my daily run after about three miles, or about a half-hour. At that point, running is not only a great idea, but a great feeling. Then I begin to think I just might keep going a little more after all. I love the temporary loneliness and the rushing quiet, and the awareness of the work my lungs and legs are doing. Running gets me back in touch with my soul. Running helps me remember I'm an animal, a body that is connected to the earth. My philosophical soul goes a little wild when I run.

But now in the office with Patrick, the doctor in me begins to explore his knee joint, to examine the wear patterns on his shoes, and to discuss how long he's had the pain. Besides addressing the mechanical factors of shoes and arch supports, I talk with him, as I do with many patients, about how his mental attitudes, in combination with the biomechanical stresses, have contributed to this injury.

When the body has to compensate for an anatomical imbalance—in his case, one short leg—the available energy (which is not unlimited) is split between maintaining balance and the goal of winning the race. The body is thrown off-balance by trying to achieve two goals at the same time. For example, at the starting line of the race, the valiant part of him is excited, saying, "Wow, this is great. Let's do it! Let's go. Only 26 miles. Look at these other people. Hey, if they can do it, so can I—I'm in good shape. At least I'll finish. Hey, what's this race going to be like today? Let's find out." The other part, the voice of the knee pain, is saying "Excuse me, but has anybody looked down

2

here at this knee joint lately? Has anybody looked inside at this bone? This bone is starting to crack."

Staying on Track

When your mind and emotions have one set of goals and your body has another, you are not in balance. A portion of your available physical energy is drained away, diverted from your mind's objective. The conflict between mind and body leads to fatigue and fatigue leads to injury because the body *doesn't care if you win a race.* Your body, you can be sure, monitors the big picture.

Good health is a matter of balance and integration in the four dimensions of your life. When you feel great, there is an abundant, ready energy in your physical body, a teasing joy in your heart, clarity in your mind and spirit, and a sense of union that is still best described by the old cliche "all's right with the world." In harmony, you function elegantly—that is, you achieve the best results with the least amount of effort.

Sports and exercise are considered healthy outlets for emotional upsets such as anger or depression. However, sports and exercise can also become an obsession or replacement for other, less successful, parts of our lives. Any of the positive qualities that athletics require can become potentially harmful, just like any other imbalance. Perfectionism, controlling behavior, anxiety, willfulness, self-criticism, and impatience grow well in the fertile ground of negative addiction.

Check yourself out. Are you feeling an inordinate amount of anxiety about your body or your racing time? Do you feel depressed even after a run? Do you resent family responsibilities that take you away from perfecting your form? Do you think your wife is being unreasonable when she says she doesn't want to eat dinner at nine o'clock every night so that you can have time to shower after your run? Emotional imbalance is sometimes very subtle: "Sure, I'll run two marathons this month. It'll be fun to see if I can do it." Sometimes imbalance even seems "justifiable": "Look, if I want to run six days a week, I'll run six days a week. Besides, you were the one that said I needed to lose weight." Emotional imbalance, or lack of perspective, results in uneasy feelings, blaming, and resentment, as well as subtle types of revenge—all of which may jeopardize not only your happiness, but also your health. Sometimes an injury is the only way to alert you to your lack of perspective.

3

Weekend Warriors

One example of lack of judgment is the fifty-five-year-old "week-end warrior" who, blinded by his desire to prove he's still able to perform, plays basketball all day Saturday after months or years of inactivity. Another example is a forty-year-old secretary who, sedentary for years, runs around a track for two months, preparing for a 26-mile run on an uphill course. These examples may seem ludicrous until you meet some of the people who limp or hobble into a doctor's office.

Remember how a baby starts the adventure of walking about the age of nine, ten or twelve months? She starts out hanging onto any convenient prop like a chair leg, letting go just a little bit, and finally, just when you turned your head away, takes a little tiny step on wobbly legs until she lands back on her bottom? A trip across the room is going to take perhaps a few weeks. Each day the little body gets up, takes a step, gets rave reviews from mom and dad, and crumples up just enough to keep her humble but undaunted. This automatic process of two steps forward and one step backward is what the pediatricians at this point call regression—just a little slowing down to give her body time to integrate the accomplishments, and keep her from overdoing her exciting advancement.

When you're fifty-five, though, you're too smart, too good at outsmarting yourself, too strong-willed to take small steps gradually. You overdo by only being able to feel or value your body when it's straining.

In the beginning, your enthusiasm for running or for a fast-paced game may only result in aching muscles which reprimand you silently the next day—if you're lucky, that is, and don't go down in a cardiac arrest on the handball court. Later on, if you become "hooked" on exercise or training for sports, you may lose sight of the healthy reasons why you run or play. You become controlled by the rigid thinking so favored by the negative ego.

Dis-ease also occurs when you lose your spiritual balance and become disconnected from others and from the Universe or God. In this state, you feel separated, superior or inferior to others, isolated. A mild case of spiritual imbalance, or warped values, is the adolescent who will "die" unless he or she has the right brand of running shoes. Without the spiritual connection to life, you lose your sense of purpose and invent false purposes, looking for outside validation. Eventually, you create failure.

Spiritual poverty also surfaces as a "me-first" attitude: egotism, selfishness and being a poor loser. For example, a patient I'll call William, a long-distance runner, suffered severe depression after an injury on the trail prevented him from running for three months. He sulked, blamed his coach, became irritated with medical advice, and belittled the winner of a subsequent marathon he was forced to sit out. Both his work and family life suffered through his period of recuperation. Life held little interest for him. He was one of the people that brought my attention to the four phases of running.

The Four Phases of Running

Through my own experiences as a runner, and from observations of my patients, I have come to distinguish four psychological stages of running which, I believe, are common to all athletes. I have patients in all four categories—The Beginning Runner, The Casual Runner-Racer, The Obsessive Runner-Racer, and the Seasoned Runner. I have seen first hand the evolution of the beginning runner into the obsessive runner-racer.

Running is a form of adult play, which means that it is voluntary and isn't seen as particularly productive although its health benefits are usually the motivating factor in the first run. Phase 1—beginning runners—run for fun, to reduce stress and to stay in shape. Running, like other sports is a special kind of play in that it involves physical prowess that is purposefully developed over time, unlike the natural unconscious physical development of children. An article by J. L. Sacks on the psychodynamics of sports mentions two motivations for adult sports.[1] Adults choose to play sports as a relief from boredom, as a means of expressing aggression and as a drive toward mastery. People who play sports are, in a way, finding the child within themselves. In using the body for running, dancing, and other forms of "play," people can regain an earlier state of spontaneity, omnipotence, freedom, safety and connection with others. Sometimes sports bring out an almost adolescent response when emotions run high because of "conflicts regarding sexuality, aggression, exhibitionism and narcissism which can all be expressed in athletics."[2] An athlete, particularly the elite athlete, who finds his or her sport to be the place where inner conflicts are being resolved may face severe depression and feelings of helplessness when injured.

Take the case, for instance, of two cyclists: Marjorie who cycles 5 miles a day to work and enjoys a ten-mile spin on the weekends, and

Melanie, a marathon cyclist who competes professionally. If Marjorie accidentally injures her leg and can't ride for six weeks, she takes it in stride, knowing she'll resume cycling when she heals. Melanie, on the other hand, may experience withdrawal symptoms such as dissatis-faction, restlessness, anxiety and fidgeting. She may become very irri-table, have difficulty sleeping, and can develop gastrointestinal symptoms. She may isolate herself from family and friends and stop communicating. To the extent that she feels "invincible," she may dis-regard her doctor's advice which makes treatment very complicated. Melanie is the type of athlete that puts exercise over everything else.

With luck, many obsessive runner-racers eventually turn into mel-low, seasoned runners, although it may be via the painful route of over-stress or traumatic injury. Seasoned runners value their running to the extent that they will not race if it means risking an injury that would limit running altogether. I am now happy to say, by the way, that I am a firmly established Phase 4 runner.

Phase 1: The Beginning Runner

You are the casual, beginning runner. You may be a bit overweight and out of shape, and are entering the sport after having had months or years away from regular exercise. You tend to be consistent in your running, yet easygoing—usually going 3 miles, four or five days a week. Your total weekly mileage is around twelve to fifteen, which fits well within the guidelines for sensible aerobic fitness. Most likely your time is about 8 to 9.5 minutes per mile.

As you continue running, you notice a gradual firming of the body, along with a loss of weight. You have more energy during the day, a bet-ter attitude, and generally accomplish more with greater ease than you did when not running. Your thoughts are clear, and you look for-ward to a relaxing run. At this stage, you seldom experience the "run-ner's high," and are not dependent on the chemicals the body produces during running, endorphins and enkephalins, that cause this feeling of euphoria. You are probably involved in other sports such as golf or tennis as well as running.

Phase 2: The Casual Runner-Racer

You are the runner who occasionally races—serious, but not obsessed about running. You average about 30 miles a week and tend to run 5 to 7 miles a day. You may even, occasionally, run a 5 or 10 km race. You will rarely train for a marathon. At this stage, you enjoy the benefits of the runner's high and use running for stress reduction. With a healthy sense of proportion, you have no qualms about taking a vacation or missing a week or two of running. If injured, you follow instructions to cut down on mileage and are very cooperative in rehabilitative programs.

Phase 3: The Obsessive Runner-Racer

You are the obsessive-compulsive runner. At this stage, you are psychologically and physiologically dependent on the runner's high and the chemicals released during the exercise. You feel guilty missing workouts or performing poorly and may choose to run rather than make business or personal appointments. You devote at least 90 minutes a day to your workout. You run under 8 minutes per mile.

You may be young, gifted, or training for a career in sports, or even headed for the Olympics. On the other hand, you may use running to escape or resolve other problems. For instance, some of you are going through a divorce, trying to lose weight, or changing your career. In personal interactions, you tend to be over-talkative and a poor listener, often impatient and critical.

Because you have trained so hard, you are prone to feel invincible, assuming that you are invulnerable to injury. You generally do not want to take responsibility for your injuries and blame your doctor or even family members if you do not recover rapidly. Irrationally, you praise your doctor for improvements one moment, and the next moment blame him or her for a prolonged recovery or for a poor performance. During recovery, you tend to become depressed, angry, and quarrelsome.

Your enforced time out from sports or running is painful and boring. You convince yourself that, unless you have a legitimate medical diagnosis, your friends or colleagues will see you as a quitter or a failure. Your recovery is most successful if you're given a strong program of physical therapy and rehabilitation, lots of reassurance, and help with redefining goals. You are clearly addicted to sports, for better or worse. Your withdrawal depression is *real*. Frank Shorter, who has been labelled as "the man who invented the marathon", exemplifies the Phase 3 runner with the statement quoted in *The Lore of Running* by Dr. Tim Noakes, "The same personality—independent, introverted, single-minded, self-reliant, self-confident, distrusting—that enabled me to excel as an athlete in full health, hindered me when I became an athlete in pain."[3]

How does the personality profile of a Phase 3 runner compare to other psychological states? Studies on negative addiction in sports by Yates and colleagues published in the *New England Journal of Medicine* found that there are apparent similarities between anorexics (people who starve themselves out of the pathological idea they are too fat) and "obligatory runners"[4] (the Phase 3 runner). However, if you are a Phase 3 runner (or the equivalent in other sports), you are not necessarily *pathological;* nevertheless, you may have some of the characteristics of the anorexics: inhibition and difficulty in expressing anger, a tendency to social isolationism, high self-expectation, high tolerance for physical discomfort, undue concerns about weight and diet, and a strong denial system about potentially serious physical ailments which lead to overuse injuries. Two other characteristics found in the Yates study, compliance and self-effacing behavior, differ from my experience of Phase 3 runners as typical Type A personalities.

At the extreme, when running becomes an end in itself, any injury which deprives a person of that end triggers a sense of great loss and mourning. To avoid the sense of loss and grief, an addicted runner will do everything possible to start running again—even before healing has been completed (as found in studies by Blumenthal and colleagues).[5] Manuel Cortez, a psychotherapist who works with many athletes, substantiated this phenomenon of mourning in a presentation to the *American Academy of Podiatric Sports Medicine:*

> In treating many dedicated athletes, I have observed the development of a mourning state similar to that associated with any significant loss upon deprivation of the exercise, usually because of injury. Most notably, this has been observed in endurance athletes such as long-distance runners. The more "addicted" these athletes are to their activity, the more pronounced the mourning process.[6]

If you feel you are obsessed by your running, you may have already experienced the sequence of responses to an injury. For example, the first stage after injury is a massive denial of the extent of the injury with remarks such as, "Just leave me alone. I'm ok. I just need to rest a minute." Even after diagnosis, the denial continues to minimize the objective clinical findings. The second stage is protest—"Why did this have to happen to me? Why now?" I have also had patients who doubted their diagnosis and demanded a second opinion (a good idea, actually, in many serious cases involving the possibility of surgery). The third stage is despair—marked by ambivalence, anger and sadness ("Nothing I do ever works. I'll never run again.") In the most extreme cases, patients in mourning over their loss of sport need psychological intervention.

Manuel Cortez says that "athletes with more obsessive personalities and those who have suffered an injury because of an overuse syndrome are more apt to develop a full-blown mourning state . . . the key is to deal with the athlete's anxiety and depression."[7]

If you consider yourself to be in the Phase 3 category, and are sidelined by an injury, it's important that you clearly define your loss. Realize how you have been using running to provide emotional well-being. Recognize that it was helping you deal with anxieties and keeping depression at bay. Talk about your loss and experience your sadness rather than deny how you feel or assume you "shouldn't" feel like this. Vent your anger (appropriately) if need be. After this process of acknowledgement, you'll be ready to move on to a level of acceptance—at least temporary acceptance. Ask for help from physiotherapists, coaches, your sports doctor or friends about re-directing your energy into another intermediate goal.

Homeopathic remedies are well suited to address the deep emotional and spiritual needs of the Phase 3 runner, as are relaxation techniques, the use of visual imagery, biofeedback, and hypnosis.

Phase 4: The Seasoned Runner

You are the runner who has surpassed the pitfalls of Phase 3. You have mellowed, become wiser, more in tune with the true needs of your body, mind, and spirit. Typically, you are more interested in casual competition rather than intense racing. You are satisfied with an 8- or 9-minute mile. You hear the birds sing when you run. If you feel a cold coming on, you stay home and read the newspaper instead of doggedly putting on the old running shorts. Even the 5 or 10 pounds you gained since your Phase 3 days don't bother you. At this stage, even if you do get an injury, you listen to your doctor's advice, you follow recovery instructions well and are philosophical in accepting some limitations. Congratulations. You have arrived at Phase 4.

If I had my competitive career to run over again, I would change some of my attitudes to injuries. I would show them more respect. Because after all, injuries weren't some unknown barrier that I was trying to crash through. Injuries were simply my body telling me that something wrong was happening. Derek Clayton (1981)[8]

What You Should Know About Over-use Injuries

Running more than five days a week increases the risk of injury by fifty percent. This statistic implies a very important consideration for your training regimen. Too much of a good thing can be hazardous to your health. Why? Even though aerobic exercise and running are preventive medicine, too much medicine equals an overdose!

Training is the process of adapting to stress. An Olympic champion, through training, performs elegantly under the most stressful situation. Training for peak performance is, by definition, a razor's edge between disaster and great results. Therefore, if you are willing to train at the highest level of competition, then be aware of the increased risk of injury and don't be surprised or hard on yourself if it does occur. There is a phenomenon, for example, of an increase in injuries just before actual Olympic trials, because athletes, in the grip of competition-itis, push themselves to their limit and go over that fine line — the line between agony or ecstasy, success or failure.

Over-use injuries are an accumulation of micro-traumas — mini-stresses — that set the stage for the proverbial "straw that breaks the camel's back." Overusing the body, taxing it consistently with little time for rest and integration of new achievements, takes a toll and ripens the conditions leading to injury. Very possibly, you will not even be aware that you are accumulating layer upon layer of stress, or that your body is not adapting to the demands you are placing on it. Then, suddenly, one morning or evening, you strain, sprain, or break something.

Most of you are familiar with the phrase, "being run down," meaning that you are, usually through fatigue and stress, in a state susceptible to illness. Overuse injury also means that there is a susceptibility present in your tendons, ligaments, muscles, joints and bones that opens the door for a variety of ills from runner's knee to a sudden trauma such as a broken leg. These problems literally force you to take a break.

During the running revolution in the seventies, I began to see an addiction to running even in non-competitive runners. I call this addiction the California Divorce Syndrome. During these years, many of my patients were women going through a divorce. I remember Madeline, for example. Thirty-seven years old and initially 20 pounds overweight, she started a running program to get back into shape after her husband left her. Her self-esteem was at an all-time low; she was angry, anxious and depressed at suddenly having to create a new life for herself.

After a few weeks of running, she began to see some very gratifying results. Her stomach flattened out, her thighs were slimmer. Her self-esteem started climbing right along with her endurance. On one visit for corns on her toes, she told me she had even started flirting a little bit with a neighbor who watched her on her daily rounds of the block. Running became her salvation. Once she got into a run, she didn't want to stop; she kept adding more mileage each week. Exhilarated, she began to think the more she ran, the more powerful and beautiful she would become. At the same time, she was procrastinating somewhat on finding a job. She was afraid of losing her new-found gains if she missed even one day a week, and actually became addicted to the chemicals released during exercise (endorphins and enkephalins) which enhance mental clarity and relaxation. She began to run longer and longer, while accumulating stress to the shin bone. Ignoring her body's warning signals of pain, she eventually came to me with a fracture in her leg, and a stress fracture on the opposite foot. She was barely able to walk, let alone run. Again, I had to address the psychological attitudes as well as treating her physically.

Mental Attitudes That Cause Over-Use Injuries
1. Pushing yourself to the limit; excessive competition with self or others (as in the week-end-only sportsman who subjects himself to unprepared-for-stress).
2. Addiction to routine without regard to conditions such as hunger, illness, injury, or sheer fatigue.
3. Putting unrealistic demands on yourself such as running when fatigued or ill, or returning to your regimen before an injury has had proper time to heal.
4. Using your sport as the only focal point in your life (getting your emotional needs met from only one source).

Training Errors

In the early part of the century, Arthur Newton, one of the most phenomenal distance runners the world has ever known, said, "Nature is unable to make a really first class job of anything if she is hustled."[9] Early on in the development of the "new" sport of running, gradual, gentle training was recognized as a key concept. Newton, in advising other rising champions later in his career, advocated setting a weekly, not a daily schedule since "you can't tell what the temperature, the weather or your own condition will be on any day." This technique of *listening* and responding to your body during training is the foundation of total fitness.

In the summary of Newton's Nine Rules listed in *The Lore of Running*, he says:

> Beginning runners start too rapidly and train too hard; they emphasize speed rather than distance, religiously following a rigid training schedule without listening to their bodies. Then, when they become racers, they overtrain, they race in training and run time-trials and races too frequently, they fail to train specifically, they do not rest sufficiently before races, and they ignore the importance of mental preparation for competition.[10]

These errors are the basis of many injuries I see in patients. One of the points I stress to racers, for instance, is to alternate the level of exertion so that they do not have two days in a row of hard workouts or long, intense runs. Alternating days of intense effort with days of rest or substitute activities such as swimming drastically reduces the risk of injury. In addition to alternating activity, I advise increasing your workouts in three-week cycles. We'll look at the advantages of cyclic over progressive training in the next chapter.

Another major training error is ignoring proper, *balanced,* exercises for strength, flexibility, and balance (see Chapter 15). In some cases, vast amounts of repetitive training strengthen, for example, muscles on the back of the legs, but leave thigh muscles in the front *proportionately* less strong. Muscle strength imbalance is a biomechanical weakness which leads to risk of injury.

Another obvious training error is competing in an event without proper preparation for that specific event. Before competing in a 10 km race, practice running a 10 km race. Always practice and simulate the event you are going to do.

Coaching Errors

"I didn't want to disappoint the coach," said Cory, a freshman in college, as we looked at x-rays of her leg fracture. "He had us running in the bleachers for crew training, and I got really bad leg pains. But, I was afraid I wouldn't make the team if I complained. I was afraid he'd think I was a wimp. You know, Dad always made fun of me if I wimped out. I guess I thought of the coach sort of like my dad."

A coach is a powerful authority figure in any athlete's life, and psychological intimidation, real or felt, can make us negate our own true feelings. Don't be persuaded to participate in a sport or activity when you know you're out of shape or out of your league. Don't let your coach push you so hard that you feel overwhelming fatigue. Be aware of a coach who only stresses the physical aspects of training, or who is only concerned about winning at all costs. Check the level of any class you start, such as high-impact aerobics, especially if you are not young, not already in shape, or if you have any history of risk factors (obesity, smoking, family heart attacks).

Poor Equipment

The running shoes that Jeremy brought into my office showed signs of great stress along the back of the shoe (the counter). That fact told me that he was putting excessive sideways stress on his heel when he ran. Poor equipment, in this case, shoes that inadequately controlled the foot, cause injury. For instance, if your foot rolls towards the inside (pronation) without a corrective device (foot orthotic), you risk a strain to the knee and upper leg.

Shoes run down. Losing the shock absorbency of the sole endangers you during running. The mid-sole of a shoe starts to fatigue between 500 to 750 miles of wear. Inspect your shoes for excessive compression. Many athletic shoes have a removable innersole or sock liner. If the liner is too compacted, it could be responsible for pain on the bottom of the foot near the heel or on the ball of the foot. Replace them with a similar shock absorbent full-length viscoelastic innersole.

Treadmill analysis has shown that running barefoot results in better form than running in soft, sloppy shoes. Select shoes according to the type of activity you will be doing—i.e., tennis shoes for tennis, walking shoes for walking, etc. On the other hand, it is not helpful, and can even be harmful, for you as a recreational or novice runner to have a pair of shoes made specifically for a competitive event. Competitive road-running shoes are usually lighter and more flexible and offer less impact protection. They are usually made so that they curve the toe in, and if you already have a tendency to roll your foot in (pronate), a competition shoe could cause a serious problem. If your foot pronates, a shoe made on a *straight* last is better than a C-shaped last. If you have a high arch, choose a C-shaped or mildly in-toed (adducted) last.

High top shoes give increased strength and control. If you have instability or muscle weakness in the ankle area, high-top shoes offer increased support. Another advantage of high tops, when running on uneven terrain, is the increased "communication" (proprioception) between nerves in the ankle and your brain. The high tops press against the ankle stimulating the nerves on either side so that muscles can respond more quickly to stabilize you. Even though the high-top shoe increases your muscle strength in the ankle by only 10 to 15 percent (over a low-top shoe), this increase may be enough to prevent a sprained ankle.

Another example of injury stemming from poor gear is a "pump bump," a painful, inflamed bump on the back of the heel caused by a poorly supportive, poorly padded heel counter (back of the shoe) which irritates the heel. For treatment, refer to Chapter 9 on heel injuries. For detailed information on shoes, refer to Chapter 3, What to Look For in Running Shoes.

Biomechanical Imbalances

In addition to coaching and training errors or poor equipment, over-use injuries stem from imbalances or abnormalities in your skeletal structure. Misalignments in your hip, thigh, knee, ankle, or feet create maladaptations that, under the repeated movements of running, cycling, kicking, jumping, etc. become painful problems. According to the Rule of Three, minor imbalances in your pelvis, leg, or foot are three times more significant during the stress of running or sports than at rest. For instance, if one leg is ⅛" shorter than the other, when you exercise, the body compensates to a degree equal to ⅜" discrepancy. An imbalance of 3 degrees in the foot of a non-athlete is exaggerated to the equivalent of 9 degrees in an athlete. Normal and abnormal biomechanics are discussed in Chapter 2.

Overuse Injuries

An underlying weakness in the body created by overuse or poor training sets the stage for the inevitable breakdown. Breaking your leg, cracking your skull, or rupturing your muscle, therefore, may look like an "accident." Nevertheless, acute trauma could be the end result of a more subtle cause: being out of touch with your body's actual state of health. Acute injuries deserve to be treated as a signal to examine your overall level of conditioning and training.

Warning Signs of Over-Use Injuries

Mental
- Inability to concentrate; feeling scattered, agitated and unproductive.
- Sleep disturbance (waking up in the middle of the night or trouble falling asleep).
- Rigidity in problem-solving (choices are polarized—everything is either black or white, with no possibility of compromise).

Emotional
- Irritability.
- Fault finding.
- Feeling of defeat or ineptitude.
- Paranoia, jealousy.
- Depression.
- Anxiety.

Spiritual
- Extreme egotism.
- Lack of concern with others.
- Lack of relationship with self, others, and the world.
- Depression, irritability or anxiety after discontinuing a sport.
- Little sense of identity beyond the sport.
- Winning at all costs.

Physical
- Stiffness and pain while exercising; if ignored, pain may continue after exercising, or may be present in normal walking. If ignored further, it eventually prevents participation in sport or normal activity.
- A feeling similar to a low-grade infection (no energy, easily fatigued).
- Frequent colds, flu, or cold sores; frequent biting of the lips, tongue or the inside of the cheek.
- Low performance even with effort.
- A resting pulse in the morning that is at least 10 beats faster than normal.

Acute Injuries Which May Warn of Over-use Injuries
- Cuts, bruises, bleeding
- Swelling
- Inflammation
- Broken bones or fractures
- Strained muscles and tendons
- Sprained ligaments and joints
- Dehydration or heat exhaustion
- Cold sweats during exercise
- Dizziness
- Uncoordination

The biggest risk for you, the active person, is not the sudden accidental injury, but the condition of susceptibility caused by the wear and tear of small amounts of stress accumulated over time. You are most likely to injure yourself when your judgment is impaired by mental and emotional blindspots such as egotism and exercising for false purposes. Training and coaching errors, poor gear, and biomechanical imbalances will expose you to both long and short-term problems.

Footnotes
1. Sacks, J.L.: "A psychodynamic overview of sport," Psychiatric Ann 9(3):13, 1979.
2. Sacks, J.L.: *Running as Therapy,* (Lincoln, NE, University of Nebraska Press) 1984.
3. Noakes, Tim, Dr.: *The Lore of Running,* (Oxford: Oxford University Press) 1985.
4. Yates, A., Leehey, K., Shisslak, C.M.: "Running—An analogue of anorexia?" New England Journal of Medicine 308:251, 1983.
5. Blumenthal, J.A., O'Toole, L.C., Chang, J.L.: "Is running an analogue of anorexia nervosa? An empirical study of obligatory running and anorexia nervosa." JAMA 252:520, 1984.
6. Cortez, Manuel J.: "Psychological Considerations," *Sports Medicine of the Lower Extremity,* ed. by Steven I. Subotnick, D.P.M., M.S., (New York, Churchill Livingstone) 1989, pp. 11-15.
7. Cortez, *ibid.*
8. Noakes, *op cit.*
9. Noakes, *op cit.*
10. Noakes, *op cit.*

Chapter 2

BIOMECHANICS: YOU, YOUR BODY, AND RUNNING

> You know, Doctor, when your foot hurts, you hurt all over.
> —Thelma (a patient, 1980)

The Mechanics of Motion: Avoiding Injury

A gold medal now hangs around your neck, you hold a bouquet of roses in your arms, and your ears ring with the deafening sound of worldwide applause. Hundreds of reporters want to know the "secret" of how you just broke a world record. You'll never be able to tell them. The peak performance, the perfection of a single well-played tennis stroke, the sublime leap into the air can be video-taped, monitored, and analyzed, and still be beyond our understanding. The body in motion is a miracle. Even the act of simply crossing the room to greet a friend is a demonstration of the magic of biomechanical functions between our brains, our hearts, our bones, and our muscles and tendons.

As a doctor I'm trained in the scientific, empirically-proven methods of prevention and healing. As a *sports* medicine specialist and runner, I also have had the privilege of knowing first-hand "what makes Sammy run." I have learned that biomechanics means more than just the sum of the mechanical relationships between anatomical parts. By merely looking at how the knee connects to the leg, I could never imagine the effortless pirouettes of the trained ballet dancer or feel the inner peace of the long-distance runner as she heads for home after twenty miles of "good" time. I have been told many times about the feeling of euphoria. I have also experienced first-hand that exquisite sense of being in touch with my center during a race or a run.

Your body is not a machine. However, you are put together with a mechanical finesse and logic which is quite breathtaking. The scien-

17

tific definition of biomechanics is the study of the working interrelationships of bones, muscles, and tendons. Quite possibly, you won't be interested in reading about something as technical-sounding as "biomechanics"—until you have a good reason to know what it means. That reason will be a pain under the knee, a pain in the ankle joint, a pain in the foot—even a pain in the buttocks! When pain interferes with your exercise routine, your sport, or your normal activities, you'll want to know the whys and wherefores of your body—and, most importantly, what you can do to regain well-being.

In order to avoid simple errors in training and the selection of gear, you should know the basics of how your body is put together. If you are a new runner, you should read this section before you run again. If you know what to look for, you will be able to avoid what some call the "diseases of ignorance." Prevention is the best medicine of all.

Running is a major component of many sports, and has come to be almost a national mania. I will be discussing primarily the biomechanics of running and walking—the distinctive activities of the human body. For example, during a run, you bend your ankle about 800 times every mile. If you weigh 150 lbs, you subject your foot bones, according to the sports "Rule of Three," to a force of 450 lbs every time you come down on the ground. The force of your shin bone pressing on your ankle bone can be more than 1500 lbs! Acceleration (running) is responsible for the increased force under your feet.

If there is any misalignment in your legs—for example, a shortness in one leg—your body compensates to balance you. Under repeated stress with no time for gradual conditioning, tightened muscles and tissues begin to bruise and tear. Pain signals an area in danger. It's that simple. The body speaks the only way it can—with pain, tension, or ruptures.

Normal Feet

The flexibility, endurance, muscle tone, and strength you had at age 10, 15, 25, or 45, or even yesterday, change silently and subtly. Developments in your skeletal structure proceed quietly, according to a programmed schedule. For example, Fig. 2-1 shows the appearance of the little bones of the foot in the unborn child, and the subsequent age (years later in the case of some bones) at which they unite for increased rigidity. Thus, in this schedule of development, the foot starts

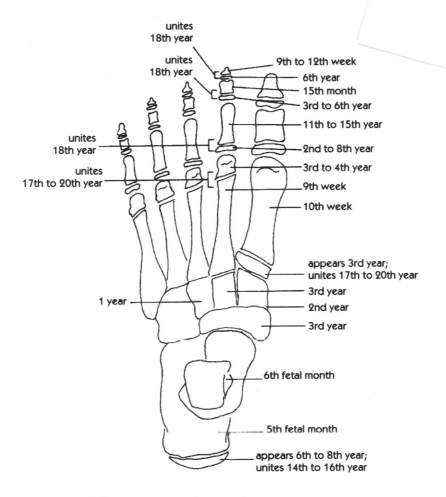

unites
18th year

unites
18th year

9th to 12th week

6th year

15th month

3rd to 6th year

11th to 15th year

unites
18th year

2nd to 8th year

unites
17th to 20th year

3rd to 4th year

9th week

10th week

appears 3rd year;
unites 17th to 20th year

3rd year

1 year

2nd year

3rd year

6th fetal month

5th fetal month

appears 6th to 8th year;
unites 14th to 16th year

2-1. When Bones Develop

out loose and flexible, gradually tying pieces together until around
the twentieth year. As you can see, little feet are soft and malleable.
This is the reason you don't buy a child a small, rigid adult shoe which
will restrict or distort normal growth.

Over the years, your foot changes according to the type of shoes
you wear, the exercise you do, and other factors like diet or disease.
Heredity plays a big factor in the problems you may develop, too, so
choose your parents wisely!

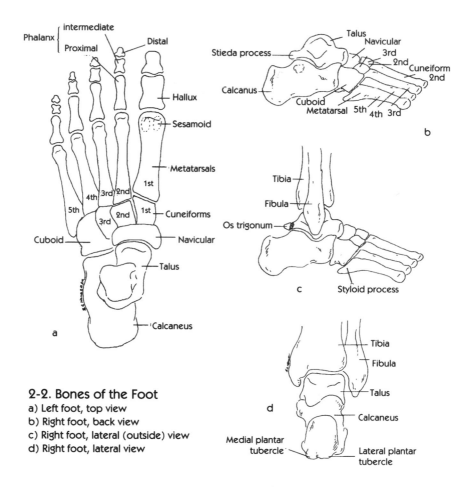

2-2. Bones of the Foot
a) Left foot, top view
b) Right foot, back view
c) Right foot, lateral (outside) view
d) Right foot, lateral view

Fig. 2-2 is a drawing of the foot bones with their anatomical names. You can use these drawings when seeking a second opinion or when trying to determine which bones are hurting you. I encourage my patients to ask questions, but many come to me sure of their diagnosis before they even see me! Fig. 2-3 shows the surface anatomy of the foot with the descriptive names of important sections.

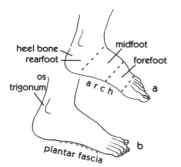

2-3. Topography of the Foot
a) heel bone, rearfoot, midfoot, forefoot, arch
b) os trigonum, plantar fascia

Anatomical Irregularities in the Foot

Short first toe (Morton's foot). If your foot looks like Fig. 2-4, you are not alone. Apes, monkeys, Greek statues and many of your neighbors also have feet like this. The potential problem for runners with Morton's foot is that the short first metatarsal bone is too mobile and does not carry its full load. It shifts the weight to other areas, causing a variety of problems. A foot orthotic (an insert in the shoe) may help redistribute the weight and alleviate the pain.

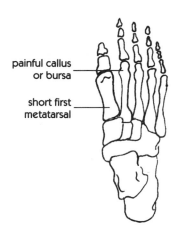

painful callus or bursa

short first metatarsal

2-4. Morton's foot or "Greek foot" (long second toe)

Long first toe (Egyptian foot). A long first metatarsal and a long big toe (see Fig. 2-5) causes jamming in the big toe joint, often leading to eventual bone spurs or arthritis. The range of motion of the big toe is limited *(Hallux Rigidus),* and there is pain with every step.

A dropped forefoot.. You may have a "dropped" forefoot, which means the ball of your foot is actually lower than your heel (Fig. 2-6e). When you run with a dropped forefoot, you land on the ball of your foot first, then rock back on the heel. This stresses the bones of the toes where they join the forefoot, creating excessive calluses and straining the muscles on the bottom of the foot. This anatomical abnormality also strains the Achilles tendon during running and fast walking. The solution is to redistribute

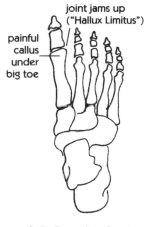

joint jams up ("Hallux Limitus")

painful callus under big toe

2-5. Egyptian foot (long first toe)

the weight with a heel lift or a foot orthotic (insert) taking the pressure off the forefoot—where a giant callus may develop.

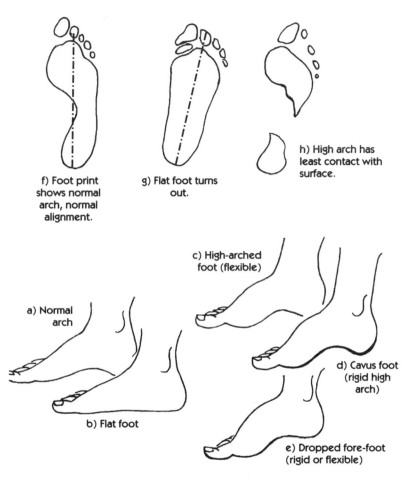

f) Foot print shows normal arch, normal alignment.

g) Flat foot turns out.

h) High arch has least contact with surface.

c) High-arched foot (flexible)

a) Normal arch

d) Cavus foot (rigid high arch)

b) Flat foot

e) Dropped fore-foot (rigid or flexible)

2-6. Types of Arches

Types of Arches

Look at your wet footprint when you get out of the shower and compare your foot with Figs. 2-6f,g,h showing the following arches:

Normal arch. 50 percent of the population has an arch that leaves a crescent-shaped space on the side (Fig. 2-6a,f). A straight line axis can be drawn between the middle of the rearfoot and the tip of the second toe. A large, unsupported space is between the end of the forefoot and the toe prints.

Flat or low arch. Twenty to twenty-five percent of the population has a collapsed arch; the whole underfoot contacts the ground and is used for support (Figure 2-6b,g). The foot is not on a straight axis, but turned outward. The flat foot doesn't necessarily cause problems unless there is also a lot of movement and looseness in the joints. The most common biomechanical problem I see in walkers and runners is weak, low arches with flexible feet which flatten out too much at contact and never have the normal arch for toe-off. The remedy, in this case, is a custom-made foot orthotic to reestablish a normal arch.

Your feet change with activity and age. With increased activity over time, your feet get longer and flatter as arches become lower. Most people find they need sport shoes a size larger than their dress shoes.

High arch. Twenty to twenty-five percent of the population has an arch so high there is no connection between rearfoot and forefoot or the forefoot and toes (2-6c,d,e,h). Also called a *cavus* arch, this foot is more rigid and poorly absorbs shock.

Sometimes the biomechanical misalignments and abnormalities are slight and very subtle, so that in everyday activities they really don't cause a problem. For instance, a high-arch foot may appear high with walking, but *flatten with running*. On the other hand, I've seen runners with a flat foot while standing and a *cavus* foot while running. Therefore evaluation of the arch in motion is often necessary to see what is really happening.

The pressure coming down on the foot, proportional to the amount of surface area, is highest on the high-arched foot. High-arched feet quickly become subject to overuse injury. With the demands of race walking and running, high arches take lots of high pressure, and are least able to absorb impact since they have so little contact with the ground (look again at the sketchy footprint of the high-arched foot). Also, high arches are relatively rigid, and as we will see, rigidity does not allow for dissipation of the shock. Not only does a high arch get more shock, it is ill-equipped to handle it. The impact then is transferred to the bones of the ankle and shank.

Wearing high-heeled shoes creates a higher arch and can lead to toe problems such as clawed toes or pain on the top of the toes. To avoid cramps at night after wearing high-heels, stand against the wall and stretch out your heel cords. Or don't wear high heels, since they are very bad for your feet.

What to do for high arches. First, look for a shoe with a very cushioned midsole and a deep toe box. The toe box must be big enough to accommodate the increased thickness at the ball of the foot. This thickness is due to the higher arch, and the tendency for the toes to claw or scrunch up (hammer toes). Another thing you must do with

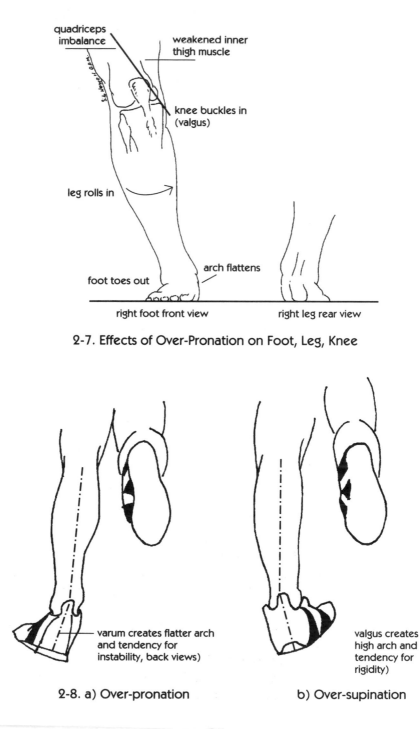

quadriceps
imbalance

weakened inner
thigh muscle

knee buckles in
(valgus)

leg rolls in

arch flattens

foot toes out

right foot front view

right leg rear view

2-7. Effects of Over-Pronation on Foot, Leg, Knee

varum creates flatter arch
and tendency for
instability, back views)

valgus creates
high arch and
tendency for
rigidity)

2-8. a) Over-pronation

b) Over-supination

high arches is to stretch the heel cord by exercising. Thirdly, orthoses are necessary to increase shock absorbency and flexibility.

Foot Function

Normal Pronation and Supination

When your foot touches the ground as you walk or run, it rolls inward (pronates) slightly in order to absorb the shock of impact. The shock absorbed by pronation, is further dissipated as the arch of the foot flattens under your weight. Besides absorbing shock, this flattening (pronation) "unlocks" the foot and causes it to be a loose bag of bones, allowing it to adjust to the surface underneath. *Normal* pronation, (i.e., non-excessive movement inward), is necessary for you to stand and support yourself. Trouble comes either when you roll inward too much or roll inward at the wrong time during contact. See Figs. 2-7 and 2-8a,b.

When your running foot is on the ground (mid-stance) (Fig.2-9a,b), it is balanced. This is necessary for maximum efficiency and safety. Once the foot is balanced, the foot has a normal arch in preparation for the next movement which is "locking" (supination). Supination enables the foot to become a lever which then propels you forward

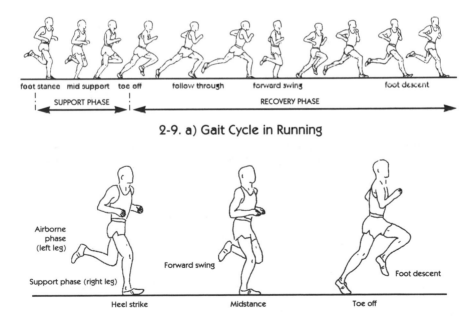

foot stance   mid support   toe off   follow through   forward swing   foot descent

SUPPORT PHASE

RECOVERY PHASE

2-9. a) Gait Cycle in Running

Airborne
phase
(left leg)

Forward swing

Foot descent

Support phase (right leg)

Heel strike   Midstance   Toe off

b) Positions of Foot in Running

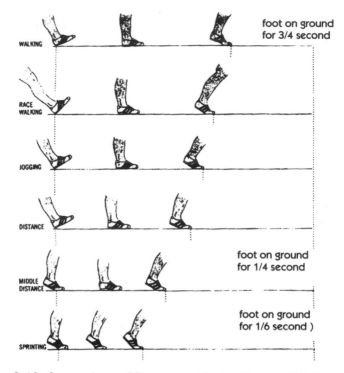

2-10. Comparison of Stance and Swing Phases of Gait
in Walking, Race-walking, Jogging, and Sprinting

into toe-off (Fig. 2-10). The foot must lock (supinate) before the heel lifts off the ground so that stress will pass straight out through the first and second toes. A flat, loose foot, like a wobbling bowl of jelly beans, has little propulsive ability. On the other hand, an overly-rigid foot (excessively supinated) during propulsion is unstable on the outside (laterally) and susceptible to sprains. A rigid foot puts more pressure on the soft tissues, creating corns, calluses, and blisters.

To give you an idea of how fast all these functions happen, studies have broken time down into thousandths of a second (milli-seconds). For instance, when you're walking, your foot is on the ground 750 milli-seconds (three-quarters of a second) (Fig. 2-10). When you're running, your foot is on the ground 250 milli-seconds (one-quarter of a second). That's a big difference. Usually, you run two or three times faster than you walk, and when you're running, heel contact can be as little as 25 milli-seconds (one-tenth of a quarter of a second). Interestingly enough, the muscles' ability to respond (reflex) takes 35 milli-seconds. So what happens? The shock, coming in faster than the body's ability to respond, cannot be absorbed. It jars the body.

In a few milli-seconds, then, the foot performs three functions:

1. On contact with the ground, the foot must pronate enough to be loose, mobile, and adaptable to a possibly uneven surface.
2. On mid-stance (when the foot is flat on the ground), the foot must be balanced and flexible, preparing to become a rigid lever for toe-off.
3. On toe-off, the foot must supinate to become rigid and propulsive.

If you have a normal foot, you land on the outside of the heel. You may notice, for instance, that the outsides of your heels are worn down on your shoes. When you run or walk fast, your feet are closer together than when you stand, which puts more pressure on the outside of the heels. Being closer together also causes you to roll in more (pronation) in order to get your shoe flat on the ground.

Hips, Knees, and Legs
Mirror Test for Hip Symmetry and Leg Length

To determine if your legs are the same length and symmetrical, check yourself naked in front of a mirror with your feet about six inches apart. Point your feet and knees straight ahead, hands on hips. If one foot is toed out and one foot is straight ahead, you have an imbalance. See Figure 2-11a.

Unlevel hips: In the same position, bend down at the knees. If one hip is up and one is down, one leg is shorter than the other. Another indicator of a short leg is uneven dimples in the buttocks. Ask a (good) friend to locate these dimples. If the dimples are not level, then you either have one leg shorter or an abnormal curve in your spine (scoliosis) which should be checked out by a doctor (Figure 2-11b).

Knees turned inward: If one knee turns inward more than the other knee, that foot may be flatter than the other foot. If both knees tend to turn inward, you probably have weak arches or a hip problem or knock-knees *(genu valgum)*.

Pronation awareness: Even though your foot does not have flat or weak arches, during running you may have a tendency to roll in too far towards the middle (excessive pronation). To get a feel for pronation so you can be aware when you run, stand with both feet straight ahead and put most of your weight on the right foot; collapse your arch as much as you can, then pronate (roll inward) your right foot. As you

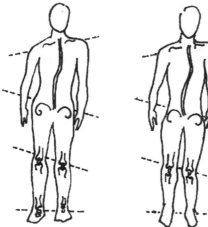
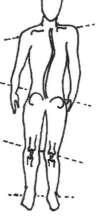
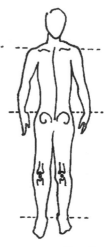

anatomical short leg   functional short leg   disappearance of functional
short leg with orthotic

2-11. Leg Imbalances: a) short leg imbalance in joints (front view)

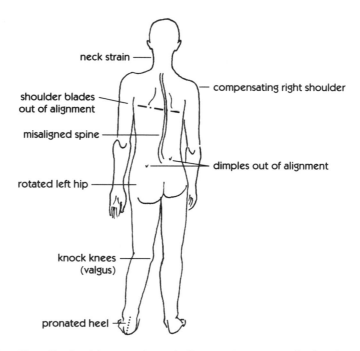

neck strain

compensating right shoulder

shoulder blades
out of alignment

misaligned spine

dimples out of alignment

rotated left hip

knock knees
(valgus)

pronated heel

b) functionally short leg creates misalignments over entire body
(back view)

collapse the right arch, notice that your right knee-cap turns inward, and the knee bends. As your right knee bends and internally rotates, so does the right thigh and hip. Pronation of the foot causes internal rotation of the leg, knee, thigh, and hip. It also causes the knee to bend inward (knock-knees or *genu valgum*) (Fig. 2-12b, page 32). This abnormal rotation in the knee, leg, or thigh is a major contributor to shin splints, runner's knee, and hip strain. It can also cause low-back pain.

The body subconsciously compensates for discrepancies in alignment. Each person makes an individual compensation, so there is no general rule of how your body might deal with, say, short-leg syndrome. Actually, to have one leg shorter than the other is not unusual in the general population, so it pays for you to check yourself for this biomechanical problem if you're having pain in the knees or legs.

One way your body may attempt to level the *shorter* side is by pulling the foot on the shorter side to the outside (over-supination). Remember how toddlers, unsteady in their gait, tend to toe-out to gain more stability? This is also true of elderly people, shuffling around with their feet pointed out.

Or your body may try to level the *longer* side by rolling it in too much (over-pronation), or keeping the knee on the long side in a flexed position to shorten it.

If you do have a short leg syndrome, have a podiatrist or sports medicine specialist diagnose your compensation pattern. A large deformity of an inch, for instance, gives the message to the body that you are falling as your foot hits the ground during running. Your foot will toe out. With a small deformity of ⅛", your body may compensate by raising your arch. Since these compensating movements interfere with the normal biomechanical function, you are beginning to accumulate tiny amounts of stress which can ultimately create an overuse injury.

How to Balance Your Short Leg

First, measure the two legs to see how much discrepancy there is. Use a tape measure to measure the distance from the outside hip bone to the outside bottom of the ankle bone on both sides. Or, put your hands on your hips to see if your pelvis is level when the back of your heels are flat on the floor. If your pelvic bones are not level, then add ⅛" blocks of wood (get them cut at a hardware or lumber store) under the heel until the pelvis is level. If your spine when level is still curved, then you have scoliosis (curved spine) and should see your orthopedist or family doctor because there will be other complications.

If you have a difference in leg lengths less than ¼" but are experiencing no pain, then you don't need to do anything. If you have been having a pain in the legs or spine, try adding a heel pad in your shoe. This can be rubber, cork, or felt.

If you have a leg that is ¼" short, put a piece of sponge rubber about ³⁄₁₆" in your heel to add height. If you have a ⅜" discrepancy, use a ½" pad. For do-it-yourself padding, you can use makeup sponge pads or a product from the sporting goods store. The pads should be worn in both running and regular shoes. If the leg is ¾" too short, you'll have to have a shoemaker build up the midsole of your shoe. A lift of more than ⅜" will have to be put on the outside of the shoe. If you build up too high on the inside of the shoe, you'll begin to lift up beyond the counter (back of the heel) of the shoe and your foot will lack stability. High-top shoes, however, would allow you to put in a fairly thick lift without a problem in the heel counter.

If the shortage is more than ¾" inch, you need to do more than just pad the heel. You also need to build up the forefoot. The rule I use is: full correction in the heel, half the correction under the ball of the foot, and half that under the toes. So, let's say you had a 1" discrepancy. You would build up the heel 1 inch, build up the ball of the foot ½" and build up under the toes ¼".

You should probably see a podiatrist who may also help you with a foot orthotic. If you are a woman with a ½" leg discrepancy, you can build up one heel of a high heel shoe ¼" and take off ¼" on the other heel, and no one will know the difference!

Biomechanical Action:
Body Parts Aligned in Motion

Running Check

To check your form, run with a friend. Have him or her watch you in front and back to see how you run, how your feet hit the ground, and your general form. If one foot is doing something different than the other foot, you have a problem.

How Too Much Pronation Affects Your Knees

Excessive rolling in of the foot to the center rotates the ankle bone (talus) which transfers the inward motion to the shank, creating a screwing motion against the knee joint which was not designed for that motion.

An example of this problem is Peter Stein, a marathon-runner who first came to my office complaining of runner's knee—pain under his right knee. The pain had begun when he'd increased to over 50 miles a week while preparing for his first Boston Marathon. This was fifteen years ago when we knew very little about biomechanics. He was training on a banked road. He told me he had no pain when his left foot was uphill and his right foot was downhill (thus his right arch was being supported by the slope of the road). When he reversed his position, however, having his right foot uphill caused his right arch to collapse and flatten, rotating the ankle and shank. This caused the knee-cap to ride to the outside of the knee bone. I gave him an orthosis for the inside of his shoe and recommended knee exercises (see exercise section for quad sets). In addition, I suggested he run uphill (not downhill) to strengthen his inner thighs (quadriceps).

Because Peter described *when* the pain occurred (e.g., on the uphill side), I was able to get a clear picture of the possible problem. I encourage runners and athletes who do serious training to keep a sports journal so that they will have a record of mileage increases, types of terrain changes, and onset of problems in case of injury or pain.

Too Much Rotation at the Hips

You may have inborn rotational imbalances or tightness about the hips. This can cause otherwise healthy feet to compensate abnormally (toe in or toe out) and hurt. For example, normally, when your knee-cap is facing forward, you should be able to rotate your knee either in or out with flexibility at the hips. If you don't have that flexibility, stretch out the hips with exercise.

Misalignments That Cause Knee Pain

Varus? Valgum? You will hear these two terms a lot in sports medicine circles, if you run in such circles! *Varus* means simply that a part of the body faces *toward* the midline. *Valgum* means that a part of the body faces *away* from the midline. There are three main areas in your leg that can have either one of these misalignments.

a. ***Tibial varum* or *valgum*.** First, take a look at Fig. 2-12a which shows the bowlegged stance. Since the lower leg bone (tibia) is pointing towards the midline *(varus)*, we call this condition a *tibial varum*. Conversely, when the tibia points away from the mid-line, there is *tib-*

31

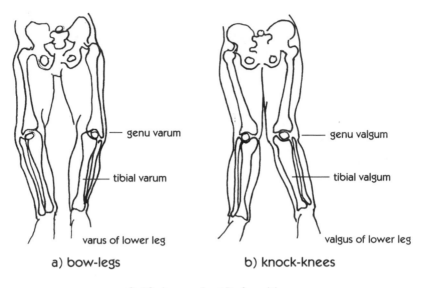

genu varum

tibial varum

varus of lower leg

a) bow-legs

genu valgum

tibial valgum

valgus of lower leg

b) knock-knees

2-12. Lower Leg Deformities

ial valgum or, more popularly called, knock-knees (Fig. 2-12b). These two abnormalities put abnormal pressure and stresses on connecting parts, which will eventually cause problems with repetitive use.

These two misalignments can be caused by congenital deformities or acquired through injury, or they can occur *temporarily* (referred to as a *functional* misalignment) as you run. *Functional varus* happens in running, even though your legs don't have anything wrong anatomically, because your legs are closer to the midline of the body. Remember that your feet get closer together when you run; therefore, running and fast walking create a bow-legged effect. Women, who typically have a wider pelvis for childbearing purposes, have more tendency for functional varus in running because they must bring their legs in to a greater degree than slimmer-hipped people. Most people are a bit bow-legged and have *tibial varum* when walking.

b. **Forefoot varus**. Just as the shank of the leg may have a tendency to turn in or out, so does the forefoot. Fig. 2-13a, b shows these two abnormalities. *Forefoot varus* can cause a foot to be too mobile, with excessive pronation (rolling inward). It leads to bunions, hammertoes, neuromas, plantar fasciitis, and even heel spurs. It can also lead to shin splints and runner's knee, and may be associated with hip or low-back strain. This is the most common foot imbalance, and is

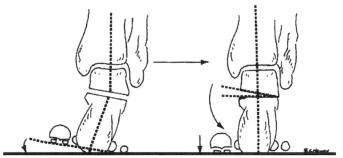

forefoot pronated in order to reach the ground

2-13. a) Forefoot Varus (right foot, rear view)

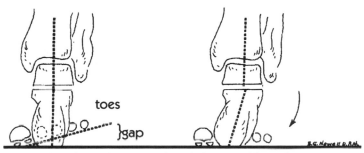

toes

}gap

in order to close gap and reach the ground foot rolls out (supinates)

b) Forefoot Valgus (right foot, rear view)

often implicated in walking and running problems. These feet will need corrective foot orthoses.

c. **Forefoot valgus**. The opposite of *forefoot varus* is *forefoot valgus* (Fig. 2-13b). This is a stiff foot with a callus on the ball of the foot, bent or clawed toes (hammer toes), and a high arch. Problems include metatarsal stress fractures, sesamoiditis, and plantar fascial strains.

d. **Rearfoot varus**. Fig. 2-14 shows a normal leg with the heel bone perpendicular to the ground and the metatarsal heads perpendicular to the heel. However, *varus* tendencies can appear in this

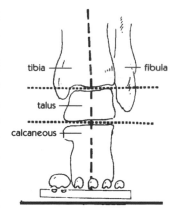

2-14. Normal Foot
to Leg Alignment
(left foot, front view)

33

area, too. In order for the inward turning heels *(varum)* to reach the ground, the arch must collapse, creating a tendency for instability—excessive pronation. This causes pain or injury commonly associated with pronation. In addition, there may be pain at the back of the heel (rctrocalcaneal bursitis or "pump bump") or Achilles tendon strains. The remedy for this is rearfoot control with a strong shoe counter.

　e. **Rearfoot valgus**. Rearfoot valgus (outward-turning heels), forces the foot to pronate to the extreme. The *valgum* creates a low arch on the inside of the foot and a tendency for flat-footedness. These heels will be helped by strong shoes with a deep, firm heel cup, and heel stabilizer foot orthotics. The rearfoot *valgum* foot is associated with pain at the outside of the ankle and foot (*sinus tarsi* syndrome), and inner-arch cramps and strains.

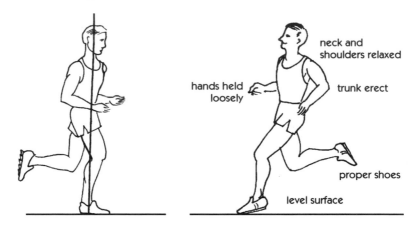

2-15. Balanced Running Form　　　　2-16. Good Running Form

Running Form

Fig. 2-15 shows the ideally balanced running body when one foot is on the ground (mid-stance). Note the line from the top of the head through the middle of the body, down the mid-point of the knee into the arch. One of my running buddies, Ian Jackson, once told me that the pelvis should feel as if it were a big bowl of water, balanced within so as not to spill over in front or back.

　Good form is shown in Fig. 2-16. The runner is erect, not leading with his head or bending back. Arms, shoulders and neck should be relaxed (check this once in a while as you run). Keep your hands loose, using no extra energy in clenching the fists, and hold a slight downward angle at your forearms. Wear layered clothing according to the temperature and, of course, proper shoes. Running on a soft, level surface is best because it reduces the shock of impact.

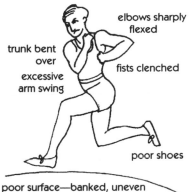

2-17. Poor Running Form

Poor form creates stress. Note in Fig. 2-17 that the runner is bent-over, swinging his arms too much, elbows too sharply flexed, and hands tightly clenched. He will be much more fatigued at the end of the run. Remember, the right arm controls the left leg, and vice-versa. A tight left shoulder may come from a right leg or foot over-use syndrome. Swimming is a good way to equalize the upper and lower body.

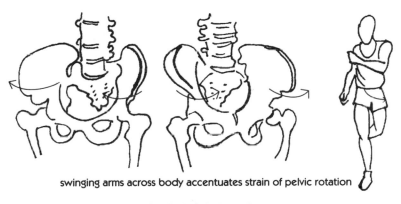

swinging arms across body accentuates strain of pelvic rotation

2-18. Pelvic Rotation

a. **Arm swing creates pelvic stress**. Take a minute to stand up and hold your arms in the flexed position (elbows bent). Swing your arms back and forth across your chest with your legs stationary. Feel how the pelvis rotates on the spine in proportion to the amount of arm swing. See Fig. 2-18.[1] Swinging your arms parallel—i.e., in the same direction you are going—is much more effective aerodynamically as well as less stressful on the pelvis. With cross-chest arm swinging, you may feel pain at the small of the back.

b. **Seesaw pelvic tilt in mid-stance**. At the moment you are standing on one leg in the middle of your running gait, the unsupported

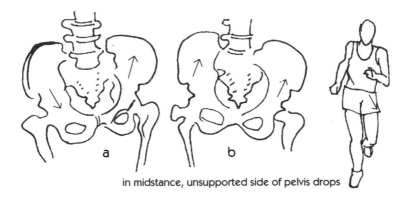

in midstance, unsupported side of pelvis drops

2-19. Pelvic Tilt:
a) Arm swing increases horizontal, side-to-side rotation.
b) When one leg is off the ground there is a shearing force as pelvis drops.

side of the pelvis drops down (Fig. 2-19)[2] creating shearing forces to both sides of the pelvic area. Overtraining (high mileage) can cause osteitis pubis—hardening and inflammation of the cartilage and bone at the front of the pelvic bone—right behind the genitals. This happens, generally, to people who have been running for a few years. Pain in the genital area must be diagnosed with x-rays to rule out stress fractures.

c. **Uphill and downhill stresses to the pelvis and hip.** As you can see in Fig. 2-20 the uphill runner is tilting his pelvis forward which limits his ability to swing his hip forward and puts greater stress on the muscles of the lower back.

The downhill runner tilts his pelvis backward, causing low back pain, especially if he already has too much curve in the spine (lordosis) (Fig. 2-21).

d. **Foot plant**. When you run, your foot should land directly beneath your knee and beneath the center of gravity. See Fig. 2-15. If you are running on a track where you can see your foot prints, check to see that each foot is landing on the track line ahead of you. Another way to check foot plant and form is to watch yourself in a mirror as you run on a treadmill. Draw a line on a treadmill, observing where your foot lands, and check yourself in a mirror.

The faster you go, the closer together your feet are so that one foot lands where the other foot was, directly on the line of progression. In leisure walking, the feet tend to be a bit turned out and operate on

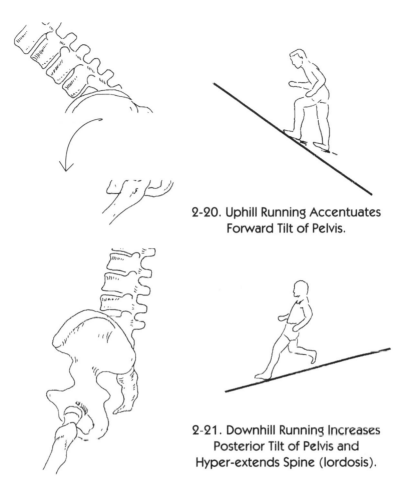

2-20. Uphill Running Accentuates
Forward Tilt of Pelvis.

2-21. Downhill Running Increases
Posterior Tilt of Pelvis and
Hyper-extends Spine (lordosis).

parallel tracks. Over-striding (when your foot lands in front of your center of gravity) wears out the heel of your shoe and creates more foot slap. When you understride, and the foot lands behind the center of gravity, you wear out the toe of your shoes. So ... watch your shoes!

Other Factors Affecting Biomechanical Function

Speed, asphalt, and concrete. The faster you go the more impact shock hits your bones and joints. To make matters worse, the faster you go the less time your foot is on the ground, so there is more force going through the foot in a shorter amount of time. As your pace increases, you are running more on the balls of your feet, and this can cause problems there and in the toes. Common problems are: inflamed nerves (neuromas), callouses, and metatarsal stress fractures.

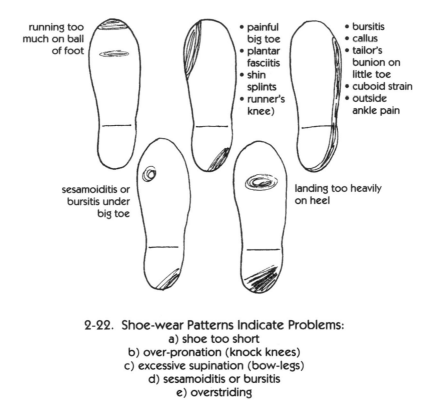

running too
much on ball
of foot

- painful
  big toe
- plantar
  fasciitis
- shin
  splints
- runner's
  knee)

- bursitis
- callus
- tailor's
  bunion on
  little toe
- cuboid strain
- outside
  ankle pain

sesamoiditis or
bursitis under
big toe

landing too heavily
on heel

2-22. Shoe-wear Patterns Indicate Problems:
a) shoe too short
b) over-pronation (knock knees)
c) excessive supination (bow-legs)
d) sesamoiditis or bursitis
e) overstriding

You need to protect your feet if you work out on hard surfaces like pavement, synthetic track, tennis courts, or in gyms. Because these hard surfaces are unyielding, your feet don't have a chance to flex naturally like they would on grass or the jungle floor. You may find that flexibility exercises are helpful in relaxing your feet and increasing range of motion.

The safest running ground is grass or a level dirt road without holes or hidden rocks. Simply running on grass can sometimes cure stressed feet. I don't advise running in the sand (unless it's the hard-packed part near the ocean's edge) because your heel sinks down and pulls on the Achilles tendon. Try to avoid running on pavement on a daily basis, and be sure that you have very well-cushioned shoes. Banked roads that twist the ankle are to be avoided, especially if you run on a gravelly, unstable shoulder.

Hills are good. Running uphill is the safest for two reasons—impact shock and weight distribution. First, the impact shock for uphill

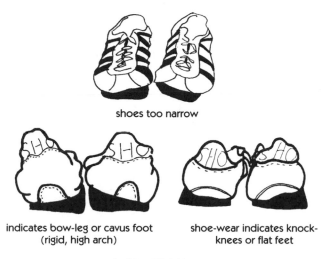

shoes too narrow

indicates bow-leg or cavus foot
(rigid, high arch)

shoe-wear indicates knock-
knees or flat feet

2-23. Old Shoes

running is only two times body weight, whereas level running is three times body weight and downhill running is four times body weight. Secondly, uphill running shifts your weight forward onto the ball of the foot, causing you less jarring shock. So run uphill, walk downhill.

Fatigued muscles don't absorb as much shock. When you have proper foot contact, you are in a state of balance above the foot, not straining to force the muscles to actively support you. Proper contact fatigues the muscles much less. Research studies with sensors placed in the leg bones, where there is no overlying protective muscle and fat, show that more stress hits the bone because of the lack of shock-absorptive muscle. Muscles, therefore, absorb as well as produce energy, thus protecting bones and joints. Fatigued muscles don't absorb shock, resulting in sloppy running form and joint strains.

Shoe-wear Check for Biomechanical Stresses

The soles of your shoes relay a lot of information about your biomechanical activity. Fig. 2-22 shows different wear patterns. Asymmetrical wear patterns indicate that something is out of alignment, just like the tires on your car. If you are malaligned, your shoes will reflect the problem. For instance, if your shoes are wearing out along the outside area, you are probably bowlegged (Fig. 2-23), and may also have a high arch. If in addition to the wear on the outside, you sprain your ankle a lot, you may need a foot orthotic.

Excessive wear on the inner area of the shoe means you are too flat-footed. If you're wearing out the front of the shoe, your shoes are too short, and if you're wearing holes in the top where your big toe is, the shoe does not have a big enough toe box.

Footnotes

1. Fig. 2-18 adapted from drawing by F. Netter, M.D.
2. Fig. 2-19, *ibid.*

Chapter 3

TRAINING FOR RUNNERS, WALKERS, AND SPORTSPEOPLE

Many shall run to and fro, and knowledge shall be increased.
Daniel 12:4

Fitness

Good news! You don't *have* to run to stay in shape. If you look the other way when runners pass you in the park, feeling guilty because you don't even own a pair of running shorts and can't stand the thought of relentlessly running and sweating on any regular basis, take heart. You don't have to run to stay in shape. I've been a runner for the past twenty years and I've written several books on the subject, *The Running Foot Doctor,* and *Cures for Common Running Injuries.* I have come to believe that running is fine if you *want* to do it. I now tell people that if they are running more than 20 miles a week, they ought to be getting paid for it. Running can be rough on the body. Unless you pay attention to how your body reacts to the stress, you may create injury instead of health.

Brisk walking, I believe, and recent studies back me up on this, is one of the most beneficial exercises you can do for total fitness. It requires nothing more than a good pair of shoes, requires little training, costs nothing, and can be done anywhere. If you walk briskly (i.e., about a 12–15 minute mile) three or four times a week, you're getting most of the aerobic stimulation your cardiovascular system needs. In combination with a good stretching program and good diet, you are on your way to vital good health.

What Is Total Fitness?

Exercise may lead to fitness but not necessarily to total fitness. The wife of one of my running friends said, "I work all day long, running to the store, mopping up after the kids, mowing the lawn. I get plenty of exercise!" Activity which is intermittent and not sustained for at least 20 minutes at 70 percent of your maximum heart rate is not the same as aerobic exercise. Regular work and daily activity can leave you feeling drained and tired instead of focused and revitalized.

The American Heart Association tells us that 55 percent of all the deaths in this country are from heart disease. Not just a problem of "older people" or men in high-stress occupations, heart disease has been on the increase for people in their twenties, thirties, and forties, including more women in high-stress occupations. Rather than being frightened by these statistics, we should be activated to do something about our health, because the risk of *heart disease can be decreased by our attention to diet and exercise.*

The advantage of total fitness is that it decreases your risk of heart attack, cancer, diabetes, and other illnesses, and increases your chance of recovery if you do fall ill. Other benefits are:

> Greater strength, stamina, and suppleness.
> Fewer aches and pains.
> Better posture and fewer back problems.
> Energy and vitality.
> Better digestion of nutrients.
> More restful sleep.
> Better ability to handle anxiety and stress.
> Better coordination and grace of movement.
> Improved appearance.
> Self-confidence.
> Clarity, better decision-making.
> Better sex.

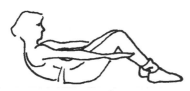

a) least difficult

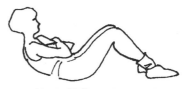

b) more difficult

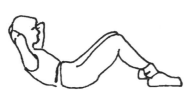

c) more difficult

d) most difficult

3-1. Levels of Difficulty in Abdominal Curls.

What You Can Do To Achieve Total Fitness

Exercise for strength, flexibility and endurance

- To test your current level of flexibility:
  a. Stand up straight, feet together.
  b. Bend slowly from the waist, knees straight. Touch floor with fingertips.
  c. If you can't touch the floor, you need some form of stretching exercise such as yoga or T'ai Chi. Do at least 30 minutes of yoga or stretching three to four times a week to remain flexible.
- To test your abdominal tone and strength:
  a. Lie on the floor with knees bent and feet on the floor. Extend arms at sides.
  b. Now try to raise your chest off the floor; keep waist on the floor for safety; hold for a count of 5 (see Figure 3-1a). Figure 3-1b, c, and d show increased level of difficulty. If you have trouble doing the raises in Figures 3-1a or b, you need to develop abdominal muscles. Do 5 curls, brief rest, 5 curls, rest, 5 curls.

Exercise non-stop for at least 20 minutes a day (cardiovascular exercise)
- Assess your current level of endurance with this 12-minute brisk walking test.

Rating:	Distance covered in 12 minutes:
World Class	Over 2 miles
Excellent	1½ to 2 miles
Good	1 to 1½ miles
Fair	¾ to 1 mile
Poor	½ to ¾ mile

- Walk briskly for 45 to 60 minutes (about 3.5 to 5 miles) at least 3 times a week.
- Run 20-40 minutes a day, 3 to 5 days a week (about 10 to 20 miles).

Eat a diet of whole grains, beans, fresh fruits and vegetables
- Eliminate all red meat, almost all fats and oils; keep poultry and fish to twice a week.
- Avoid sugar, processed foods, and foods with additives.

Drink ½ gallon of water a day
- Drink mostly filtered or spring water.
- Avoid soft drinks and coffee.

Keep your weight in a reasonable range
- Avoid going on and off diets to lose weight.
- Maintain the basic diet above; with exercise, excess weight will melt off with time.

Eliminate smoking
Moderate alcohol consumption
Release unhealthy stress and poor attitudes
- Stay in touch with how your are feeling.
- Listen to your body. Do what you need to do to feel balanced.
- Take time each day to still the mind, rest, and reflect.
- Be playful.

Training Tips for Walkers

Training? For walking, our basic form of movement? You bet! Walking is the safest, easiest on the body, and most practical exercise, other than swimming and cross-country skiing. But before I talk to you about some guidelines for walking, I want to share a quote from Brenda Ue-

44

land's *If You Want to Write* who wrote, at the age of ninety-three, about the creativity that she felt when she walked.

> For me, a long five or six mile walk helps. And one must go alone and every day. I have done this for many years. It is at these times I seem to get re-charged. If I do not walk one day, I seem to have on the next what Van Gogh calls "the meagerness"...the "depression." After a day or two of not walking, when I try to write I feel a little dull and irresolute...when I walk grimly and calisthenically, just to get exercise, to get it out of the way, then I find I have not been re-charged with imagination...but when I look at the sky or the lake or the tiny, infinitesimally delicate, bare, young trees...when I say "I am free," and "There is nothing to hurry about," I find then that thoughts begin to come to me in their quiet way.
>
> It is the little bomb of revelation bursting inside you. I found I never took a long, solitary walk without some of these silent, little inward bombs bursting quietly: "I see. I understand that now!" and a feeling of happiness.[1]

In vigorous walking every muscle of the body is used. The calories burned in brisk walking are almost equivalent to those burned in running since increased speed doesn't automatically burn more fuel. Rather, the energy used depends on the distance traveled. Walking gives the heart the best workout, lowers blood pressure, firms your body, and lowers the triglyceride levels in the blood.

To get the most out of walking, walk briskly rather than amble, stroll, or saunter. President Harry S. Truman said, "Walk purposefully. Walk as though you have some place to go." At any level, walking has its benefits in increasing circulation and clearing the mind; however, studies in sports medicine have given us some guidelines on how to exercise for the greatest benefit to our cardiovascular system.

Start Slowly. Assess your fitness by taking the Rockport Fitness Test:

1. Measure a mile where you can walk with few interruptions such as stop lights.
2. Walk the mile as fast as you can.
3. Record your time to the nearest second. Most people walk between 3.0 and 6.0 miles per hour so it should take 10–20 minutes to walk the mile.
4. Record your heart rate immediately at the end of the mile (it begins to slow very quickly after you stop running). Count your pulse for 15 seconds and multiply by 4, then record this number. This gives you your heart rate per minute after your test walk.

You can write to the Rockport Walking Institute to get their pamphlet which shows fitness levels based on the time and heart rate after walking a mile.[2] The pamphlet gives graded walking programs that allow you to progress in weekly mileage according to your starting level.

If you are unaccustomed to physical activity, start with a pace of about 2 miles an hour for 20 minutes, and increase your speed and distance over a period of weeks.

There are two reasons to pay attention to your heartbeat rate. First, too fast a rate for too long a time can create stress, exhaustion, and other damage leading to increased risk of injury. Secondly, the quality of your performance and the ability to achieve your goals depend on an optimum workout *for you*.

Exercise at 60 to 75 percent of your maximum heart capacity.

Here is how to determine your safe pulse rate for exercise. The highest possible human pulse rate is 220.

Subtract your age from 220 (let's say you're 45)

$220 - 45 = 175$. That is your maximum; however you should only exercise between 60 to 75 percent of your maximum, so multiply 175 x 60 for your exercise rate of 105. To get a 10 second pulse count at this target rate, divide 105 by 6 = 17 beats.

Do conditioning stretches before and after walking.

The warm-up stretches in Chapter 15 should be done for 5 to 10 minutes. If you haven't time to do them both before and after walking, it's probably better to do a set afterwards. To warm up without the stretching, just start walking at a slower pace and then after about 10 minutes, start a brisk pace.

Attain a brisk speed.

You can increase your cardiovascular fitness by 8 to 15 percent by walking briskly three times a week for 30 minutes. When you can walk about 4 miles an hour and can still carry on a conversation while walking (you're breathing fairly hard, but not out of breath), you're probably at your target heart rate of aerobic effectiveness.

Steady as you go.

Consistency is the key to getting the benefits of walking. You need to burn 2,000 calories a week. This means that you have to maintain your ideal heartbeat rate (60 to 75 percent of your maximum heartbeat rate) for 45 minutes to an hour, three to five times a week.

For a person in reasonably good health, a normal walking pace is somewhere between 3.0 and 3.5 miles per hour. A speed of 3.75 to 4.0 miles per hour is considered a brisk pace, and speeds up to 5.5 miles per hour are not unusual. Anything below 3.0 is slow.

You will find it fairly easy to walk 4 miles in an hour (a 15-minute mile) after a few weeks of conditioning. This will burn off 400 calories each time—2,000 calories in five days!

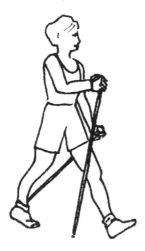

3-2. Exerstriding with Rubber-tipped Ski-poles.

"Exer-walk."

Exerstriding is a new form of overall body exercise that uses rubber-tipped ski-poles while walking or running.[3] The upper body muscles are strengthened as you use the poles to help propel you forward. 20 to 50 percent more calories are burned each minute than with simple walking. Abdominals are exercised, and your cardiovascular workout is higher. Risk of injury is reduced because all the muscles share the workload (Fig. 3-2).

What to look for in a walking shoe.

The question I am most often asked by patients, friends, and other doctors is "What shoes do you recommend?" Although the foot, during walking, lands with only one and one half times the force of body weight, as compared to the force of three times body weight in running, good walking shoes are a must. This is particularly true if you are heavy.

Good Socks

Don't forget that socks are part of your gear. The major requirement of socks, whether they be 100 percent cotton or a cotton/orlon blend, is that they keep the feet warm (or cool depending on the climate) and dry. They should be absorbent and should not bunch up causing friction or irritation. This is particularly important if you have diabetes or poor circulation because you are more susceptible to infection if you develop a blister. If you have a problem with athlete's

---

A Checklist for Walking Shoes

- Buy a shoe with a firm heel counter (back of shoe) that cups the heel and controls any tendency to roll inward during heel strike.
- Buy leather or leather-and-mesh construction which provides support and allows for good ventilation.
- Buy a light-weight, not bulky, shoe.
- Make sure that there is a roomy toe box to allow the toes to spread comfortably during the push-off phase of the walking stride.
- Be sure there is a well-cushioned heel to soften the heel-strike; the heel should elevate the back of the foot only slightly higher than the front.
- Look for a protective, *shock-absorbent* sole.
- Be sure there is substantial arch support to prevent foot fatigue.

---

foot (itchy rash between toes), change socks two to three times a day. Make sure that you wear socks that "wick" well (soak up moisture). Walking sockless will ultimately soak your shoes in a highly potent level of sweat which may mean you walk alone!

Training Tips for Runners

"Should I have a physical exam before beginning a running program?" I often hear this question, and have included these guidelines to help you make your decision:

If you are:

Under 30. Check with your doctor if you have a cardiac condition, hypertension, weight problem, heavy smoking habit, diabetes, high blood cholesterol level, breathing problems, irregular pulse, joint or back problems, family or personal history of any heart problems.

Over 30. See your doctor before starting any vigorous exercise program. Your exam should include a review of medical history, electrocardiogram, blood pressure, serum cholesterol, and a discussion of your jogging or running program.

Over 40. See your doctor before starting any vigorous exercise program. A stress test on a treadmill with electronic devices recording heartbeat and other body functions may be recommended by your doctor.

Note to women. Walking, jogging, or running during menstruation may help alleviate cramps. It can also be helpful during pregnancy when done under a physician's supervision. Check with your obstetrician/gynecologist.[4]

Warm-up—Cool-Down

Are you the type of runner who would rather increase the actual amount of time spent running, and hedge by cutting down your warm-up or cool-down time? Don't do it. You risk more injury by cutting back on the warm-up, and it's not worth it.

If you absolutely can't do the warm-up, then do 10 minutes of medium-to-brisk walking before you start running. But be sure to finish the run with 9 minutes of stretching. Refer to Chapter 15 for warm-up exercises.

Cyclic vs. Progressive Training

Like Madeline, the divorcee who literally jumped into running to regain her shape and her self-esteem, many new runners want instant results. They start off too rapidly and train too hard. With overtraining they become irritable. If you are over-concerned or anxious about your performance, you could be pushing yourself too hard. *Train, don't strain.*

There are two kinds of training methods for runners. The first is progressive, which means that each week the intensity and duration of the workout increases. With the progressive method, you start running, say, 5 miles a week, increasing a mile or two each week, until you are going about 20 miles. Without intervals for rest between increases, you are at risk for accumulating unadapted stress. A steady climb in mileage with no periods of recuperation stresses your body. Therefore, progressive training often leads to injury.

Ely, forty-two, for example, began jogging twice around his block and added a block each week, until he was running 2 miles. When he was running 5 miles, his heel began giving him trouble.

Here's what happened. Ely's increasing mileage (starting when he was not in good shape to begin with) gave the message to his bones that he was going to be exercising. In the fourth week the bones, in preparation for building more mass, first decreased in thickness. Ely kept right on running every day, adding more stress to the bones during a time of calcium reduction, eventually creating pain and small cracks in his leg bone at the fourth week.

To prevent a progressive build-up of continuous intensity and stress, I recommend that you use the *cyclic* training method which takes into account such physiological changes as bone mass. Whether you are at a beginning, advanced, or professional level, you will find this system builds a superior, and healthier track record.

The cyclic method, as the name suggests, allows your body to adapt to increased demands in a rhythmic, harmonious way. With the cyclic method, you work out at your appropriate level for 3 weeks. During the fourth week, you switch to another activity which works different parts of the body, resting those under stress. This method of cross training allows the running muscles to stay flexible and toned—well-prepared for an increase in duration in the fifth week. The cyclic method also allows the bones to recover, minimizing the likelihood of stress fractures. This method of training allows the body to adapt naturally to stress, adds variety to your program, and helps you avoid staleness.

How To Use the Cyclic Method of Training for Running

First Week:	*Easy:* run your preferred goal three times
Second Week:	*Moderate*: run your goal four times
Third Week:	*Harder:* run your goal four or five times
Fourth Week:	*Easy:* switch to cross-training (reduced running, biking, swimming, walking, golf)
Fifth Week:	*Easy:* increase your goal by ½ to 1 mile or 5 minutes every 3 weeks; run three times
Sixth Week:	*Moderate:* run your new goal four times
Seventh Week:	*Harder:* run four to five times a week
Eighth Week:	*Easy:* switch to cross-training
Ninth Week:	*Easy:* increase your goal by ½ to 1 mile or 5 minutes—run four times

In addition to the above schedule of training, take into consideration your age and any risk factors for heart disease before you start exercising regularly. The risk factors are smoking, obesity, high cholesterol, and a family history of heart disease. If you have risk factors, take an exercise stress test at your doctor's office or have her or him refer you to an exercise cardiologist.

Breath

You are at the correct level of exertion when you are not out of breath when you are exercising, but as soon as you increase your pace you find it difficult to sing, talk, or hum. This level will be about 70 percent of your heart rate, which is ideal for running or other aerobic activity.

If you can, breathe in through the nose and out through the mouth. As you do this, visualize your breath coming up from the earth, past the front of your legs, back through your abdomen, up over your head. Then mentally exhale the breath down past your chest and back out the abdomen. The visualized breath describes a figure-eight around the body. I've found this meditation helps me get past that 30-minute warm-up period before running is really enjoyable.

Anaerobic Work—When You're Running Out of Breath

Anaerobic exercise means that you are working at a level higher than 90 percent of your heart rate. The word anaerobic literally means "without oxygen," and indicates that you're using the oxygen stored in your body. Unless you are an athlete training for competition, you should not be working at this level. Without proper training and conditioning, you are at greater risk of fatigue and injury.

If you play a sport that requires you to run hard—to work hard enough that you are out of breath—then you need to train anaerobically. You should not work anaerobically (do interval work) until you can run comfortably for one hour.

The first week start cautiously, let's say, ten 100-yard dashes, working at 80 percent of your maximum. The second and third weeks run ten 100-yard dashes at 85 percent. At the fourth week, change to five 200-yard dashes at 80 or 90 percent. Try for a quick rhythm and a long stride. Stay relaxed. You won't be breathing easily, but you shouldn't be bending over gasping for air after each sprint. You can play around with this, but you'll find that when you go back to running aerobically (not out of breath), you will have increased your aerobic threshold and will be able to run at 75 percent of your capacity.

Sleep

Sleep earns its name as the great restorer. I know many of you fight for time to run and are also fiercely involved in your work. Cutting corners on sleep is definitely asking for trouble. Sleep is a vital key to staying on track and to curing your over-use injuries. Your brain, especially the frontal lobe, is very active during sleep as it processes information from your waking day. If you're training more or running more, you need more sleep, so be sure to stay tuned in to what your body wants—probably between 6 and 9 hours. It's best to get into a conditioned sleep pattern—that is, go to bed about the same time every night and get up at the same time.

Physical Tips for Sensible Exercise
- Either stretch your leg muscles before a run, or begin the run by fast walking for 10 minutes before running. Stretch for at least 9 minutes after the run.
- Use cyclic training—increase duration or pace during the third week. During the fourth week, switch to walking, swimming, biking, tennis.
- If you are very tired at exercise time, take a nap instead.
- If the weather is bad, stay home and read a book.
- If you're hungry, eat (wait at least 3 hours before running).
- If stiff or achy, stretch longer than usual, go for a swim, do yoga or take an easy walk.
- If after 15 minutes into a run you still feel lousy, stop and walk. Remember, this is for fun! This is playtime, so be playful and enjoy your exercise.
- Be attuned to your body's level of energy, apathy, or contentment—listen to the wisdom of your body.
- Be sure your level of competitiveness is appropriate and directed by realistic goals.
- Be aware of how your routine affects family and work.
- Be open to spontaneous opportunities for fun and exercise beyond your own routine—be flexible.

What To Look For in Running Shoes

Jack had an old pair of army boots in the garage, and he thought, what the heck, they still seemed to fit. Why not use them to run? After all, they were good, sturdy boots.

Obviously, Jack had never seen the list of injuries that can result from running in footwear that is "fifty per cent worse in rearfoot shock absorption, 100 percent less flexible, and more than 200 percent less shock absorbent in the forefoot than an average training flat." This is how one study described army boots.

If the Shoe Fits, Wear It

There really is no answer to "What is the best running shoe?" If the shoe fits *you,* and fits you for any biomechanical problem you may have (for example, excessive rolling in of the foot), and is appropriate to the kind of running *you* do, then buy it. Remember, running is a uni-directional sport: the foot goes forward, straight ahead, unlike multi-directional activities, such as tennis and aerobics, where the foot goes sideways as well as forward. A running shoe is designed for uni-directional exercise. There is a shoe, by the way, which is called a cross-trainer which is made for all types of sports. Improvements in the design of running shoes in the last decade have dramatically decreased the incidence of certain injuries such as Achilles tendinitis, heel bone damage, and knee problems.

Dr. Peter Cavanagh, author of *The Running Shoe Book,* and director of the biomechanics lab at Penn State University, suggests the following guidelines for buying running shoes based on lab tests he conducted for *Runner's World.*[5]

The Shoe Search Chart

Fill out the following Shoe Search Chart by answering questions about your old shoes, your feet and legs, your injury history, and your running style and running habits. Follow the explanation of each point at the end of the chart, since you may not know what this "foot jargon" means. Fig. 3-3 on page 57 shows the parts of a running shoe.

Note: A varus wedge is a built in correction of 5 degrees in a shoe.

Point 1: Examine Your Old Shoes

OBSERVATION	INFERENCE	CHECK IF APPLICABLE
Heel Counters:		
Turn inwards:	You probably pronate excessively Rearfoot control is important Could try varus wedge	_____
Turn outwards:	May have rigid foot type. Avoid varus wedge. Look for a good heel counter but other rearfoot control properties not critical.	_____
Generally battered:	Look for a better heel counter in your next shoe.	_____
Uppers:		
Leather uppers badly stretched:	May need a wider shoe, but leather may be essential to give your foot the space it needs	_____

OBSERVATION	INFERENCE	CHECK IF APPLICABLE
Hole above the big toe:	Needs a higher toe box.	_____
Uppers in bad condition:	Your running style and habits are hard on the shoe. Avoid mesh uppers. Go with well-made nylon weave (taffeta).	_____

Midsole and Wedge:

Hard and brittle:	You waited too long before buying a new pair of shoes. Plan to run fewer miles in the next pair.	
Uneven compression on inside and outside edges:	You need a more substantial material in the midsole and wedge. May have to sacrifice shoe weight.	_____

Outsole:

Rear outside corner badly worn:	Probably a rearfoot striker. Make sure new shoe scores well on rearfoot impact and sole wear tests.	_____
Front outside edge badly worn:	Probably a mid or forefoot striker. Forefoot impact is important and good wear chacteristics under ball. (Note: not measured by *Runner's World* wear test)	_____
Right-left shoes wear differently:	May suggest leg length discrepancy or dynamic asymmetry in style.	_____

Fit and Comfort:

Often had black toenails:	Need higher toe box.	_____
Numb toes while running:	Need wider shoe.	_____
Pressure points in forefoot:	Leather upper may help.	_____

Point 2: Look at Your Feet, Legs, and Body Weight

Foot type:

Normal foot:	No worries on this score.	
Rigid high arch:	Problem foot. Good impact properties essential. Shoe must allow motion so poor rearfoot control could be a positive feature. Also get a flexible shoe. You may need additional heel lift and professional attention.	_____
Flexible high arch:	Still look for good shock absorption.	_____
Flexible flat foot:	Still needs all the support it can get. Good rearfoot control. Supportive upper. Try varus wedge. May need professional help.	_____
You wear an orthotic:	See special needs for orthotic wearers in Chapter 12.	_____

WHAT TO LOOK FOR IN RUNNING SHOES

OBSERVATION	INFERENCE	CHECK IF APPLICABLE

Rearfoot alignment:

Rearfoot valgus: Pronate in standing, probably even more extreme in running. Rearfoot control important. Try varus wedge. _____

Rearfoot varus: Avoid varus wedge. _____

Rearfoot-forefoot imbalance: May need professional help if severe. _____

Foot size and shape:

Unusual "bumps" on foot: Leather uppers will adapt to unusual shape. _____

Left and right feet are different lengths or widths: Fit larger foot. Lacing pattern which will take up slack on smaller foot important. In extreme cases may need to buy 2 pair to get 1. _____

Leg Alignment:

Bow-legged Varus wedge OK. _____

Knock-kneed Avoid large flare. _____

Both may need professional help.

Body Weight:

Male over 170 lbs. Female over 140 lbs.: Avoid racing flats. _____

Point 3: Consider Your Injury History

Knee Injuries: Rearfoot control important. Avoid excessive lateral flare. _____

Heel Spur Syndrome: Look for good rearfoot impact, good rearfoot control, good flexibility, but good torsional stiffness. May need heel pad. _____

Shin Splints: Good impact properties are important and good rearfoot control. Make sure your training habits are sound. _____

Stress Fractures: Good impact properties are important as well as flexibility for "march" fracture. _____

Achilles Tendon Problems: Good heel raise. Low penetration into shoe (part of rearfoot control). _____

Ankle Sprains: As low heel as Achilles will allow. Avoid varus wedge if inversion sprain. _____

Point 4: Consider Your Running Style

Point of first contact with ground:

Rearpart of shoe: Both rearfoot and forefoot impact properties are important. Also rearpart wear should be good. _____

OBSERVATION	INFERENCE	CHECK IF APPLICABLE
Middle or fore-part of shoe:	Forefoot impact properties are particularly important. Also good wear in region under ball.	_____

Foot motion during midsupport:

Stay on outside border:	Avoid varus wedge. Look for good heel counters, firm midsole.	_____
Tend to flick heel toward midline:	Will lead to excessive wear under ball of foot. Look for good forepart wear but baffles may be necessary to alleviate leg pain despite their poor wear properties.	_____

Point 5: Consider Your Running Habits

Running Surface:

Road running:	Good impact properties essential.	_____
Wet roads:	Traction important particularly for racing.	_____
Trails and uneven surface:	Good tread pattern, good rearfoot control.	_____

Competition:

Average runner:	Needs heavier, more stable shoe, not racing flats.	_____
Elite runner:	Needs lighter, more flexible shoe.	_____

Environment:

Hot and humid:	Breathability (permeability to water vapor) is important. Broad mesh with thin permeable lining would be good. Air circulating insert an advantage.	_____
Cold weather:	Get waterproof uppers with no vents. May also need additional insert to insulate foot from cold sole.	_____

Point 1: Examine Your Old Shoes

If you are a new runner, you don't have any old running shoes to look at, so go on to point number 2. If you have old shoes examine them for the following points:

Heel Counters

First, stand the shoes up side by side on the edge of a flat surface and look at the backs of the shoes (heel counters). If the counters are leaning inward or outward, there has been a greater strain on the counter than it could handle. The most usual direction will be inward

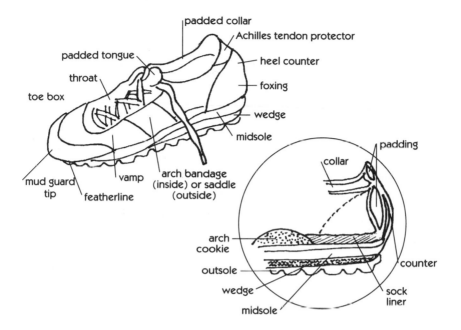

3-3. Parts of a Running Shoe

(Fig. 2-23) which means that you probably overpronate. If so, look for a shoe with **good rearfoot control**.

If your heels are slanting outward (Fig. 2-23), you may be very susceptible to ankle sprains, because you are running on the outside of your feet. You probably have a rigid foot which does not adapt well to the variety of surfaces you encounter. Avoid shoes with a varus wedge which can cause your foot to tilt even further out, increasing the likelihood of ankle sprains or foot or leg pain. A varus wedge is a built-in correction of 5 degrees that is thicker on the inside of the heel and tapers to the outside. Instead of an actual wedge, some shoes now have stronger rubber on the inside of the heel and softer rubber on the outside to achieve the same correction. The shoe table in the annual October issue of *Runner's World* will tell you if a shoe is built with a varus wedge, or you can ask about this in an athletic store with knowledgeable sales people.

Either way, if the counter is badly deformed, has cracked, or is very soft, make sure you choose a shoe which has enough stiffness in the back.

Uppers

Now turn the shoes around and look at them from the front. Look at the toe box for clues as to whether the shoe was wide enough and roomy enough (in height). If your shoes are leather, they have deformed in the directions in which your foot applied force. If they were nylon, which does not conform, the constant force together with abrasion may have caused the uppers to rip away from the sole in the ball area.

If the sides are bulging over the sole, your shoe is too narrow. You must get a wider shoe next time. When you shop, remember that European brands tend to be narrower than American shoes. Since there is little standardization of sizing in the shoe industry, the size in your next shoe may vary from what you've been wearing.

If you have any unusual anatomical features on your foot, a leather upper is a must. Be wary of shoes which have a leather upper sewn onto nylon taffeta. The nylon will not allow the leather to take the shape of your foot.

If your uppers are in relatively good condition, even though other parts of the shoe are badly worn, you may want to purchase the same type of shoe again. If you are hard on the uppers, don't buy nylon mesh shoes, which are not as durable as nylon taffeta or weave.

Leather shoes are the most durable, but need a bit more care and are a little heavier. Look for a shoe with strong, well-stitched uppers. The best have double stitching at major stress points. If you buy a nylon shoe, make sure it is reinforced with leather all around the featherline (the junction of the upper and bottom). This will relieve some of the wear on the nylon. Many runners feel nylon is the best choice since it doesn't harden or crack from exposure to rain and sun. Nylon is cooler, dries faster, doesn't chafe the foot and doesn't need breaking in. The best shoes have suede reinforcements around the stress points— toe, heel, and laces. Shoes that have plastic rings around the lacing holes will hold up better under tight, repeated lacing.

Midsole and Wedge

If the midsole and wedge of your old shoes have become hard and brittle, you aren't getting the shock absorption you need anymore. You definitely need new shoes. Look also at the heel and ball areas to see if the material has compressed more on one side than another.

Outsole

Wear patterns on the outsole are indicators of both running style and shoe quality. Shoes don't wear out where the most pressure is, they wear out where the most motion occurs between the shoe and the ground.

If you are a rearfoot striker, it is likely that the back outside edge of the shoe will be worn off diagonally much more than the forepart (see Figure 2-22e). If so, look for shoes with *good sole wear and rearfoot impact properties.* If you are buying a shoe with a waffle sole, make sure it has a built-up area or wear bar on the part that you wear down.

If the wear is mostly on the front outside part of the sole, you're probably a midfoot or a forefoot striker. A waffle sole will wear down faster than a homogeneous sole. This may be so extreme for a forefoot striker that, after a few hundred miles, the rest of the shoe will be in perfectly good condition, but the outsole useless.

Fit and Comfort

How did your old shoes feel? Did you get blisters? Were your toes ever numb after a run, or did you get black toenails? If the shoes gave you many miles of injury-free running, you probably can buy the same shoe. It might still be a good idea, however, to read through the next points.

Point 2: Look At Your Feet, Legs, and Body Weight

First determine if you have a normal, flat, or high-arched foot. One way to do this is to wet your foot and then walk across a dark, smooth surface so that a clear impression of the sole is left. You can also draw around your feet while standing on a piece of paper. Compare the print with those in Fig. 2-6. If yours is a **normal arch,** you probably need no extra support unless you're doing high weekly mileage and need support to help balance the foot. The range of shoes you can wear is quite varied.

A **high-arched** foot is a rigid foot with little flexibility and little ability to dissipate shock. Most likely, you'll need a custom-made arch support. There are different types of high arches, but the major distinction is between the rigid and the flexible.

A **rigid high-arched foot** (also called a *cavus* foot) has a limited range of motion in both flexion and extension (up and down movements), but particularly in supination and pronation (leverage and shock absorption). The difficulty with the rigid high-arch is that it cannot absorb shock the way a normal foot can. High arches need shoes with exceptional shock absorption. Because the high-arched foot is already rather restricted, it's better in a shoe with less rearfoot control. I sometimes tell runners who have high arches to take a file and get rid of flared heels on their shoes in order to allow a little more flexibility.

A **flexible high-arched foot** is subjected to tremendous pressures during running. Since the arch supports that come with shoes are not going to help you much, I suggest you get an additional insert which will take the shape of the foot and provide support. Again, exceptional shock absorption is important.

If you have a "dropped forefoot" where the front part of the foot is lower in relation to the heel (Fig. 2-6e), you need a shoe which has a large height differential between the forefoot and the rearfoot. You might also need a heel pad.

A **flat foot** may need considerable help or none at all. This type of foot lies flat on the ground, and pulls the rearfoot into a pronated position, creating stress on muscles and bones. A very low arch may need a custom-made orthotic. Like the high-arched foot, flat feet can be either rigid or flexible.

The **flexible flat foot**, too adaptable and unstable, causes the most problems. Look for a straight-lasted shoe to give more support. Make sure the shoe has enough room for an orthotic if you need one, and that the rearfoot control is strong.

An intermediate solution to arch supports, incidentally, is available in over-the-counter products by Spenco, Dr. Scholl's, Fredonic, and Lynco to name just a few. I advocate getting a temporary orthotic to make sure it is going to work for you, since a custom orthotic can cost $300 to $350, and temporary ones are about $65. If you run 15 to 20 miles a week, you definitely need a permanent orthotic if you have a foot problem. Another temporary solution is to tape your foot for support.

Rearfoot and Forefoot Alignment

If you were to draw a line through the midline of the back of your heel, and the line pointed towards the midline of your body, you have rearfoot valgus (2-13b). Or, conversely, if you were to draw a line through the midline of your heel and it pointed away from the body, then you should stay away from shoes with a varus correction.

Substantial imbalances between your forefoot and rearfoot require professional help. A heel counter should extend high enough to cup the heel even if you put inserts in your shoes. Make sure there is padding on the inside of the heel counter, as well as at the top of the heel.

Size and Shape of Your Foot

Check the top of your foot for any unusual bumps or projections, especially where the big and little toes meet the forefoot. If you do have knobs or bumps, remember that nylon uppers are not going to conform to these irregularities and will continue to irritate them as long as you wear the shoe. Leather uppers are a must for abnormally shaped feet.

It's a good idea, before you go to the store, to measure both feet. If one foot is larger than the other, buy a pair of shoes to fit the larger foot. If the feet are significantly different you may have to buy two separate pairs of shoes in two sizes.

Shoes are constructed on a form called a "last." The last of the shoe refers to the shape.

Straight-lasted shoes are good for flat or low arched feet. If you also have bunions or trouble with your toes, a straight-lasted shoe will put less pressure on your toes.

C-shaped-lasted shoes are helpful if you toe-in.

Board or stiff-lasted shoes are good for very flexible feet.

Slip-lasted shoes are good for a high-arched rigid foot. Slip-lasted is most flexible and grips the heel better.

Combination-lasted shoes are good for forefoot flexibility in the front for toe-off, and have cardboard in the back for hindfoot stability.

Anatomical-lasted shoes have a cupped indentation for the heel to help keep the heel's fat pad in place. This is particularly helpful for heel spur syndrome.

Your Legs

Two leg problems may affect your choice of running shoe—bow legs and knock knees. If you have either condition, you should be able to see it in the mirror. Bow legs, the more common problem, results in excessive pronation and if severe, you'll need professional help. If it's not so severe, you may be able to use a shoe with a varus wedge, although the rearfoot control may not be sufficient for your needs.

If you have knock knees, you definitely need professional help, especially if you are having pain or are going to increase your mileage. There is no shoe on the market that caters to this problem.

Your Body Weight

Racing shoes are not a good idea for men weighing more than 170 pounds or for women over 140 pounds. The heavier you are, the more important is cushioning.

Point 3: Your Injury History

The proper shoe is a blessing to a runner. A good shoe is not, however, the only factor in injury-free running as we have seen. Sometimes a change of shoe is exactly the answer to a running problem, but more often, it's not that simple. Let's consider some of the injuries you might have had, and see how they relate to your choice of shoes.

Knee Injuries. As we have seen in our chapter on biomechanics, most knee injuries are the result of misalignment and overuse. There tends to be a gradual onset of pain.

Pain around the kneecap seems most likely to be shoe-related. Shoes that allow the foot which overpronates to continue its motion without resistance will be adding to the problem. *Rearfoot control* is vitally important if you have a history of knee injury. Most knee problems are not impact injuries. If a shoe is rated high for a soft and compressive midsole, this fact is bad news for the knee. Excessive flare at the heel should also be avoided by runners with knee pain. Many clinicians feel that flare will, if anything, exacerbate any pain, particularly on the outside of the knee.

Heel Spur Syndrome. If there is pain underneath the front edge of the heel bone whenever pressure is exerted, you need a shoe with *good rearfoot impact absorption*. In addition, a shoe that provides resistance to twisting along the long axis of the shoe will probably be helpful. The *stiffer* the shoe, the better it will be for heel spur syndrome. Heel pads will be useful for symptomatic relief. Good arch support can help, so make sure your shoe can accommodate an orthotic.

Shin Splints. Usually if you pronate excessively, you work the tibial muscles harder. Therefore, a shoe which controls rearfoot motion will be extremely important if you have a tendency for shin splints (pain in the shank of the lower leg). Make sure that impact absorption is also adequate.

Stress Fractures. When shin splints are allowed to progress untreated, there is a danger of developing a stress fracture on the front bones of the lower leg. Stress fracture is definitely a result of unabsorbed impact which accumulates over time. Forefoot impact must be adequately cushioned, and if you are a rearfoot striker, you need cushioning in the heel as well. When you look over the table of forefoot impact values in the latest October issue of *Runner's World,* give a high priority to this rating. Stress fracture is also related to shoes that are too inflexible; however, even though racing flats are flexible, they generally do not have the forefoot cushioning that is needed to protect against stress fracture.

Achilles Tendinitis. One source of Achilles tendon problems could be the differences in heel and forefoot height among various shoes you wear to run during the week. If, for example, you have one pair of shoes for training with a substantial heel raise, your Achilles tendon won't be stretched as far as it will be when you wear another pair of shoes with a lower heel and flatter sole, such as a racing shoe. The lower heel causes more stretching of the tendon leading to inflammation of the tendon. Try not to make sudden changes in your shoes once your foot has adjusted to a certain pair. If you have Achilles tendon problems, generally, you need to wear a shoe with a higher heel raise.

Ankle Sprains. If you habitually sprain your ankle (and don't have runner's knee), wear a shoe with flared heels to make foot placement more stable. If you tend to sprain your ankles on the outside, avoid shoes with varus correction. If you don't have an Achilles problem, you may be better off with as low a heel as possible. This reduces the risk of turning the ankle.

Point 4: Your Running Style

Determine which part of your foot hits the ground first (do this at your most common training speed). If your heel contacts the ground first, you are a rearfoot striker. If so, you need both rearfoot and forefoot impact cushioning to protect the length of your foot plant.

If you land more on the midfoot to forefoot, then you need forefoot cushioning. If you run on the outside of your foot, don't buy a shoe with a varus correction. Look for a shoe with a strong heel counter.

Do you snap your rearfoot towards the midline of the body (abductory twist) when you run? If you do, your shoes may reflect it in excessive wear under the ball of the foot. You'll need a shoe that wears well on the sole. Twisting will wear down waffle soles faster than a flat sole, but the waffles may ease the effect of the twisting at the knee and ankle joints. Start with a flat sole, but if this is a change for you, watch during the first few runs for knee pain.

Point 5: Your Running Habits

Terrain. Where you run is a big consideration in choosing a running shoe. If you run on roads and concrete, be sure to choose a shoe for its impact properties (that is, if you don't care about the relatively heavier weight). If you run on irregular surfaces, and have a tendency to sprain your ankle, high heel counters and flared heels help stabilize you over rough terrain. Rugged all-terrain shoes really help in this instance. Good traction is necessary if you are going to encounter wet, slick surfaces. If you're going to be racing, you'll want shoes that will perform well no matter what the weather turns out to be the day of the race. Generally, a flat sole is the best for running.

A strong rubber outer sole is usually between ⅛" and ¼" thick. If your sole is more than ⅜", it probably won't bend enough at toe-off. Soles have a life of 750 to 1,000 miles before they become too compressed to adequately absorb shock, so remember to check them after a few months.

The mid-sole will have one or two layers of soft but firm material that allows the shoe to bend where your foot bends. Air-bladders are used by Nike and other companies to prolong the lifetime of the mid-sole. The shoes that last longest have polyurethane in the mid-soles. If you wear orthotics (devices inserted into the shoe to correct foot problems), then buy a shoe with a removable in-sole so you can replace it with your orthotic.

Be aware that on a rainy day deep tread can pick up a great deal of weight from mud. Smaller tread could give you the same amount of traction, without collecting debris. There are add-on traction devices for snow running.

Temperature. Nylon mesh with a broad knit is best for high temperatures and humidity. However, if there is an impermeable lining underneath a wide mesh, it will prevent any cooling effect. You might even need an insole which will allow air circulation underneath your foot. In a leather shoe you can cut some ventilation holes without damaging the uppers too much. Leather or nylon weave is good for cold weather.

Support. While the forefoot of the shoe needs flexibility for push off, your shoes must provide firm support from the front part of the arch to the heel. This is the shank area, and should not bend more than a few degrees. If you're small and don't weigh a lot, don't buy shoes that are really stiff because you'll have trouble toeing-off. You'll pull your Achilles tendon when you force your foot to bend. Children, because their feet are still soft and malleable, should not wear a small adult shoe. Women who have a "man's foot" may wear a man's shoes, as long as it's not too stiff. A men's size 7 is a women's size 9.

Don't use your running shoes to play sports like tennis, racquetball or basketball, which are multi-directional activities. Your running shoe, with its uni-directional design, will not let you make the quick moves and changes of direction; in addition, you risk breaking down the heel counter.

Heel Lift. A shoe's heel lift should be between ½" and ¾" higher than the front of the shoe. This increases the shock absorptive ability of the sole as well as preventing straining of the Achilles tendon. The heel should be curled a bit to help you roll forward into your stride after heel-strike.

Evaluating What You Have Learned

By now you should have filled out your shoe search chart according to what you observed or what you know about your old running shoes, your feet and legs, your past injuries, your running style, and habits. You will have a list of notes about recommendations for each area or problem (e.g., "good rearfoot control" or "must have impact cushioning").

If you still cannot figure out what you need, make the best analysis you can. Go to a running shoe store and ask if you can take a few pairs to your podiatrist's office. It's helpful to see a doctor who has a treadmill and video camera so that your running can be analyzed on slow motion. Most stores will cooperate with you, allowing you to return those shoes which are not going to be used.

Remember, a higher price does not automatically mean a better shoe, but good shoes cost more because of the research and development of the such engineering factors as orthopedic heel counters, shank support, arch supports, and sole flex.

Buying the Shoes

Go to a store that specializes in running shoes—staffed by sales people with running experience. Take your checklist, running socks and an orthotic if you use one.

Try on both left and right shoes. There should be a space the thickness of your thumb between the end of the shoe and the end of your big toe. Try on several pairs with different types of construction to compare fit and feel before making your choice.

Inquire as to the store policy on returns of shoes that are defective. The best store gives an instant replacement, instead of sending defective shoes back to the factory—you don't want to be without your running shoes for six weeks!

Wear your new shoes around the house for a couple of days just in case you find that you want to take them back—at least they won't have been worn outside in the dirt. The worst thing you could do is run a race in a new pair of shoes. Run the first few times in the shoes at an easy pace. You can rip out the arch cookie if it feels uncomfortable, or replace it with something else.

During the first 50 miles or so listen carefully to your body. If the new shoes have caused an ache or a pain that won't go away, you may be forced to stop using the shoes and switch to another pair, at least temporarily. If some part of the shoe rips or tears, or the stitching comes apart, take the shoe back if you don't think it's something you caused to happen.

Enjoy your new shoes, and congratulate yourself on taking the extra time and effort to give yourself the best.

What You Should Know About Orthotics

The Greek word ortho literally means straight, upright and correct. An orthotic is a bio-dynamic device that fits into shoes to accomplish two things:

To insure that the foot moves correctly through the various phases of walking or running (which include heel contact, whole foot contact, and toe-off), the orthotic functions like a *rudder,* to help the foot in proper follow-through.

To *support* the foot, encouraging it to find the best position as it moves, it enables the foot to communicate and align with the rest of the body. The body is then balanced above the foot in mid-stride as well as when the foot is on the ground. It's like a pair of glasses that help you see better.

There are two types of orthotic. Soft, temporary supports are made on the initial visit to a podiatrist, to give you an idea if an orthotic is going to help. They conform to the foot by normal body heat and pressure. Generally inexpensive, they range between $35 and $65, and will last from three months to a couple of years depending on what type of material they're made from.

Permanent orthotics for specific activities or sports will be made from a cast of the foot, and sent to an orthotic lab for fabrication. Prices range from $250 to $350, and most have a guarantee against breakage.

Different sports require different orthotics. An orthotic for running may not be appropriate for playing tennis because it's too controlling, and wearing it for everyday use could be uncomfortable because of the degree of tilting or canting built into it. Orthotics vary in length, stiffness, and amount of control depending on what activity will be done.

A half-length orthotic stops well behind the toes, and primarily supports the arch. It's good for limited walking and standing. A three-quarter length orthotic gives a little bit more support, and helps control the foot while the heel is off the ground. It's effective in shoes with higher heels, as it relieves pain under the metatarsal heads by taking the pressure off certain points.

Generally the rule is to use the most *flexible* orthotic that will be effective for the problem. *Semi-rigid* orthotics can help control various degrees of over-pronation and other biomechanical problems. *Rigid* orthotics are usually only used for very flat feet which need a lot of support.

Control is provided by a rearfoot and a forefoot post, respectively. For uni-directional sports, such as running, a rearfoot post and a forefoot post may both be used. For multi-directional sports, less rearfoot control is needed, to allow more side to side motion, as well as less forefoot control. For sports such as golf, no rearfoot control is needed, and forefoot control may be minimal. Usually the main concern is for arch support.

Footnotes

1. Brenda Ueland, *If You Want to Write,* (Sant Paul, MN, Graywolf Press), 1987.

2. "The Rockport Guide to Fitness Walking," Rockport Walking Institute, P.O. Box 480, Marlboro, Massachusetts 01752.

3. Exerstrider Products, Inc., P.O. Box 3313, Madison, WI 53704.

4. "Guidelines for Successful Running," American Academy of Podiatric Sports Medicine Running Committee, 1729 Glastonberry Road, Potomac, MD, 20854, (301) 424-7440.

5. Peter R. Cavanagh, *The Running Shoe Book,* (Mountain View, CA, Anderson Press, Inc.), 1980.

Chapter 4

CONVENTIONAL
TREATMENT

Some people think that doctors and nurses can put scrambled eggs
back into the shell.
—Dorothy Canfield Fisher

Fractures, stress fractures, injuries from accidents, physical deformities
like bunions and hammertoes, congenital deformities (short-leg syndrome), are often best treated by western orthodox medicine. If you're
in an accident, go to the emergency room of a hospital. Save your life
with emergency medicine, and then you can think about alternatives
and homeopathic remedies!

Major diseases such as cancer, diabetes, and various life-threatening diseases are often best treated by western medicine. However,
some chronic conditions like asthma or arthritis may actually be worsened by dependence on antibiotics, steroids or prolonged use of anti-
inflammatory medicines, so investigating homeopathic remedies and
alternative methods is worthwhile.

If you injure yourself in sports, and don't know if you need a specialist, go to your family doctor first. He or she will give you a referral
if your problem merits a specialist. You can also ask for a referral from
any other physician you see. It is perfectly acceptable to consult with
doctors before deciding to have them treat you.

To help you understand some of the differences between specialists, I have listed different types of orthodox medical practitioners (alphabetically).

Orthodox Medical Specialists

Cardiologists. These physicians, trained in American Medical As-
sociation-approved universities and hospitals, specialize in problems of

the cardiovascular system (heart). If you are in a high risk category for heart disease with any of the following factors: are a smoker; are very overweight; have a family history of heart disease; are over 30 and are starting exercise for the first time; have had any heart problems prior to starting an exercise program, you should see a cardiologist first before starting to run or play sports.

Family doctors. The family doctor is a general practitioner who is a good first step for any medical problem. They can give you an overall physical examination if you are going to start an exercise program, and can also give a diagnosis of a general medical condition. If your problem involves a knee or spinal injury related to exercise or sports, your family doctor can make a preliminary diagnosis. Family doctors will be able to refer you to a specialist if the problem needs this kind of expertise.

Internists. These physicians are M.D.'s who specialize in diseases of the internal body such as diabetes, ulcers, gastro-intestinal problems, and communicable diseases.

Neurosurgeons. These doctors are M.D.'s and are highly trained. They perform spinal surgery and treat serious back and head problems. They often work together with an orthopedist.

Orthopedic surgeons. These doctors attend four years of medical school and then do a general surgical residency after internship. They are specialists in musculoskeletal problems. They treat problems of the knees, hip, back, neck, or any other skeletal condition. Generally, a serious back problem requires the expertise of these specialists. It's best to see them for serious fractures other than ankle and foot fractures. They are also trained to treat serious diseases, such as cancer, which require surgery.

Osteopaths. Osteopaths have a doctor of osteopathy degree or M.D. and undergo the same training as a medical doctor, but they are taught to do manipulative medicine (putting misplaced bones back into place). Most osteopaths (but not all) tend to have more liberal attitudes toward alternative treatments.

Pediatricians. These physicians specialize in the diseases of children. If your child has a sports-related injury, take him or her to your regular pediatrician first. If there are complex problems involving the spine, back, groin, hip, legs, or knees, ankles or feet, the pediatrician will refer you to a specialist.

Physiatrists. These practitioners are M.D.'s who specialize in physical medicine and rehabilitation and are experts on the musculoskeletal system. Sometimes called orthopedists without scalpels, they are exceptional healers who combine medical training with sensitive touch to diagnose and treat acute and chronic back problems. Some work with sports injuries and some are rheumotologists. There are not many of these specialists in practice, but you might find one in a veterans' hospital or in a big rehabilitation center. If you have severe or chronic pain problems, it may very well be worth your while to track down one of these doctors. They also work in conjunction with many specialists such as physical therapists, occupational therapists, and masseurs. Refer to Chapter 20 for more information.

Podiatrists. These doctors attend four years of podiatric medical school. They also do internships and residency training. Podiatrists specialize in problems of the lower extremity. Since they are medical doctors, they can admit patients to a hospital, and are qualified to do surgery on the foot and leg and to treat non-surgically on other conditions. Since podiatrists do not perform knee surgery, see an orthopedist for serious fractures and knee problems.

Radiologists. These physicians are M.D.'s who specialize in diagnosis with x-rays and magnetic resonance imaging.

Other Sports-related Specialists

Certified athletic trainers. Athletic trainers are usually associated with high school or college teams. They can perform first aid and refer to other specialists.

Exercise physiologists. These people are research-oriented and have a Ph.D. degree. They study the physiological changes that go with exercise. Their research on such fields as electrolyte imbalance, the cardio-vascular system, and other sports-related areas is very important for sports medicine. They are found in major medical centers, and sometimes work directly with athletes.

Physical therapists. These practitioners undergo training for three to four years to learn rehabilitation, muscular restructuring, movement exercises, and the use of a variety of therapeutic equipment. They usually work under the supervision of an M.D.

Sports psychologists. Sports psychologists are specialists in working with the stresses involving competitive sports. They offer techniques and guidance such as helping athletes to focus on achieving goals, letting go of excessive goal-setting, and alleviating psychological stress. They work with individuals, teams, and with children who have disturbances related to sports.

Diagnostic Techniques

Conventional medicine excels in the technical diagnosis of illness and injury (listed alphabetically):

Bone scan. A bone scan injects radioactive dye into the blood stream. The dye concentrates in the bone in an area of increased inflammation. Similar to the CAT scan, a bone scan will show a stress fracture three weeks earlier than will an x-ray. Bone scans are best for detecting hard-to-find inflammation in the body. A bone scan would be used for diagnosing stress reaction of bone, stress fracture, bone tumors, and infection.

CAT scan. Computerized axial tomography—a CAT scan—is very good for revealing skeletal and bone problems. It will show a stress fracture three weeks before an x-ray will. It is also superior to an x-ray in showing cysts and lesions within the bone, such as in the ankle joint. CAT scans are also used for diagnosing cancer.

Lab tests. Bloodwork and urinalysis may need to be done in sports-related injuries to rule out arthritis or gout and evaluate other conditions such as:

Anemia, which means you don't have enough iron in the blood which can cause fatigue.

Electrolyte balance. Electrolytes include various salts such as potassium, sodium, and chloride which are needed for metabolic balance. Electrolyte levels can be depleted by heavy training.

Cholesterol level which indicates whether your blood vessels are clogged with this fatty deposit. If so, blood flow is restricted causing high blood pressure. Your doctor will advise you about your walking and running program. Walking and running help increase the ratio of the "good cholesterol" which helps eat up the "bad cholesterol."

Dehydration is another condition which will be evaluated by urinalysis.

Infection, such as mononucleosis which causes fatigue. You may, for example, think you're tired because you're running too much but, in fact, you may actually have an infection. Over-training can also bring on mononucleosis.

Allergies can often be detected by lab tests.

Hypoglycemia, (low blood sugar) has symptoms of constant hunger, fatigue, dizziness, and poor concentration.

Hyperglycemia (too much sugar in the blood) which is usually present in diabetics. Symptoms are increased hunger, thirst, and heavy urination in the evening. Both hypoglycemia and hyperglycemia are helped by moderate walking and running.

Thyroid deficiency can make you slow and sluggish, with a tendency to gain weight; skin and hair are dry or brittle. A hyperthyroid condition makes you lose weight, feel nervous, and act scattered. Both conditions are improved by exercise. Moderate exercise levels off many imbalances.

Blood in the urine, which sometimes happens to runners and must be checked out by a medical doctor. This is called "runner's hematuria" and can be caused by dehydration, kidney infections if you're worn down, or after bladder trauma. It also is associated with red blood cell damage if you over-train.

MRI (magnetic resonance imaging). Magnetic resonance imaging forms a picture of the body based on the resonance of the hydrogen atoms in various tissues. It is useful for looking at soft tissue, whereas the CAT scan is better for looking at bone. MRI is very useful for detecting injuries, for example, in the Achilles tendon, posterior tibial tendon, ligaments, or various organs. If you have a problem in the Achilles tendon which x-rays haven't picked up, an MRI will usually show the lesion if it's present. A sports medicine physician uses MRI for looking at the knee menisci (the cartilage within the knee joint), soft tissue such as the spinal cord or the brain, and intervertebral disc disease in the back. It will show cartilage anywhere in the body, and is particularly effective on the ankle.

Ultrasound. This process is used for soft tissue and for tendon problems. Ultrasound can detect disease, degeneration, or rupture of the Achilles tendon.

X-ray. X-ray is used primarily to look at bones and structure. It shows the outline of soft tissue but is not the definitive tool for soft tissue. People often ask me about the effects of x-ray and how many x-rays are "too much." While radiation does accumulate during your life, harmful buildup from yearly check-ups, foot x-rays, chest x-rays, or dental x-rays is *usually* not a problem. When you do get x-rayed, you should be given a lead shield to protect the rest of the body from absorbing rays. Do not get an x-ray if you're pregnant. In the 1950's many people were x-rayed too often and should not have more.

Gait and motion analysis devices. Computerized gait analysis has become feasible even for walkers and recreational runners. These machines give you feedback as to the quantity and quality of your biomechanical balance. Performance and training errors can be found and corrected very easily through videotaping and motion analysis. This type of analysis is helping athletes to set new world records. It also keeps amateur and recreational athletes healthy and free from biomechanical imbalances that lead to energy depletion.

Thermography. This process scans the body, and locates hot and cold spots to detect changes in body temperature. Thermography is useful for finding areas of inflammation, strain, or injury. It is often used in diagnosing back disease, or pin-pointing inflamed areas. It also helps to differentiate emotional problems from organic problems. Thermography can be used to scan a leg with shin splint pain for possible stress fracture, although the diagnosis is not as definitive as a bone scan.

Chapter 5

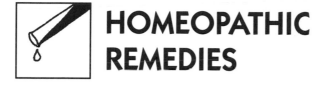 # HOMEOPATHIC
REMEDIES

Homeopathy cures a larger percentage of cases than any other system
or school of medicine.

—Mahatma Gandhi

My patients tend to be very curious with a real interest in their treatment. With my first two books, *Cures for Common Running Injuries*
and *The Running Foot Doctor,* I literally had patients come into the
office holding one of the books telling me, "I think I have the same
thing as Peter Stein!"

In those days, I had not yet been introduced to homeopathy. But
since then I have found it to be so useful in sports injuries that I am
very excited to share it with you. In order to help you understand what
homeopathy is and how to use it, I have tried to answer some of the
common questions I hear every day.

"What is homeopathy?"

The basic philosophy of homeopathy is that the body has an innate
capacity to maintain health and the ability to reestablish balance if
disease occurs. Homeopathic remedies help to heal the body by *enhancing the defensive responses of the immune system.* Because they
work *with* the body (as opposed to *against* the body's symptoms as
conventional medicine does), the remedies are intended to be an am-
plification of the body's natural order and healing processes.

This system of medicine uses remedies that are made from natural
substances (animal, vegetable, and mineral) diluted to very small
amounts. These medicines are manufactured according to strict phar-
macological methods and are safe and non-toxic with no side effects.
They are commonly sold without prescription and have been in use
throughout the world for about two hundred years.

The crucial point to understand about homeopathic medicine is that remedies are given to aid the body's efforts to heal itself. *Homeopathy treats the patient—not the disease.* In contrast, conventional drugs are generally prescribed to control or suppress symptoms. As a result of this suppression, the body's immune system cannot fully perform its function, and the disease may be driven deeper.

The fundamental principles of homeopathy to remember are:

- The body is a self-regulated system with the innate capacity to heal itself.
- The natural healing processes of the body can be enhanced by giving an ill person extremely dilute doses of substances that in large doses would cause similar symptoms of illness when given to a healthy person (this is the "Law of Similars" explained below).
- A person who is ill must be treated according to the specific and unique symptoms he displays. It is the *person* who is treated, not a specific illness.
- Treatment must take into account the mental and emotional states of the ill person as well as the physical symptoms.
- The substances used for remedies, when prepared by a strictly controlled procedure, become more and more potent as they undergo a specific process of progressive dilution.

"How does homeopathy work?"

Symptoms are the body's defense mechanism. A homeopath observes the symptoms and behaviors of an ill person, and questions his or her reactions to different conditions in order to find the correct remedy. Unlike conventional medicine which treats symptoms, not causes, homeopathic medicines help the body strengthen organs and systems so it can defend itself. Let's take two examples to demonstrate this difference between the two systems:

Ann has a headache every day at 4 p.m. Her M.D. gives her a quick physical exam and prescribes Tylenol for the pain. He says he can't find anything wrong and that she should call him if her headaches get worse.

Jan has a headache every day at 4 p.m. She goes to a homeopath who asks her many questions about the stresses in her life, what's she's been eating, and other questions about her general environment and her specific disposition in different circumstances. He asks her to describe the kind of headache she has and when it started, what makes it feel better or worse, and so on. He takes extensive notes about her replies and finds that not only does she have headaches, but she isn't sleeping well at night and feels very anxious. He consults various homeopathic reference books (called the *Materia Medica*) and gradually narrows down to one or two remedies which best matches what she has told him. He gives her one dose of a remedy in the office and suggests she pick up a vial of the remedy at the pharmacy to use for the next few days.

In Ann's case, the doctor's goal was to stop the pain of the headache. In Jan's case, the doctor's goal was to give her an overall picture of her condition, and pick one of a number of possible remedies to restore her system to well-being.

When you are exposed to stress or infection there are usually several or many bodily responses. For instance, there may be an inflammation, a fever, a cough, or a rash. These signs indicate that there is a "fight" going on inside the body and that the body has activated its defense system in order to maintain balance. A fever, for example, is a form of resistance to a bacterial or viral infection. Recent research by physiologist Matthew Kluger and his associates at the University of Michigan Medical School has shown that a fever increases white blood cell mobility and activity and aids in the natural production of interferon, an antiviral substance. The homeopathic approach does not try to suppress the fever. Instead, the homeopathic method uses a medicine which in a healthy person would cause the unique symptom of fever that the sick person is experiencing. To find the correct remedy the homeopathic physician asks such questions as: "What time of day did the fever begin? Is there thirst with the fever? Does the fever make the patient feel chilly?" Essentially, the homeopathic approach uses all outward indications as well as reactions to conditions to determine *how* the patient is sick. Homeopaths believe that to suppress a fever with aspirin or other powerful drugs actually *reduces* the body's capacity for healing.

Another example is the mucus produced with a cold. The body uses mucus to carry away the waste products of the infection. Since the body is ridding itself of waste, the homeopathic point of view is that it's not logical to suppress the expectorating process with cough medicine. Suppression of the cough does nothing to help the true healing process, and, in fact, inhibits the natural defensive actions. Many allopathic (conventional) physicians agree and don't prescribe expectorants.

The Law of Similars

The foundation of homeopathy rests on the "law of similars." To support the body's immune system, a remedy is given based on the principle that like cures like. This law states that a substance that causes symptoms in a healthy person, will, in specially prepared tiny amounts, cure a sick person who has those same symptoms.

The discovery of the law of similars was made by Dr. Samuel Hahnemann about two hundred years ago. However, the principle that "like cures like" was not new even then. It had been known and used by healers in other ages before Hahnemann's time—for example, by Hippocrates, the father of medicine, in the 4th century and by Paracelsus, the Swiss physician and alchemist, in the 15th century. Today orthodox medicine uses vaccines (small doses of disease-causing substances) to immunize the body against illness. However, conventional medicine, while using the law of similars in vaccines, does not share the other fundamental principles of homeopathic medicine—that is, the use of tiny, safe amounts of medicines, and treatment of the mind and body as a unified whole. Another demonstration of the law of similars is found in elementary physics. You may recall that placing a weakened magnet next to a similar pole of another magnet will recharge the weakened magnet over time. Like recharges and heals like.

The homeopathic use of the law of similars has produced a remarkable array of effective natural remedies. The healing properties of remedies have been found by extensive testing of substances on humans over two hundred years in many countries, and close observation of their specific reactions. This method of finding which remedy cures which symptoms is called "proving." The repetoire of hundreds of homeopathic cures is called the *Materia Medica,* and is the reference source for homeopathic physicians.

Hahnemann was the first person to test substances to see what symptoms they would cause. Doctors of his day assumed, for instance, that quinine cured malaria because it was bitter and astringent. He questioned this assertion because other medicines that were bitter and astringent did not cure malaria. He took doses of quinine and developed all the symptoms of malaria—intermittent fever, burning, chills, trembling—and thus "proved" the similar symptoms of malaria. Thus was born the term homeopathy—"homeo" meaning similar and "pathy" meaning suffering.

Homeopathy Treats the Mental, Emotional, and Physical Levels

Another important homeopathic principle is that illness is a disharmony or dis-ease of the mental and emotional states as well as the physical state. Remedies are selected to match the overall characteristics of the individual, emotionally, physiologically, and mentally.

Holistic treatment is not new or even "new age." As Socrates said in 500 B.C.: "There is no illness of the body apart from the mind."

Since mental, emotional and physical factors are taken into account, homeopathic treatment is, by nature, comprehensive. The treatment is based on very specific reactions and conditions. Thus, homeopathic treatment is extremely individualized.

Medicines are not selected on the basis of a generic disease state such as "headache." Instead, the homeopathic approach takes into account what kind of headache the person has. Let's say one person gets a sudden, violent headache all around the head like a band. His head feels like it will burst, especially getting up from the bed. He's restless, fearful and thirsty. He gets worse as evening approaches, and he hates being in a warm room. This person's symptoms matches the remedy *Aconite* perfectly.

Another person also has a pounding, bursting headache that comes on suddenly like the *Aconite* patient, but sports additional characteristics: a throbbing pain accompanied by a red, hot, flushed face, indicates the appropriate remedy is *Belladonnna.*

Yet another person with a migraine-like headache with blurred vision, profuse flow of saliva, and some nausea would match the remedy *Iris versicolor.*

Because each person has a different complex of symptoms and other conditions affecting bodily functions, treatment must be chosen individually. Homeopathy offers different remedies for different types of "headache," "flu," "coughs," and so on. This method of individualized treatment is very different from the way most of us use conventional medicines. Conventional drugs are advertised as panaceas for coughs, colds, headache pain, and back pain. With this type of advertising so prevalent in our culture, it's only natural that you may be tempted to look for homeopathic remedies that are "good for" certain ailments, and you may very well find a remedy that works consistently for you.

On the other hand, you may find that no one remedy will be right for all colds, sore throats, bruises, or backaches. In the sections on injuries such as runner's knee and sprained ankles, I have indicated remedies that generally seem to work to heal those specific injuries. However, other conditions might indicate a different remedy. In order to choose the correct medicine, you need to look very closely at your individual charactcristics (i.e., what makes your injury feel better or worse; whether you're restless or tired after movement; whether you prefer being outside in the cool air or inside a warm room).

If you have not used homeopathic medicines before, you may find these questions strange. Why does it matter if you like the window open at night when you sleep? Why does it matter if you feel better at the seashore rather than in a hot, dry climate?

The answer is that the body is a living system with a wide range of responses to the environment. Each of us is different. The answers to these questions will lead a homeopath (and you, if you are self-prescribing) to a number of possible remedies, one of which will most closely match your condition. You may have to try a few to find the right one.

"Is there proof that supports the principles of homeopathic medicine?"

Yes. First there is the strong empirical proof from the everyday use of homeopathic remedies for over two hundred years in the *Materia Medica.* In addition, there are also clinical and laboratory studies that show the effects of homeopathic remedies (as well as other microdose substances) on living systems such as immune cells, bacteria and seedlings. Lastly, new scientific theories about the nature of energy and matter are compatible with the principles of homeopathy. But first, what is the empirical evidence (i.e., observed from experience)?

Empirical Evidence. Some of the most impressive large scale uses of homeopathic remedies happened during the last century when epidemics of serious diseases were rampant. Those who took homeopathic medicines survived in significant numbers over those who were given the conventional medicines available at the time. It is unlikely that this significant difference was due simply to the placebo effect.

Remedies are also found to be effective on both infants and animals—neither of whom are very susceptible to the psychological nuances of the placebo effect. Remedies given to infants have produced almost immediate results in common childhood problems such as teething, fevers, colic, and even neurological disorders. Many veterinarians use homeopathic remedies to treat animals, and much has been written about using remedies on domestic pets, cattle, and horses.

In this book, I have included some of my own empirical proof based on the stories of my patients who have been improved by the use of homeopathic remedies.

Clinical Studies. In his book *Discovering Homeopathy: Your Introduction to the Science and Art of Homeopathic Medicine,* homeopathic educator Dana Ullman reviews some of the important studies which have been done on homeopathic medicine. In double-blind studies, remedies proved effective in such diverse health problems as the control of allergic reactions, the improvement of burns from mustard gas, and the relief of rheumatoid arthritis. In one study of rodents that had been injected with cancer cells, homeopathic remedies were shown to prolong their life by 52% longer than rodents who were given placebos.

Ullman notes that in human studies where no improvement from remedies was demonstrated, the remedies were given without considering specific, complex individual histories, which directly defies the fundamental law of similars. Therefore, by demonstrating that remedies *don't* work when they are not matched to symptoms, the evidence actually supports the principle of the law of similars upon which homeopathy depends.[1]

Laboratory Findings. The idea that microdoses of a substance can have any effect on living systems is increasingly being investigated by researchers inside and outside the field of homeopathy. Ullman cites evidence published in *Science News* that small doses can actually have increased strengths:

> Chemists who work for the U.S. Government's National Bureau of Standards and who knew nothing about homeopathy noted that when they shook [vigorous shaking of the dilute solution is also done in the manufacture of remedies] the coupled molecules of nitric oxide, the units did not weaken and break into parts, but rather developed stronger molecular bonds. One can theorize from this research that the homeopathic process of dilution and succussion (shaking) may actually create superstrong molecules, perhaps superstrong medicines.[2]

Fertilizers potentized with homeopathic remedies have been put on yeast cultures and wheat seedlings in laboratory experiments. Both the yeast and the seedlings fertilized with these extremely dilute substances showed increased growth rates.

In 1988, the prestigious scientific journal, *Nature,* published some revolutionary findings by French researchers Benveniste and colleagues who were studying the "micro-dose paradox." These studies, repeated independently by several laboratories, showed significant responses in blood cells that were treated with an extremely dilute substance. The dilution of the substance used in this study exceeded even the chemical constant known as Avrogadro's number in which no molecule of a substance is present. Even though the scientific rigor used in the experiments was irrefutable, the publishing of this information continues to raise hackles in some conventional scientific circles who claim that such dilute substances cannot possibly have an effect.

A subsequent, as yet unpublished, research study confirming Benveniste's results was performed by Dr. Glen Rein, a bio-electromagnetic researcher and director of Quantum Biology Research Lab in Palo Alto, California. He used human immune cells to test the efficacy of homeopathic *Aconite* and observed similar functional changes as those found in Benveniste's study (one of which was the peculiar phenomenon of "peaks and troughs" which occurred as the solution became more dilute). Thus he confirmed that dilute substances (much beyond Avrogadro's number) do have a biological effect at the cellular level. In fact, the effect was even more pronounced the more dilute the substance.[3]

Homeopathic remedies may have unique abilities to help cells detoxify. One important finding from clinical trials on rats was published in the journal, *Human Toxicology.* The research showed that microdoses of arsenic (in potencies as low as 7 and 14x) helped the rats to eliminate toxic doses of arsenic they had been previously given. This seems to be an exciting avenue for more research in light of our current environmental hazards.

Current Scientific Theories. Since homeopathy is based on the premise that the body has an inherent capacity to maintain health, it fits in very well with current theoretical scientific thinking that sees living systems as self-regulating. This capacity for self-regulation and self-healing in life forms has been examined and written about by such authors as Erich Jantsch in *The Self-Organizing Universe* and physicist Ilya Prigogine in *Order Out of Chaos*. The work of other investigators such as stress expert Dr. Hans Selye also recognizes the importance of working *with* the body's natural responses to imbalance —again supporting the basic premise of homeopathy.

The fundamental homeopathic principle of treating an *individual* is also in alignment with current scientific reasoning that living systems are extremely sensitive and adaptive. For example, more and more information is coming to light about the effects of ions in different environments, the geothermal effects on brain chemistry, and the metabolic processes that may underlie food cravings. A homeopath asks the question "Do you feel better in the evening or in the morning?" in order to select an appropriate treatment. Scientific data shows there *are* daily rhythms, ebbs, and flows within the body that affect mood and energy.

Homeopathic medicine is seen by some advocates as a potentially major contributor to a new comprehensive medical approach to treat some of the currently "incurable" problems of immune deficiencies, viral diseases, and environmental allergies.[4]

As we have seen, homeopathy works at a very subtle level with microdoses. At this level of dilution, the medicines are best understood, not by our standard Newtonian physics (i.e., more chemical = more effect), but by a whole new model of physics. In *Vibrational Medicine,* Richard Gerber, M.D. makes a case that conventional medicine is based on a Newtonian viewpoint in which the human body is a complex *machine.* As a machine, the body is given conventional drugs to affect chemical changes in body processes at the cellular level. This linear type of medicine, which relies on rather gross chemical effects (as compared to subtle energy changes), does not seem to be the way the body really heals. Gerber believes that medicine is moving away from the Newtonian concept and towards an Einsteinian view point of the human being as a multidimensional organism with complex regulatory energy fields. In this model, where effects are produced in energy fields or patterns, homeopathic remedies fit perfectly.[5]

Gerber says, "The homeopathic approach utilizes minute quantities of medicinal substances to create therapeutic physiological changes through subtle-energy field interactions." Towards that argument he cites new research such as done by Dr. Bernard Grad of McGill University in Montreal on the effects of subtle energy on seedling growth-rates.[6]

Homeopathy, then, is an empirically proven system of highly individualized medicine that seems to coincide with emerging technical research and theories regarding the processes of living systems.

"Does it work for any problem, including the flu and a broken ankle?"

Yes. There are four ways homeopathy can be used for health:

- **First aid**. One way to use homeopathy is for first aid treatment to relieve the pain and trauma of injury.
- **Acute illnesses**. Remedies can be used for the treatment of a myriad of short-term ailments such as colds, flu, sore throats, ear aches, diarrhea, and hangovers.
- **Chronic conditions**. Remedies can be used to relieve the pain and symptoms of chronic conditions and old injuries. Remedies may correct some conditions, and prevent further damage and degeneration of other conditions. This type of homeopathy uses what are called "constitutional remedies," deep-acting medicines best taken under the guidance of a trained homeopath.
- **Promotion of overall health**. The homeopathic approach embodies a whole philosophy of preventing illness and building a stronger, healthier bodily constitution.

"How are homeopathic remedies made?"

Sometimes people confuse homeopathic remedies with indigenous medicines also made from herbs and flowers and other natural materials. Many of these natural medicines are also effective for certain conditions, but they are completely different from homeopathic remedies.

Homeopathic remedies are made under a strict set of rules whereby animal, vegetable, and mineral substances are dissolved or ground into fine powders and progressively reduced by a specific procedure of serial dilution that reduces the quantity of the active ingredients to an infinitesimal amount. Serial dilution means that the active ingredient, say a dose of *Belladonna,* is mixed with nine parts of distilled water, and shaken vigorously; one part of this solution is again mixed with 9 parts water, shaken vigorously, and so on to the desired strength. This process of dilution with shaking is called "potentization." The substance becomes more and more potent as it is diluted.

The most common strengths are 3, 6, 9, 12, and 30. When a homeopathic medicine is labeled *x* or *d,* this means it was diluted 1:9. For instance, when a remedy is labeled 30x, this means it was diluted 1:9 and vigorously shaken; then diluted again 1:9 and shaken; and this procedure was repeated 30 times. When a homeopathic medicine is labeled *c,* this means that the medicine was diluted 1:99. The higher strengths of 200, 1,000, 10,000, 50,000, and 100,000 require a homeo-pathic physician's prescription.

"How can such dilute substances have any effect?"

For many of my patients, the idea of remedies with such infinitesimal ingredients is sometimes very hard to understand. Traditionally, we think in terms of "more" as equivalent to "stronger" or more effec-tive. In the case of homeopathic remedies, less is more.

I find it interesting, by the way, that homeopathic remedies, in be-ing so dilute, seem to be following an essential law of nature—that less is more. The correlates of this principle are found, for example, both in architectural design (form follows function, that is, nothing extraneous is added to the form beyond what is needed for proper function) and in the rigorous mathematical principle of "elegance" or "an elegant sufficiency" in equations denoting a simplicity that is fitting or correct.

There are, of course, many theories that attempt to explain how such a dilute substance can effect a healing response. Luckily, healing does not depend on our understanding of these sub-molecular pro-cesses! They work, but we still don't understand how they work. One theory proposes that these dilute remedies pass more easily through physiological boundaries of blood cells, and even through cellular and nuclear membranes.

Another theory proposes that because the remedy is "similar" to your symptoms, it resonates with you. As it resonates, it amplifies the healing message to your body. This theory says that we have a life force (vital energy) that can be described as a pattern and that our pattern can be affected by a similar pattern that "resonates" with us. Dana Ullman uses a music analogy. We know that resonance in music means that when we strike a C note on the piano, the C notes in other octaves resonate and vibrate.[7] In the same way, our energy is affected by a resonating energy within the remedy.

Another metaphor for this concept of resonance is what happens when a car starts to skid during a turn. To regain control, the best action is to turn *into* the skid—to go *with* the direction of the car's movement.

"How are homeopathic medicines different from conventional pharmaceutical drugs?"

The main points to remember about the differences between homeo-pathic and conventional medicines are these:

- Homeopathic remedies are different from conventional drugs in that they work *with* the body's immune system to enhance the capacity to heal, rather than working *against* the symptoms that your body has produced to fight an illness or an injury.
- Homeopathic remedies, composed of infinitesimal substances, stimulate the specific organ complex to do the healing, rather than overcoming the disease process with large amounts of chemicals as is done by conventional medicines.
- Homeopathic remedies resonate with the particular symptoms of the individual, whereas conventional medicines are administered regardless of the individual's particular constitution.
- While highly potent when matched to the right set of symptoms, homeopathic remedies are non-toxic and have no side-effects unlike antibiotics, steroids, and cortisone drugs.
- Classically, homeopaths give only a single remedy for a condition, as contrasted to conventional medicine which may prescribe one drug for high blood pressure, another for diabetes, and still others for symptoms that keep arising (often from the side effects of the drugs themselves). This keeps the body more free from many cross-cutting strong substances.
- A homeopathic remedy is taken only until improvement occurs, unlike some conventional medicines which are prescribed for a set length of time.
- Compared to conventional medicines, homeopathic remedies are very low in cost.
- Homeopathy works best in a clean body—i.e., a diet low in additives, toxins, fat, caffeine, and free of tobacco, pollutants, and invasive drugs with strong side-effects. It cannot be as effective on a wildly toxic constitution bombarded by poor diet and prescription drugs. Children, for example, do very well with homeopathic remedies because their systems are usually relatively pure.

"Why does homeopathy make sense?"

If symptoms are a defense of the body, it's logical to look for a substance that helps the body's defense. Homeopathic medicines are prepared from substances that produce actual disease symptoms in humans. Therefore the natural healing response of the body is triggered, so that balance can be restored. Furthermore, the medicines are targeted for very specific individual reactions and needs. Homeopathy's approach is holistic and balanced rather than specialized and fragmented; it seems to follow other basic laws of nature. As a form of subtle energy, the homeopathic remedy fits into the emerging model of Einsteinian physics where matter is equivalent to energy. Remedies are non-toxic, safe and economical. Homeopathic medicines make sense most of all because they work . . . and often very quickly.

"How do you know it's working?"

Obviously, you know a remedy has worked when you start feeling better. Many cases of homeopathic cures have a dramatic conclusion. Such was the case with Jim Bouton, former pitcher for the Yankees. During practice in Portland, Oregon, the day before a game, he was stricken with an asthma attack, which immediately took him off the field and into bed. Despairing of being able to play the next day, and fearing that this setback would be the end of the season for him, he asked the team's trainer, Dr. Steve Katz, to look him over.

Dr. Katz gave him a homeopathic remedy for asthma. "I couldn't believe it," he said, "Steve gave me some little white pills—I think it was *Ipecac.* Two hours later, I was ok. I was actually breathing like a normal person. You have to understand, asthma attacks had always lasted five to ten days for me. I had never had one go away this quickly. Well, the next day I pitched. I'll never forget it. I felt like my concentration and focus were even better than usual. It felt like a miracle—and I pitched a winning game, by the way." In Jim's case, his asthma flared up again in the space of several months, but after taking the remedy a couple of more times, the breathing problems disappeared altogether.[8]

Treatment with homeopathic remedies is by no means always so dramatic and immediately conclusive. For example, time is a big factor in sports injuries involving bone fractures or stress fractures. In these cases, there is a mandatory four to six week period during which new bone cells are produced and breaks are knit back together. However, there's a good chance that homeopathy may speed healing. Such was the case with Ian Romansky.

Putting Ian Romansky Back on the Court

Ian was a high school basketball star who had been having increasing pain over his outer ankle bone. Both he and the coach thought it was "just" tendinitis or a strain. So he played on.

The pain got worse—and jumping (landing on the ball of the foot) was particularly painful. By the time I saw him, he had had the pain for two weeks. X-rays showed no obvious fractures. But when I vibrated a tuning fork next to his ankle (to test for stress fracture), there was even more pain. My diagnosis, therefore, was stress fracture with tendinitis.

I told Ian he could not run or jump for a few weeks while his bone healed. Both the coach and Ian were very upset because the school's playoff games were only a month away. "How long will he be out?" the coach asked me. They both groaned loudly when I told them bone usually takes six weeks or longer to heal. They asked me if anything could be done to speed up the healing.

"Well, maybe homeopathy could help," I said, "and we could try physical therapy with electrical stimulation. That may increase the healing and decrease the stiffness."

Ian complained of pain that was worse with motion, worse with touch and better with a tight Ace wrap and ice packs. For those symptoms I gave him *Bryonia*. Later on he developed stiffness which was worse when he first moved the joint, but better after he moved around a bit. He was very restless, but moving around made him feel better. His ankle was better with heat and worse with cold. At that point, I took him off the *Bryonia* and gave him *Rhus Tox*.

During the next stage he developed an aching in the bone for which I gave him *Symphytum*. That worked well. In four weeks he was able to run, jump, and shoot baskets. X-rays showed that the stress fracture was healing well (there was a healing callous surrounding the bone inside, which acted as a natural splint). I put Ian in an air cast, and made orthotics for his shoes. I told him to practice as long as he had no pain. His team won the playoffs!

Generally, physical therapy and electrical stimulation may speed healing by a week. But in Ian's case, I believe the homeopathy speeded the healing by an extra week.

In many cases, the healing effects of homeopathic medicines like *Arnica* may be quite obvious.

Sue Miller's Story

Sue Miller, thirty-two, is a runner and occasional racer who uses *Arnica* and *Arnica* ointment for the sore, bruised feeling after long runs. "Usually it takes me about a week to recover from a marathon," she told me on the phone, "but if I take *Arnica* right afterwards, I don't get much pain or bruising. Later in the week, if I feel stiff I take *Rhus Tox*. I love these remedies!"

In other cases, where a long-acting remedy like *Silica* is used for overuse injuries or for a general feeling of listlessness, the effects are more gradual. A long-acting remedy could bring increased vigor over six to eight months.

Pat Bannister's Year of Healing

Pat came to me with a painful bunion. She was trying to walk for exercise, but told me, "I really want to walk, doctor, but some days I just don't have the energy. I just feel so tired all the time. I know I should get exercise and it makes me feel kind of guilty. Besides," she sighed, "my bunion hurts, and that's another reason I resist walking." She had been diagnosed by another doctor as having a systemic fungal infection called Candida plus chronic fatigue syndrome.

Pat seemed to me to lack spark or fiber. The image she reminded me of was a shaft of wheat that lacked a stalk; she was like a plant that's drooping. She brightened for a moment and said, "That's exactly how I feel. Like a droopy plant!"

She said that she tended to be sickly and get colds a lot. She was chilly in general and fairly inactive. Her personality type was shy but somewhat stubborn. She appeared to go along with other people's ideas, but when it got right down to it, she would go her own way.

I told Pat that we couldn't do surgery on her bunion until she was stronger in her overall health. I thought surgery would be too much of a drain for her at this point. After considering all her medical history, symptoms and personality type, I decided she was a *Silica* patient. *Silica* is the element that gives the strength to a shaft of wheat, and like a limp stalk, she seemed to be lacking vitality and strength. I gave her a single dose. She left and I didn't see her for one year.

She came back to see me and told me she'd had quite a year. After I had given her the remedy, she'd gotten very sick—much sicker than she'd been. But ... after about three months, she felt better than she'd ever felt in her life!

She confided to me that after she had gotten so sick, she had been really angry with me. "I kept thinking—I came to you, and you didn't even fix my bunion. You gave me a remedy and I ended up getting worse!" She had chosen to disregard my caution as she left the office that day, that if she started to get worse, to give me a call. I explained that sometimes a remedy will initiate an "aggravation" of symptoms, which means you get worse before you get better. But she had felt so angry and hopeless by that time, that she didn't even call me. At any rate, I thanked Pat for reminding me that I need to make myself more clear on this point with patients. We are postponing her bunion surgery until she feels really ready to undergo it.

"I've heard that sometimes after taking a homeopathic remedy a person gets even sicker. Why is that?"

It's true that sometimes a remedy will induce an aggravation of current symptoms. I have mentioned both Pat's case above and the case of my son who felt sicker after taking a dose of *Mercury* for his severe bronchitis. Both of them got worse before they got better.

The idea of an aggravated symptom becomes logical when we take into account that the remedy is working by the law of similars—the remedy which mimics the disease has enhanced the symptoms in order to stimulate healing. The body experiences a surge of the symptom which, in turn, activates the immune system response.

Keep in mind, however, that this aggravation of symptom is rarely observed in injuries; it is much more observable in ailments or chronic conditions.

"Who uses homeopathy?"

Homeopathy is used by many people in England, France, Europe, and in America. The beauty of this system is that it is so accessible. Many health practitioners have adopted homeopathy as part of their practice. These healers include medical doctors, physician's assistants, nurse practitioners, naturopaths, chiropractors, body workers, and the general lay public. Hopefully, you will become one of the users of this system.

"Is there a specific benefit from using homeopathy for sports and exercise injuries?"

For you, the walker, runner, or athlete, homeopathic remedies offer a valuable resource for self-care. Instead of spending time and money going to a doctor for every little cramp or scrape, you can handle many minor ailments and injuries yourself. Even though serious injuries may require conventional medical care, nevertheless, homeopathic remedies can be kept on hand in a "survival kit" for first aid and for use in certain acute (short-term) conditions.

Even if you continue to see a conventional medical doctor who does not prescribe homeopathic medicines, you can increase your treatment options by using some of the remedies suggested in this book. As a podiatrist and as a runner, I am delighted to be able to recommend remedies that are virtually without side effects and that support your body's own best defenses. To use a sports metaphor, I like to think of homeopathic medicines as another member on your "inner healing team."

A Homeopathic Headstart for the Sportsperson

Whether you are an exercise walker or an Olympic contestant, homeopathic remedies, such as *Arnica,* may reinforce your stamina when you are competing or training strenuously.

A good illustration of this is a story I heard from Whit Reaves, an acupuncturist and homeopath in Boulder, Colorado. One of his patients is Cindy Staiger, a cycling champion who won the 1988 Race Across America. This is the most grueling cycling endurance event in the world, and at 3,000 miles exceeds the Tour de France by a 1,000 miles.

Reaves followed Cindy by car across America for 11 days as she pumped her away across the states. "She was on the bike for 21 hours a day, sleeping only about an hour and a half a day," he said. "Every 8 hours she took a dose of *Arnica* (a remedy for trauma, pain or recovery). I gave her *Mag Phos* for muscle spasms and did a little acupuncture on her during rest breaks to help her relax. Before this race, she had done constitutional acupuncture and herbs to help her knees, so she took the race pretty well. She won. She didn't have any knee or leg problems afterwards at all."

Equally as important as acute relief of symptoms is the great effectiveness of homeopathy at stimulating deep levels of lasting health with what are called "constitutional remedies."

A Typical Office Visit

Karen, a young, divorced mother and a dancer, came to me with low back pain. She had been referred by her doctor, a man I had previously treated for his own low-back pain. He hoped I could help Karen, too. We talked a little bit about the onset of her problem and how long she'd had it.

I asked her when her back got worse. She sighed a little, thinking, and said, "It seems like it gets worse right after I talk to my ex-husband." Probing deeper, I asked how she has resolved her divorce, and she answered, "I feel like I'm always walking on tip-toes with him. For example, last week I was afraid if I didn't give in about his choice of my daughter's school, he'd cut off our child support." This statement told me important information—that her emotional state is clouded by fear, fear of loss of support, which is most likely being translated into a low-back problem. The mind and heart will always find ways of expressing their needs, and if emotions are not expressed openly, physical symptoms will do the talking.

It seemed to me that anxiety was going to be a key symptom in the choice of her remedy (even though she came in complaining of low back pain and did not mention anxiety to me). I began thinking of remedies which fit an anxious patient, as I continued my history taking.

My questioning of Karen proceeded into other areas, such as what foods she likes. "Sweets, of course. Doesn't everybody? I don't eat a lot of greasy stuff, though. I always cut the fat off any meat. I eat a lot of cheese, and scrambled eggs because they're easy to fix . . . and, I eat a *lot* of peanut butter sandwiches," she said sheepishly. I asked her if she's thirsty a lot, and she said, "Not really." Her food preferences were further clues that I would use to select a remedy.

Does she wake up in the middle of the night at a certain time? "No, but often I can't sleep because of the thoughts going around and around in my head." Does she prefer to be warm or cool? "Oh, I hate the heat in summer. That's why I like being in the Bay Area!" When I asked whether she kept her feet uncovered at night, she laughed. "Why, as a matter of fact, I do. I just can't stand to sleep in a warm room; I always keep a window open at night—luckily, I sleep on the third floor."

My portrait of Karen continued to grow as she told me about her job as an administrator for a child care center. "You know, my job there is really to keep everybody happy. . . . I like it very much. Although sometimes I could just cry when I see a child I suspect isn't being treated well at home. It's a real emotional see-saw sometimes. That's why I need to do my dancing. It's such an emotional outlet for me."

As we continued talking, she told me how she keeps trying to decide whether to leave her present job and pursue a career in teaching dance. "I can't seem to make up my mind. One day I feel one way and the next I feel almost the opposite! I feel so wishy-washy." With this statement I felt I had a keynote symptom for *Pulsatilla,* since changeability is a prime factor in this remedy. *Pulsatilla* is made from the windflower, and like the plant swaying in the breeze, *Pulsatilla* patients experience variable emotional states and physical symptoms. They are often young women with sweet and sensitive dispositions with a tendency to want to please others. However, before I made a final decision, I wanted to go over my notes, distilling the information, and comparing it against the *Materia Medica* reference books that contains descriptions of hundreds of remedies.

After taking her history (which took about 40 minutes), I examined Karen for physical imbalances. I checked her back and hips for signs of short-leg syndrome (one leg shorter than the other). I looked at the soles of her shoes for wear patterns that indicated an unbalanced foot and leg. I looked for other physical clues that suggested the need for an orthotic. We also discussed her exercise routine, as well as her current dance training.

After assessing all the factors I learned during Karen's visit, I gave her a pair of temporary orthotics to correct a tendency to over-pronate. I also prescribed a stretching routine for the abdominals. Lastly, I gave her a dose of *Pulsatilla,* adding that she should take a dose of 6x pills twice a day until the back problem goes away.

When I spoke to her a few months later, she seemed different. She had come to some career decisions, she said, and had become more clear-cut and decisive in her dealings with her ex-husband. Her back was no longer a problem as she learned to listen to her feelings— not store them in her back muscles!

"What if I have a sprained ankle plus a cold? Will one remedy help everything or should I take a couple of them?"

The classic rule in homeopathy is to use a single remedy at a time. Usually, a single remedy is selected to initiate healing so that its effects can be seen clearly. Generally, I don't recommend taking more than one remedy in a short span of time. I have seen several cases of one remedy curing multiple problems, but this is usually a constitutional (long-term) remedy and not an acute remedy (short-term).

On the other hand, if one remedy is taken and does not improve the condition within a short time, then another remedy may be tried. For example, if *Arnica* is taken for a painful wound but no improvement is forthcoming, you may have to try *Bellis* or *Sulphuric Acid.* If a remedy is taken for a constitutional problem, and there are no signs of improvement—no mental or emotional improvement, no relief of the immediate symptom, and no aggravation of a symptom, then you must look for a remedy which matches your condition more precisely.

If you are under the care of a homeopathic physician and he or she is treating you constitutionally (e.g., for a chronic condition), don't take any other remedies for an acute situation (e.g., sore throat, influenza, etc.) unless you check with your homeopath first. The symptoms you are experiencing may be arising out of the healing that is in progress from the constitutional remedy. Sometimes only a single dose of a remedy is given during a period of several months.

"How come most homeopathic remedies are taken 'until better'?"

When signs of healing are present, the remedy is no longer needed. To continue to take the remedy after you *get well* may invite the remedy to "prove" out with you—which means that you begin to create the very symptom you were curing. With homeopathic remedies there is no need to become obsessed with massive amounts of drugs or medications once the healing process is well-established.

"Why isn't homeopathy more widely used today if it's been around for 200 hundred years?"

At the turn of the century about 15 percent of American medical doctors were homeopaths. Few people realize that the American Medical Association was formed in part as a response to the founding of the American Institute of Homeopathy two years earlier. Doctors in the AMA were hostile to homeopaths. Boundaries were drawn. If a member of the AMA simply consulted with a homeopath, he was punished or expelled.

Not only did homeopathy have to exist alongside hostile physicians, but changing lifestyles brought about a new way of "doctoring." First of all, as people became more mobile, there was a shift away from long-standing community and familial relationships. Secondly, AMA medicine became specialized, and developed a strong partnership with powerful pharmaceutical firms. Diseases were dealt with as separate, pathological phenomena apart from general well-being.

Further damage was done when medical funding was denied to homeopathic colleges (there were about twenty at the turn of the century) because of pressure from the AMA and the drug companies. One by one homeopathic schools closed or were converted to conventional medical curricula.

But, as we know, the tides of understanding may go out, but they also come back in. During the last two decades, there has been an active search for a simpler, less consumeristic approach to health and medicine. The revolt is firmly entrenched as we move into the decade of the 1990's, and open our minds and hearts to a wealth of alternative ways to be and stay healthy.

"A friend of mine said she took a homeopathic remedy and nothing happened. She doesn't believe in it."

Once in a while people tell me about someone they know or someone they heard about who "tried homeopathy, but it didn't work." These stories don't surprise me. The effectiveness of homeopathy is only as certain as the person choosing the remedy. Remedies must be chosen according to the principle of the "law of similars," which means that if symptoms are not correctly observed, the correct (or matching) remedy may not be chosen. In that case, "homeopathy doesn't work." The key to successful treatment is the careful observation of the patient's condition and symptoms.

"How can I start using homeopathy?"

Call Homeopathic Educational Services in Berkeley, CA (see Chapter 20) to find a homeopath in your area, or look in the yellow pages of the phone book for practitioners. For chronic conditions and serious problems, it is best if you're under the care of a homeopath, who can take your case, give you a constitutional, and listen to any specific ailments you may have.

For small aches and pains, minor injuries, and many common infections and diseases you can educate yourself about homeopathy and begin to use it.

Most of us have a medicine chest stocked with bandages, aspirin, antacid, cough medicine, alcohol and the like. By learning the fundamentals of homeopathy and having a "homeopathic medical kit" or first-aid kit on hand, you can increase your ability to treat yourself and your family when minor health problems arise. For relatively little cost, you can purchase a starter kit from various clinics and pharmacies which I have listed in the resource guide in Chapter 20.

"What main points should I remember when I use homeopathic remedies?"

- Depending on your injury, select one remedy that best matches your present symptoms. Look for a *keynote* (special or unique) that will help you differentiate one remedy from another.
- For first aid and self-care use whatever potency (6, 9, 12, 30) you have in your medicine kit. Doses of over-the-counter homeopathic remedies are measured in x (1:9 dilution) and c (1:99 dilution). The rule of thumb is that stronger potencies are used

95

when you are more confident about the accuracy of your prescribing.

- For first aid, if a remedy is not effective within 2 to 6 hours, select another one.
- Discontinue taking a remedy as soon as you feel better.
- Touching remedies can contaminate them. Drop pills into your mouth directly from the cap of the bottle. Unless specifically directed, don't swallow the pills. Instead, put them under the tongue so they can be absorbed by the mucous membranes.
- Sometimes coffee interferes with the healing powers of the remedies. Just to be on the safe side, don't drink coffee—not even decaffeinated coffee—while taking homeopathic treatment. Black tea is no problem. Also, certain medicines such as *Nat Mur* may be counteracted by mint-flavored mouthwash or toothpaste. Check with your doctor.
- Keep remedies out of sunlight; keep them away from household cleaning products, perfumes or other open bottles of homeopathic remedies as they may be easily contaminated by other odors or air-borne substances.
- While under treatment with homeopathic remedies, don't use anything with camphor in it, such as Vicks' VapoRub, as camphor antidotes remedies.
- Don't have any dental work done if you are taking homeopathic medicines without first checking with your homeopath since it may antidote the action of the medicines.
- Homeopathic medicines can be safely used with conventional medicines. Ask your doctor for dosage advice. In some cases a drug may antidote a homeopathic remedy.
- Store the medicines in their original bottle; don't transfer to another container. Properly stored, they last indefinitely.

Footnotes:

1. Dana Ullman, M.P.H., *Discovering Homeopathy: Your Introduction to the Science and Art of Homeopathic Medicine,* (Berkeley, CA, North Atlantic Books,) 1991.

2. *Ibid.*

3. G. Rein, *The Use of Cultured Cells in Characterizing the Nature of the Subtle Energy in Homeopathic Remedies,* Proceedings of the First International Society for the Study of Subtle Energy and Energy Medicine, (Golden, CO), 1991.

4. Ullman, *ibid.*
5. Richard Gerber, M.D., *Vibrational Medicine,* (Santa Fe, NM, Bear and Company), 1988.
6. *Ibid.*
7. Dana Ullman, interview, 1990.
8. Jim Bouton, interview, 1990.

Other Reading:

Boericke, William, M.D., *Pocket Manual of Homoeopathic Materia Medica,* 9th ed., (New Delhi, B. Jain Publishers), 1984.

Cummings, Stephen, M.D. and Ullman, Dana, M.P.H., *Everybody's Guide to Homeopathic Medicines,* Los Angeles, J.P. Tarcher, Inc., 1991.

Farrington, E.A., M.D., *Comparative Materia Medica,* (New Delhi, B. Jain Publishers, Pvt. Ltd.), 1988.

Fisher, Peter, "An Experimental Double-Blind Trial Method in Homeopathy: Use of a Limited Range of Remedies to Treat Fibrositis" *British Journal of Homeopathy,* 74 (1986): 142-147.

Fisher, P., Greenwood, A., Huskisson, E., Turner, P., Belon, P., "Effect of homeopathic treatment on fibrositis," *British Medical Journal* 1989 vol. 299, pp. 365-6.

Gibson, Douglas, M.D., M.B.,B.S.,F.R.C.S., *Studies of Homoeopathic Remedies,* (Bucks, England, Beaconsfield Publishers, Ltd.)

Gibson, R.G., Gibson, S.L.M., MacNeil, A.D., et al., "Homeopathic Therapy in Rheumatoid Arthritis: Evaluation by Double-Blind Controlled Trial," *British Journal of Clinical Pharmacology,* 9 (1980): 453-459.

Lilienthal, Samuel, M.D., *Homoeopathic Therapeutics,* (New Delhi, B. Jain Publishers), 1986.

Kent, James Tyler, M.D., *Lectures on Homoeopathic Materia Medica,* (New Delhi, B. Jain Publishing Co), 1984.

Kent, James Tyler, M.D., *Repertory of the Homoeopathic Materia Medica and a Word Index,* (London, Homoeopathic Book Service), 1986.

Panos, Maseimund B., M.D. and Heimlich, Jane, *Homeopathic Medicine at Home: Natural Remedies for Everyday Ailments and Minor Injuries,* (Los Angeles, J.P. Tarcher, Inc.), 1980.

Vithoulkas, George, *The Science of Homeopathy,* (New York, Grove Press, Inc.), 1980.

Chapter 6

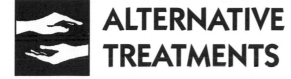 **ALTERNATIVE TREATMENTS**

> Let that which is unknown become known!
> —Kahuna teaching

Many Paths to Health

Many patients ask me "Is there anything else I can do for my injury?" I am happy when patients take the attitude of actively participating in their recovery, and I encourage you to do the same. Ask questions. Don't be afraid to call some of the teachers and practitioners of the disciplines described in this chapter and discuss your goals for physical and mental health. Remember, your present condition, whether it be an illness, an ailment, or an injury has something to teach you and is pointing to a new direction. You can make the most of this time to explore and discover, and perhaps you will come upon a method, a teaching, a teacher, or a treatment that will change your life.

True healing takes place only with a change of consciousness. There is a saying which goes, "Change is the only constant there is." We are always changing. Our bodies are completely renewed every seven years since every cell of our body is replaced periodically. Change is not optional. We are going to face it every day. We have the choice of resisting it or embracing it. I like to use the following two models for the change process as taught by Lazaris:[1]

The Loop of Perfection

Let's say, as an example, you injure yourself during training. You feel terrible about it. You immediately feel guilty or perhaps you blame someone else. You're angry, frustrated, hurt, or humiliated. You make the decision that next time, you'll do it "perfectly." This is living in the past, always returning to the problem or injury and reworking what went wrong. In this mood of regret or resentment, everything you do centers on trying to perfect the past, thinking, "Maybe this time I'll be a better person." When you live in the past, however, it's very hard to get well. The loop of perfection looks like this:

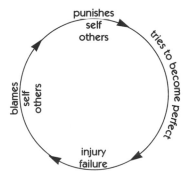

6-1. Loop of Perfection

The loop of perfection is an addictive-compulsive cycle from which no growth is possible. In the loop of perfection, you are always becoming more of who you *were*. However, there is another way to change: the path of freedom.[2]

The Path of Freedom

You injure yourself. Instead of blaming yourself, you acknowledge that you have some responsibility in the events leading up to the injury, even though you may not be aware of all the implications. As you go through the varied emotional responses, you allow yourself to experience them—"I'm really mad." "I'm hurt, I feel awful." Sooner or later you forgive yourself, recognizing that your injury could happen to anyone, that you're not perfect, and that you were never meant to be perfect. In this climate of acceptance you begin a true understanding. You gain insight into how you may need to do things differently in the future. In this process, change is open-ended, freeing you to become more of who you *can be,* not more of who you were in the past.

All of us have beliefs and attitudes, thoughts and feelings, choices, and decisions which are the raw materials with which we create what we call "reality." As an individual, you shape these energy patterns with your imagination, desires, and expectations. What you intend and anticipate usually comes into being. Therefore, if you want to change, you have to change your beliefs. You change everything by changing your beliefs and making different choices. This dynamic of change looks like this:

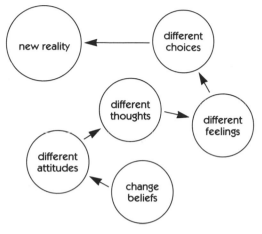

6-2. Path of Freedom

Every time you go for walks, go for a run, meditate, eat well, laugh, and enjoy your life you are giving a message to your subconscious about your renewed committment to health. This committment is the powerful intention that fuels your life.

Depending on your condition or problem, there is a veritable wealth of choices of supplemental or primary care practitioners. Exploring new treatment paths can open up whole new perspectives from which to view the human body.

Manipulation and Body Work

Acupressure and Shiatsu

Acupressure is the method of putting very firm pressure on acupuncture points and meridians (lines of energy flow) with the fingers. The goal is to stimulate or slow down imbalances of energy and to work with muscle knots. In my experience, acupressure helps to relieve tension, stress and pain, but the results are not as long-lasting as those of acupuncture. It is, however, a safe form of self-treatment.

Shiatsu, a form of acupressure, views the human body as a microcosm of the universe, with organs of the body governed by the Five Elements—Fire, Earth, Metal, Water, and Wood. For health, no one element should be dominant or deficient in relation to the others. This

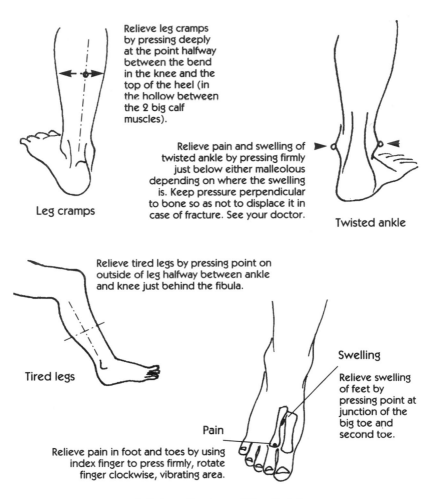

Relieve leg cramps by pressing deeply at the point halfway between the bend in the knee and the top of the heel (in the hollow between the 2 big calf muscles).

Leg cramps

Relieve pain and swelling of twisted ankle by pressing firmly just below either malleolous depending on where the swelling is. Keep pressure perpendicular to bone so as not to displace it in case of fracture. See your doctor.

Twisted ankle

Relieve tired legs by pressing point on outside of leg halfway between ankle and knee just behind the fibula.

Tired legs

Swelling

Relieve swelling of feet by pressing point at junction of the big toe and second toe.

Pain

Relieve pain in foot and toes by using index finger to press firmly, rotate finger clockwise, vibrating area.

6-3. Leg, Foot, and Toe Points

view is also shared by Five Element acupuncture. Disease is believed to result from unbalanced, blocked energy that is either too devitalized or too active. A Shiatsu therapist will assess your illness or condition on the basis of how it manifests in your daily life, and how your body responds to it. Diagnosis is made through observation, listening, questioning, and touch. As with other body work, there may be a powerful release of emotions during or after a session.

Figs. 6-3 through 6-6 show some acupressure points to press in the foot, leg, knee, hip and hand for pain relief—and even to reduce the burning of sunburn.[3]

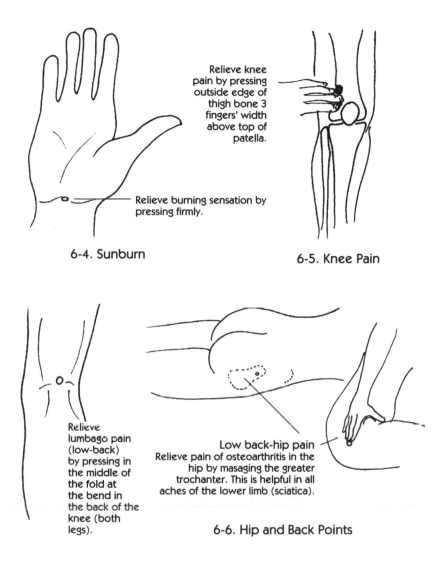

Relieve knee pain by pressing outside edge of thigh bone 3 fingers' width above top of patella.

Relieve burning sensation by pressing firmly.

6-4. Sunburn

6-5. Knee Pain

Relieve lumbago pain (low-back) by pressing in the middle of the fold at the bend in the back of the knee (both legs).

Low back-hip pain
Relieve pain of osteoarthritis in the hip by masaging the greater trochanter. This is helpful in all aches of the lower limb (sciatica).

6-6. Hip and Back Points

Acupuncture

Acupuncture, an ancient system of oriental medicine requires a skilled practitioner and is not a self-help treatment. The acupuncturist evaluates the body's total constitution, assessing the interplay of the qualities of a person's energy—qualities of feeling, appearance, sensation, activity, and motivation. Diagnosis is made on the basis of interpreting the *quality* of the pulse (rough, jumpy, leathery, wiry, slippery), observing various external conditions, including the tongue, eyes, and skin, and taking into account how one responds to the environment. Acupuncturists want to know such things as whether your symptom feels better with heat or cold, whether you feel better in the morning or evening—even how you feel about your work and family. Since balance in life is the primary concern, acupuncture takes into account all aspects of your physical, emotional, and spiritual health.

Treatment consists of stimulating specific points on the body to change disharmony into harmony. The acupuncture points lie along invisible paths of energy called meridians; there are fourteen main meridians and about two thousand acupuncture points. In the ear alone, for example, there are over a one hundred points with reflex connections to other organs and parts of the body. Needles of hair-like thinness made of stainless steel are sterilized, and cannot transmit infections. Inserted only 1 or 2 milli-meters, they cause almost no pain.

Many chronic injuries, neuromuscular problems, or musculoskeletal conditions respond beautifully to acupuncture treatments. Stiff shoulders and necks, headaches, and backaches including sciatica can be treated with good results. Cyclists, for example, who have spasms in the neck and shoulders or swelling and irritation of tendinitis and bursitis may be helped with this treatment.[4] For general vitality and healing, acupuncturists may also recommend herbal medicines or dietary advice.

While acupuncture excels in releasing and realigning blocked energy, I still recommend that you have a conventional western diagnosis for sports injuries such as runner's knee, back pain, groin pain, and other possibly serious medical conditions before undertaking acupuncture treatments.

Alexander Technique

The Alexander technique consists of a series of alignment lessons on how to retrain your body out of its bad postural habits. Gentle manipulations, breathwork, and realignment techniques are given on a one-to-one basis or in a class by a trained teacher.

The goal of the technique is to help you become aware of how you habitually hold and use your body in restricting, tense, and unnatural ways, and to relearn the correct way to stand, sit, move, and breathe. The course of instruction or treatments is individualized to your own body so that it's difficult to say what you can expect in your sessions. Individual sessions last about a half hour to 45 minutes, three times a week in the beginning. After reconditioning is established sessions are usually done once a week. A series may last from twelve visits to several months, depending on the seriousness of the postural problem.

This technique was developed by F. Mathias Alexander around the beginning of the 20th century. Alexander, an actor who was having trouble with his voice on stage, began to investigate how his posture and skeletal alignment were creating blockages in his ability to use his throat and voice. He came to realize that many of the things which feel "normal" to us are actually negative habits which must be un-learned before we can substitute better habits. He felt strongly that the body must be attuned from both a physical and mental standpoint.

During a lesson, the teacher gently manipulates different areas of the body. At the same time the student is taught to give verbal messages to the body such as, "Neck free, head forward and out," or "Back, lengthen and widen." Students are taught how to release individual tensions from different areas in the body.

One of the important lessons learned with this technique is to rec-ognize the "clutching" tense reaction that we fall into when we have a big project to complete or some other major "goal" to achieve. Re-ferred to as "endgaining," this common reaction to striving too hard is corrected so that energy and breath can flow more effortlessly.

Through this gentle movement and persistent suggestion to break old habits, muscles begin to let go. Patients report that they experi-ence everyday activities from a whole new feeling of lightness and even exhilaration.

The Alexander technique is useful for many chronic physical prob-lems such as asthma, ulcers, hypertension, tension headaches, low-back pain and rheumatoid arthritis. Since the technique improves overall alignment and release of tension, it is an excellent discipline for athletes and active people.

Applied Kinesiology/Touch for Health

Applied kinesiology is a method of diagnosis and treatment devel-oped by chiropractor Dr. George Goodheart. It is now used by a wide range of health professionals including chiropractors, osteopaths, acupuncturists, and dentists as an adjunct to their practice. Touch for Health was subsequently developed for self-care, using some of the main techniques of applied kinesiology.

These two methods are built on the idea that the body has an in-nate "knowing" of what is wrong with it—of what weakens or strength-ens it. Muscle testing accesses a wealth of specific information as to

> Remember, just because a conventional doctor tells you that surgery or potent drug therapy is the only answer, this may mean that he or she simply has no other method to offer, not *necessarily* that surgery or drugs are the only options.

physical and nutritional deficiencies, or emotional and mental rigidities. Following the discovery of problems and blockages, massage or electro-stimulation is done on lymphatic points to improve the flow of energy.

There are about twenty different branches of applied kinesiology. Chiropractors use it to test for structural problems while some nutritionists and homeopaths may use it to test for food allergies or homeopathic dosage levels. Interestingly enough, when foods are placed in the mouth or in the hand, muscles respond by becoming weaker or stronger according to the body's recognition that the particular food is healthful or detrimental.

Psychologists use applied kinesiology to determine where a person is carrying emotional stress. After working on an emotional issue with a patient, the muscles are again tested to see if the matter has been effectively resolved. Therapists who specialize in learning disabilities and dyslexia work to dispel blockages in acupuncture points to help children synchronize and harmonize neurological reflexes.

Points on the body that have become blocked are analogous to a tripped circuit-breaker that turns off when overloaded. This can occur from the stress of an emotionally-charged event, build-up of scar tissue, inadequate or excessive nutrition, over-training, or using a faulty athletic training technique.

Although no scientific research has been done to validate the results of applied kinesiology, I have heard of some interesting anecdotal stories. In one such case, Dale Sveum, a baseball player with the Milwaukee Brewers, had broken his leg in 1988 and continued to experience a lot of pain in the ankle. He was out of play for a year and the team was considering having to let him go. After one session of applied kinesiology he had no more pain or discomfort and went back to playing ball that same week.[5]

The self-help method, Touch for Health may improve the flow of lymph which feeds and cleanses the cells of the body. Students are taught to clear neurolymphatic points with gentle self-massage in basic classes. You can read more about this technique in *Touch for Health, a Practical Guide to Natural Health* by John F. Thie.

Chiropractic

Chiropractic treatment has existed since 1895, when it was developed by American healer David Daniel Palmer, who discovered the power of spinal manipulation. Often referred to as "drugless" therapy, the method primarily treats mechanical disorders of the spine and the joints. It can benefit a variety of ailments such as slipped discs, strains, joint problems, lumbago, and neuralgia. Some patients have also found relief for migraines, headaches, asthma, arthritis, and some chest pain. However, certain symptoms for which you might be tempted to see a chiropractor should have a careful medical diagnosis. For example, a leg cramp while walking (as opposed to a cramp while in bed) may indicate a narrowed or blocked artery. If not making reasonable improvement, check with your family doctor or homeopath. On your first visit, a chiropractor will take a chiropractic history, and give you a physical examination. (X-rays are usually taken of the injured part of your spine while it is bearing weight. Full body x-rays should normally be avoided.)

A chiropractor will treat your condition by adjusting joints and realigning bones and spinal discs that may have popped out of their normal position. The manipulations, done on a special adjustable table, are normally painless, although they may create a noise during the movements. This noise comes from bubbles of nitrogen that form inside the joint cavities in response to the adjustments.

The doctor of chiropractic has a well rounded medical background. They are considered primary care health care providers and are drugless practitioners. They believe the body is a self-healing mechanism which has an innate force within in it which may be blocked when there are spinal malalignments. These chiropractic subluxations respond well to adjustments which are specific to the area of fixation. There is ample medical evidence that chiropractic treatment is both effective, and cost efficient for low back pain as well as a variety of musculoskeletal problems. Regular chiropractic treatment may keep your energy flowing and improve your health.

As with all medical specialists, if you are not doing well with one, seek the attention of another and get a second opinion. If a chiropractor is not solving your problems seek the attention of an osteopathic physician or orthopedist. Before considering back surgery get the opinion of one or more chiropractors.

Although orthotics (correctional devices) from a chiropractor may

---

Go To An Emergency Room For:

- A neck injury followed by vomiting or difficulties in speaking or swallowing.
- A neck pain which spreads to the legs.
- A back injury with the inability to urinate.
- Severe head and neck pain which makes looking downward intolerable.
- A neck problem with dizziness, which may indicate a stroke. See your family doctor first.
- Any serious medical problem.

---

be useful for a specific problem, they are not generally biomechanically suitable for a sports problem. If in doubt, see a podiatrist.

Heller Work

This method of structural integration, an outgrowth of Rolfing, also employs deep tissue manipulation. The system was developed in the 1970's by Joseph Heller, the first president of the Rolfing Institute.

Since Heller work is not offered as a specific treatment for a specific injury, the most appropriate client is the person with tendencies for overuse, biomechanical imbalances, and dynamically imbalanced muscles (e.g., where the hamstrings in the back of the leg are stronger than the quadriceps in the front of the leg).

The treatment is less passive than other forms of structural integration. For instance, if the practitioner is working on the knee joint, the client may be asked to move his leg while the manipulation is being done. The Heller worker talks to the client during the session, asking about what emotions are occurring as the work goes on. In this interactive way, the client gains information and insight about his mind-body relationships. Body patterns, such as a caved-in chest, are recognized as physical responses to emotional traumas or fear; in the case of a caved-in chest, for instance, the person is probably unconsciously holding himself in a protected position.

Treatment usually consists of eleven sessions, as compared to the ten of Rolfing. Because breathing is considered the most fundamental aspect of health, the first session concentrates on the ribcage. The client might be asked the question, "What inspires you?" The point of the question is that inspiration, the act of drawing air into the lungs, also refers to what draws in spirit to us—what inspires us. Each session addresses the emotional and spiritual levels as the body work progresses.[6]

A person's daily movements are reviewed and analyzed, and the client is instructed as to how to find his natural balance point to enhance and retain the hands-on work of structural integration. The eleventh and final session is a review to encourage the client to manage and regulate his body according to where the balance point is. An exercise plan may be given and follow-up sessions may be indicated.

Reflexology

An ancient Chinese technique, reflexology is enjoying a renaissance as an effective and safe method for vitalizing the body and improving an amazing variety of conditions. The theory behind reflexology, is that there are zones on the soles of the feet that communicate with internal organs. The painful sites indicate congestion, dis-ease, or imbalance in corresponding organs. Studies have confirmed that this connection between parts does exist.

Treatment by a trained reflexologist is done lying or sitting. A slow, systematic kneading of the foot and ankle will uncover problematic areas which are gently, but firmly pressed by the fingers and thumbs. Usually, the massage of a painful site is a "good kind of hurt." Reflexologists recommend the method for prevention of disease as well as for specific intervention; the whole body benefits from a general toning as congestion is released, and circulation and lymphatic drainage is improved.[7] A session lasts about 40 minutes. You should begin to experience a change in your condition after about three weeks of bi-weekly sessions. Serious imbalance or disease might take up to thirty visits. During the treatment period, the body is detoxifying, which may bring on symptoms such as increased urination, acne, aching joints, sore throat, diarrhea, or a cold. These kinds of symptoms should be regarded as a good sign; they are often the way the body releases toxins.

Some highly trained reflexologists are able to manipulate displaced bones in the feet back into place. Interestingly enough, adjusting bones in the feet may heal related problems in the ankle, leg, thigh, pelvis, or back. Although this specialized type of reflexologist who moves bones may be very hard to find, the benefits for those who want to avoid surgery may be worth the effort of finding one.

As a self-care method, reflexology is best used by the layperson for general toning and relaxation. For athletes and for those who are active, learning the basics of reflexology could be a useful self-care technique for maintaining health. Sinus conditions, for instance, tend to make the toes very sensitive to touch, and one particular toe may be very painful. Reflexes to the left side of the head are on the left foot and vice versa. However, don't try to treat yourself or anyone else who is quite ill or frail. Do not perform home treatment on anyone with varicose veins, thrombosis, phlebitis, or ulceration of the feet.

Rolfing

Named after its founder, Ida Rolf, Rolfing is a deep-tissue therapy that manipulates the connective tissue of the body to release long-held patterns and bring the body back into alignment. The goal is to balance the body so that it works with the least effort in conjunction with gravitational forces. The premise in Rolfing is that the connective tissue of the body is a plastic, malleable material capable of being reshaped. The ideal body is imagined as a pillar from which hang the rib cage, limbs, and pelvis—the parts working with (not straining against) the gravitational forces.[8] Rolfing is concerned with the integration of body structures, not just with posture per se.

Not regarded as a therapy for a symptom, Rolfing emphasizes body awareness as well as structural change. Rolfers do not work on acute symptoms such as a sprained ankle where there is swelling and inflammation.[9] These conditions are best treated by conventional medicine and homeopathic remedies. However, for those people with a tendency for joint injuries in ankles, knees, hips, and low back or for athletes with severely tight hamstrings muscles, for instance, the deep manipulation of tissue can help.

The work of re-structuring the body's soft tissue is typically accomplished in ten sessions, each of which has a particular purpose. Scar tissue and adhesions (where tissues have stuck together) from accidents and injuries are broken up; the aim is to "reorganize" relationships of muscles, ligaments, and fascia in limbs, pelvis, shoulders, back and neck to encourage new postural alignment and movement. The person is taught the most efficient way to use his or her body considering the limitations, liabilities, and virtues of that particular body. Breathing patterns are analyzed and discussed to increase oxygen for enhanced metabolism and energy.

People who have been Rolfed report that they experience more flexibility, better respiration, elimination of musculoskeletal pain, as well emotional benefits. While Rolfing has had a certain reputation as a painful method because of the deep tissue level of the work, current practitioners claim the system has undergone modifications so that results can be achieved without a high degree of pain. Rolfing is being used by many professional athletic teams and individual athletes, including dancers, runners, cyclists, and gymnasts, as people turn to drug-free alternatives to enhance performance and maintain health. Rolfers, incidentally, generally recommend that athletes have their sessions in the off-season of their sport so that the body has time to integrate the new structure, sense of balance, and timing.

In my experience, Rolfing may bring good results for chronic muscular disorders; however, I am not entirely convinced of the *lasting* benefits of Rolfing, although Rolfers themselves believe that the body needs only occasional re-structuring. In my opinion, many cases of biomechanical imbalances, while helped by Rolfing, still require corrective foot orthoses.

Rosen Work

The bodywork technique known as Rosen work recognizes that emotions, feelings, or psychological patterns are held or locked within the physical body. Developed in the 1940's by Marion Rosen, a German physical therapist, this kind of bodywork uses firm, but gentle massage to release chronic muscle tension, and to bring about awareness of old emotional wounds. Practitioners work to release knotted muscles, tight chests, raised shoulders, or rigid backs that come from past emotional trauma or pain.

This work may benefit people who have chronic patterns that contribute to overuse injury. Rosen work is effective for poor form that doesn't respond well to coaching and training. It is particularly effective with people who have over-developed muscles and have carried tension in habitual patterns for years. Practitioners note that sometimes a literal interpretation of a body stance indicates a belief or attitude. For instance, a dancer who exaggerates her posture may be expressing the need to "stand up to the world."[10]

Rosen workers will talk to you about your past while massage is taking place to determine the kinds of life decisions that might be creating disharmony within the body. Unlike deep structural integration or massage, Rosenwork aims at releasing deep layers of emotional pain. Because the method encourages the discovery and integration of emotional material, you may gain insights into rigid thinking patterns or compulsive behavior that cause you to rigidify physical stances.

Rosen work is interactive and presumes the patient is interested in personal change but needs support. An emphasis is put on breath work. There are Rosen workers in most metropolitan areas of the United States and a large following in Sweden.

Sports Massage

The healing power of sports massage is becoming increasingly more well-known in the competitive world of sports. Developed in the Eastern bloc countries in the mid-1970's, sports massage techniques have found their way into many American professional teams. There are now over two hundred certified sports massage therapists working in this country.

Sports massage is given either before or after an event. For instance, a triathlete will get a pre-event massage on the neck, arms and wrist to prevent cramping or injuries during the race. Therapists say that the massage warms up connective tissue, increasing blood supply. After the event, a massage alleviates some of the soreness and cramping resulting from the micro-trauma done to muscles, helping to prevent an accumulation of damage that may lead to over-use injury.

What makes sports massage different from any other massage?

First of all, the goal is to keep the highly-trained athlete as close to peak condition as possible without going over the edge into over-use injury. It's particularly effective for muscles used over and over again. Therapists recommend its use in baseball (for shoulders and back), for cycling (thighs, back, shoulders, and neck), golf (back and shoulders), rowing (back and shoulders), running (back of legs and thighs), and skiing (legs).

Therapists use *compression* to spread the muscle fiber and increase circulation, *trigger point therapy* to apply direct pressure to sensitive points in the gluteal and hamstring muscles, and *cross-fiber friction* to loosen muscles in a sideways direction.[11]

Trager Work

Differing from the types of massage that dig deeply into the muscles, Trager work uses gentle, rocking, rhythmic movements to promote an altered state of awareness of the body and to release tension patterns. A Trager practitioner "talks" to the muscles of the patient during a session, using mental communication in conjunction with physical patterning to establish lasting healing. This psychophysical massage was developed by Dr. Milton Trager more than fifty years ago as an adjunct to his medical practice.[12] A Trager practitioner works with a combination of long, sweeping motions and shorter, swiveling-type movements which bring a sense of relaxation and peace. It is not a painful treatment.

Proponents of the technique point out that it works well in sports because of the emphasis on moving efficiently and freely. A pilot program in Austin, Texas, headed by coach John Pearcy, uses Trager massage with runners and triathletes; he feels that this bodywork increases the efficiency of the body, enhances recovery from competition, and keeps athletes more limber and loose. Other advocates of this method talk about the effortless quality of mental relaxation that comes from being "Tragered." They feel that when used together with proper coaching and training methods, this form of body work contributes significantly to high performance. Some athletes, particularly tennis players, find that the system helps back problems associated with over-efforting in the movements involving serving and volleying; tennis and golf pros recommend Trager bodywork to their students as a supplement to coaching. Other athletes describe a releasing of tight jaw muscles, and a freeing of shoulders, ankles, and calves. Chronic low-back pain or old back injuries are particularly well suited for this treatment.

An advantage of the gentleness of the Trager technique is that it sometimes succeeds in relaxing muscles that would be overstimulated by harsher, more invasive massage which might create further tension. The Trager "rocking pattern" seems to confuse or overcome a spastic muscle pattern. Some athletes have claimed that Trager work gave them a calmness and centeredness during the stress of competition. Professional marathoners have reported that tendinitis problems have healed more quickly following a series of Trager sessions.[13] However, as I have said before, be sure that you have any orthopedic problem properly diagnosed before starting any alternative treatments.

Movement Practices

Aikido

Aikido, a forty-year-old form of self-defense, was founded after World War II in Japan by Professor Morihei Ueshiba. His guiding principle was that winning at someone else's expense was not really winning. The movements in Aikido are meant to divert harm to one's self while not inflicting permanent injury on an aggressor.

The name Aikido is composed of three syllables:

AI which means "to meet, to come together, to harmonize."

KI which means "energy, spirit, mind," and "spirit of the Universe."

DO which means "the way."

Therefore, Ai-ki-do means "the way of harmonizing with the spirit of the Universe." It is a practice for understanding earthly life through the study of the energy flow of the universe. To study this art is to build character, to learn to walk the spiritual path with practical feet.

The most unusual aspect of Aikido, as an art of self-defense, is the concept of contacting the energy of your opponent and blending with it, rather than fighting him with conflict and force. The ideal of Aikido is not to defeat your enemy, but, rather, to be in harmony with him spiritually and physically. Aikido is sometimes called the "art of non-resistance" or the "non-fighting martial art."

Practice is done with partners (whereas in T'ai Chi work is usually done solo). You learn how to yield, how to lead and guide another person's movements—how to throw an opponent through non-resistive techniques. Most important for the practice is a flowing flexibility and a stable balance. The goal is to be in complete control of the mind and body, to maintain a calm, alert posture. The continuous and flexible motion which originates in the belly is like the performance of a dance. Most of the joint techniques, such as those applied to the wrist or elbow, flex the joints in the direction of natural bending. They are in harmony with natural flexing. There may be some pain in resistance during practice, but no permanent harm is done to the joint.

Because the philosophy promotes non-conflict, there are no tournaments or matches. Students attain mastery through periodic tests or ranking for more advanced belts which take into account character, diligence and training attitude. Aikido is an excellent practice for all-round strength and flexibility, but done incorrectly, and sometimes inadvertently, you can hurt yourself in Aikido. High falls can be hard on the back; knees can be easily stressed in Aikido, as in any martial art.

Chi Gong

There are hundreds of forms of Chi Gong, a Chinese practice of energy work which has been done for over three thousand years.[14] A movement form which works with the "chi," the core energy of the body, Chi Gong exercises are part of the martial art T'ai Chi. Chi Gong releases the energy of the body so that it can circulate freely. Lower level work involves breathing exercises; advanced levels teach how to access energy with the mind. Mind is the direct link to energy, and students are taught how to increase their inner power. Practice is done daily.

Feldenkrais

Moshe Feldenkrais, the Israeli physicist behind this system of mind-body re-education, never referred to his work as therapy, but as learning. He proposed that the rigidities and disharmonies of our bodies are not so much an illnesses with a specific label, as they are the product of faulty learning. Trained as a physicist at the Sorbonne, he came to develop his unique and profoundly simple methods to heal his own crippling knee injuries from playing soccer. He believed that lasting improvement in flexibility and comfort comes from making better use of our brain, rather than, as is so commonly believed, in "working hard" to better a condition. Using the brain to restructure the mind-body connection, he demonstrated, worked for the highly trained athlete as well as for the person crippled by cerebral palsy.

A basic premise of the method is that we live in four possible states: asleep, awake, conscious, and aware. Increased consciousness develops through insights and perceptions which lead us further to the state of awareness, where our insights can be put to use. Therefore, awareness is the *experience* of the change in mind-body connection, not just an intellectual understanding of what change is like.

Feldenkrais retraining has two components. One component is the work done by the individual in changing his or her awareness. For example, in the seminars called Awareness Through Movement, pupils (not patients) learn to replace, in a playful and non-cerebral way, habitual ineffective movements. Feldenkrais practitioners believe that a physical distortion exists in the brain as literally as in the vertebrae.[15]

The key to change, in this system, is in affecting the motor system which alters the patterns in the motor cortex of the brain—thus disseminating changes throughout the nervous system. The core of the work is accomplished through deceptively simple and often slow movements. A foot is flexed and extended. Minute attention is given to such movements as turning the head to one side. The aim of the teaching is to free the brain from the habitual in order to free the body. Learning is approached as discovery, rather than as a rote experience. New movements become automatic and unconscious, replacing the old unconscious patterns. Changes in strength and flexibility of the skeleton and muscles, as well as profound change in self-image and quality of life are the potential results of the work.

The other component of Feldenkrais work is called Functional Integration, a manipulation of the body by a practitioner. People are treated for deformities, injuries, congenital illness, and a variety of physical problems with an emotional foundation. Feldenkrais work can awaken a body treated as a machine to new sensory awareness, and is a good antidote to the training athlete's achievement orientation.

T'ai Chi Chuan

T'ai Chi Chuan is an ancient and venerable Chinese martial art practiced with the goal of attaining physical well-being as well as peace of mind. It is very popular with older people, and is done daily in China in public squares. Nowadays, you often see T'ai Chi practitioners practicing in public parks. Popularly known as a method for self-defense, T'ai Chi is, in its entirety, a philosophy of life. Athletes in other fields study it to increase their stamina, flexibility, coordination, elegance of movement, and to increase concentration. More than a physical exercise program, T'ai Chi teaches specific movements, principles of energy dynamics, and body alignments, all of which lead the student to self-discovery and self-confidence. The goal of T'ai Chi is tranquillity. The person learns how to resist nothing, thereby enhancing the dynamic flow of the body's vital force. Resistance, in this case meaning blockages in energy, can cause disease.

I have recommended T'ai Chi to several patients, especially for low-back pain. The results have been impressive. I practice this method myself and find it, paradoxically, relaxing *and* energizing, and good for my overall balance. Practice is often done outside in the natural elements for 20 minutes or more. It can be done at any age; some people have taken it up in their seventies.

Yoga

Yoga is a four-thousand-year-old Hindu philosophy of health and balance. The sanskrit word yoga means "union" referring to the union of the individual with the divine. In the west and in Europe, the popular notion of yoga is a series of complicated-looking physical postures. Actually, physical yoga, called hatha yoga, is only one part of this comprehensive teaching. Other aspects of yoga include breath control and meditation (including one type called karma yoga which is meditative mindfulness while working). The goal of yoga is self-realization.

Yoga sees the world as permeated by a subtle form of energy called "prana" similar to the idea of "chi" in acupuncture and T'ai Chi. Prana flows along channels (the equivalent to acupuncture meridians), and is concentrated in centers of energy called "chakras." Disease results from blocked energy. The goal of the postures is to unlock the energy flow. Some yogis are capable of consciously directing prana to parts of the body to revitalize and regenerate them.

Yoga has a wide range of benefits for people of all ages, and can be helpful in the prevention and treatment of a wide range of disorders including musculoskeletal, respiratory, digestive, nervous, and psychological conditions. I highly recommend it for runners, walkers, and other athletes. The stretching postures provide the key to the flexibility and limberness essential for the balanced, injury-free runner or athlete. Because training for sports is so intensive, the muscles of the body become very shortened. The muscles in the back of the legs in runners, for example, are chronically tightened. Without flexibility, an athlete is not truly fit.

There is no sense of hurry or competitiveness in the philosophy of hatha yoga. The postures (called *asanas*) are done only to the point where there is stretch, but no strain. Each asana is held at this point for a few counts, as the muscles are given a chance to lengthen slowly, releasing tension and stress. The movements are done at a quiet, relaxing pace with few repetitions. Some of the complex postures take as long as a few months to accomplish, as the body limbers and loosens with regular practice. If you have run for years without doing any serious stretching, you may be astounded at how inflexible you are. The pleasure that comes with the gradual lengthening of the muscles in the legs, spine, hips, and arms is well worth the time spent. Some of the postures where the feet are in a position higher than the head—for instance, the shoulder stand—reverse the effects of gravity, allowing all the internal organs to be stimulated. Starting yoga while young and maintaining a practice (which is easy because once you feel the effects of yoga you don't want to discontinue doing it) definitely decreases the aging process.

Some athletes have described a feeling of "weightlessness" and ease in everyday activities once they have developed more fluidity in their body through yoga. Overall vitality, strength, and range of motion increases, and athletic performance is enhanced as well.

Yoga is also a good counterbalance to the competitive outlook of running and sports. Practicing these asanas regularly gives you quiet time for letting thoughts slip away. Doing the physical postures is an-

117

other form of meditation and helps cut through obsessive thought patterns and unrealistic goal setting. Yoga can easily be done at home, and there are good books and video-tapes available for self-study; however, in order to be sure you are achieving the postures as they're intended, it's probably best to start your practice with a good teacher. Half an hour a day is sufficient for the average person, but if you have a chronic condition, you may want to practice for an hour or more. Doing yoga may also reduce the time you need to sleep.

Therapeutic Yoga

Biomechanical muscle imbalances resulting from old injuries or poor training may be corrected under the guidance of a trained yoga practitioner. Since this type of correctional work requires special training beyond normal yoga classes, be sure to discuss your problems thoroughly with a teacher and determine if he or she has the experience you need.

Mind and Energy Work

There is a growing movement toward developing methods of healing using subtle energy. While scientific research is still in its infancy with energetic healing, I feel strongly that these methods have much to offer us. Chronic conditions from old injuries and acute sports injuries can be helped enormously by psychic healing. You may wish to use these practitioners to augment your conventional treatment.

Healing with Energy

Therapeutic Touch is the practice of directing healing energy toward a wounded or diseased person. This practice of hands-on healing was brought out of the "closet," so to speak, by a gifted therapist, Dora Kunz.[16] Professor of Nursing Delores Krieger, who coined the term therapeutic touch, brought it into the clinical setting of New York hospitals.[17] Her research demonstrated that therapeutic touch significantly increased hemoglobin levels; subsequently, the method has become very popular within the nursing profession.

Although therapeutic touch is in the same general field as faith-healing and spiritual healing, it is a secular practice and its proponents don't believe that faith is the major factor in the way it works.[18] It is based on the concept that the world is a dynamic, inter-connected whole. Disease is seen as disorder and disharmony, not just in the physical body, but in the entire bioenergetic field surrounding the body.

Therapeutic touch aligns itself with emerging scientific field theory.

Nurses report very real physical effects from using the method on patients: pain relief in arthritis, wounds and terminal diseases; reduction of swelling; and enhancement of bone knitting. The anxiety and stress of prolonged terminal illness is also greatly relieved.

In a session, the practitioner centers his or her energy to open and clear the channel of universal life energy, and establishes the *intention* of healing. The assessment of the patient's condition is done by passing the hands around the energy field without physical contact. The field of a healthy person will be sensed as smooth or evenly distributed. The field of an unhealthy person will elicit feelings in the practitioner of "blockages," congestion, deficiencies (a drawing in or hollow feeling), or imbalanced energy flow. Sometimes there is a sensation of heat or "pins and needles."

Treatment consists of balancing the energy field with stroking, clearing motions, much like smoothing a rumpled bedspread. Sometimes the hands are applied directly to an area, usually with one hand in front and one in back. Throughout the session, the practitioner visualizes the patient as being "whole."

In therapeutic touch, the ability to direct healing energy through the hands is not seen to be a special gift, but an inherent ability of the human being. However, some people do seem to be more effective than others in hands-on healing, and in those ranks, of course, are psychic healers.

One such healer, Matthew Manning, makes the point that faith, or belief in the healer, is not always the main factor in his success.[19] He has found that some people who come to him with absolute faith that he will be able to cure them, unfortunately, are not always cured. Others who are initially skeptical of Manning, but who have been referred by physicians who have exhausted conventional treatment for their patient, are helped.

Manning also stresses that it is unrealistic to expect to lead an unhealthy life and expect to be healed if the root problems are not addressed. Therefore, he includes lifestyle counseling, as do many other alternative therapists, as part of the treatment. He feels that the person must take responsibility for changing his or her own life.

Most legitimate psychic healers also emphasize that rarely does psychic healing achieve a total cure in one session. Miracle cures are less than one in 10,000 says Dr. Thelma Moss, a leader in the psychic healing movement. Dr. Moss is among many researchers who have documented the transfer of energy between living systems and established the existence of bioenergetic fields. With psychic healing, there may be a complete cure (rare), an improvement or cure over several sessions, or a stabilization of a progressive disease (staying the same and not worsening).

Holoenergetic Healing, a term meaning "healing with the whole force," was coined by healing researcher, Dr. Leonard Laskow, originally an obstetrician and gynecologist. An unusual encounter brought energy healing into his life.

He happened to be at a conference where he shared a room with a man who had testicular cancer that had metastasized to his lungs. The man awoke moaning with pain in the middle of the night, and was having trouble breathing. Laskow asked if there was anything he could do, and the man said, "Anything."

Laskow's spontaneous response was to put his hands on either side of the man's chest. He began to visualize a radiant ball of energy coming from his head, coursing through his heart, and flowing out his hands into the man's body. He imagined the ball of light between his hands, continuing to meditate on the light for a awhile.

In a few minutes, the man began to breathe more easily. He said the pain was gone. During the next few days the man experienced no more pain. The experience was so profound for the doctor that over the next few years he decided to investigate the phenomenon with another colleague. He wanted to find out if the occurrence of healing could have been explained by the placebo effect (which means that a certain percentage of patients get well even if they are given a harmless substance). In controlled laboratory experiments he directed *an intention of healing* to bacteria which had been given various amounts of an antiobiotic which, of course, is supposed to kill bacteria.

What he found was that *his intention to "love" or "heal" the bacteria prevented their destruction by the drug to a quantifiable extent.* Since bacteria cannot be affected by the "placebo effect," he demonstrated that energy was, indeed, being transferred to these organisms, which allowed them to resist the killer drugs.

In further studies he measured the transference of energy between humans, and found that a person receiving thoughts of love and compassion from a group had an energy field almost four times larger than a person who was not the target of the healing energy. The receiver also mentioned subjective feelings of "a wind rushing past me," or "I began to feel really happy."

In *Healing with Love,* Laskow explains that our physical body is actually a field of energy which has taken a particular form. Physicists have proven that matter and energy are interchangeable; that matter is energy that exists in the form of vibration. The physical body, then, is a dense manifestation of an energy field. Furthermore, our body is surrounded by *other* levels of energy patterns (subtle energy fields) which have a less dense vibration, but which influence our body.

Dr. Laskow says, "The fields surrounding our bodies reflect and represent our emotional and mental states as well as our physical bodies ... there is a "balance" between a thought form and a physical form. A vibrating negative thought form, such as hatred, can constitute part of a standing wave; the other part (physical form) might be a tumor ... they are in balance." Therefore, healing must break up the negative thought pattern, replace it with a new form (trans-form it) and bring about a new healing homeostasis that is aligned with one's spiritual purpose, natural order, and harmony.

Reiki is an ancient form of natural healing by energy transference. Advanced training for Reiki work proceeds by degrees of mastery through a series of attunement processes. Practitioners who have been empowered in a direct lineage from the master, Usui, distinguish their teaching as the "official Radiance Technique."

Practitioners recommend Reiki for a variety of conditions, and suggest using it even for first aid (cuts and burns) after, of course, cleansing and conventional first aid. Reiki healing has been known to work for colds, flu, pain, and stress.

If you are interested in a good listing of research in the area of psychic healing, I suggest the very readable book by Michael C. Moore and Lynda J. Moore, *The Complete Handbook of Holistic Health.*[20] In choosing a psychic healer, it's very important to get references if you can. Be wary of people who guarantee results, who suggest giving up conventional treatments, or who work only in seances.

Hypnotherapy

Hypnotherapy is very useful for getting to the root of fixed ideas that we carry from earlier events and traumas. By creating a state of mind where normal, conscious thinking is suspended, a therapist can elicit information that can reveal amazingly useful information to the client.

Far from being a state where one is asleep, hypnosis is actually a heightened awareness to previously unconscious material. A trance of varying intensity or depth is induced, but the person is aware of words being spoken; the awareness is focused on the inner state rather than on outer stimuli. Classical hypnotherapy, as used by Sigmund Freud, for example, uses a pendulum, a light, a spinning object, or the sound of the therapist's voice to induce the trance. The therapist, once the subject is relaxed and "under," gives suggestions to achieve a desired therapeutic result such as removing a pain. This type of authoritative therapist and passive client is not seen as much today as more interactive forms of hypnotherapy.

Dr. Milton H. Erickson some thirty years ago developed a more interactive hypnotherapy which reduces resistances on the part of the client. The client's own unconscious provides the answers to problems or the resolution of blocks.

Hypnotherapists feel that most psychological as well as many physical symptoms result from the way people cope with life's demands. Often specific events cause us to react or make a decision that becomes a fixed postulate which we use in other situations without thinking. We act in a rote way, not a creative and fresh way. We become stuck and fail to grow as individuals. We cannot understand why we do not feel fulfilled. The hypnotherapist may be able to help us identify these decisions which are now no longer appropriate for our lives. I've found this process helpful for some of my patients who are athletes with performance anxiety or fixed ideas about their ability to succeed in events.

Meditation and Breathing Exercises

Meditation can be combined with breathing to enhance vitality. Through concentration on breathing, normal functions of the body are slowed down and the mind is stilled from its constant chatter. For example, during normal waking activity, we use a rapid brain wave pattern called beta; beta brain wave is associated with rather rapid breathing. By slowing down the breathing pattern, we move to the alpha brain waves, which are better for remembering data, clarity of thought or studying, and healing. Finally, when we breathe very slowly, the brain waves slow down to the delta frequency, considered to be a transcendental state offering great relaxation and stress release.

Meditation is the practice of training the mind to bring our thoughts into focus—by letting the thoughts go through the mind unimpeded. Gradually the mind becomes quiet, breathing becomes deeper, and the body is in a state conducive to relaxation and healing. Studies have shown that the heart rate, blood pressure and metabolism can be lowered with meditation. It can help headaches, nervous stress, high blood pressure, phobias, and anxiety. Meditation can be a very useful practice for high-performance athletes who are continually under the stress of competition.

In the beginning of meditation, you will notice the constant thoughts and repetitive stream-of-consciousness chatter in the mind. Meditation allows you to release these thoughts without judgment or without giving them further power, and to continually practice re-aligning the mind to its quiet center—the inner self. When the mind calms, the true self can be felt. At this point, you have more power to decide what is really important in your life.

The powerful effects of meditation are not limited to the time in which you sit relaxed and centered. By meditating on a daily basis— sometimes 15 to 30 minutes is enough—you will find your problem-solving ability, your ability to plan and focus the mind (to do one thing at a time, and do it well) is greatly enhanced. Research has even found that people who meditate are better able to respond quickly to a threat-ening situation, to perform better in competitive events, and to recover more quickly once the challenge has passed.

When I want information about a problem, for instance, I often meditate using a focused method. I sit in a relaxed position and bring my mind to the process of breathing, focusing on inspiration and ex-piration. After a few minutes, I focus on a single idea, issue or goal. I take note of the ideas that pop into and out of my brain which may or may not have anything to do with the idea. Sooner or later my focus sharpens and I get the information I'm looking for.

Focused running and walking is a very pleasant and refreshing ac-tivity. During this active, dynamic form of meditation, the focus is on running (or walking) form—on the swinging of the arms, the posture, the breath, or on the smooth rhythm of muscular exertion. You may simply focus on your movements, and on the spirit that animates your body.

During focused running and walking, you may experience vari-ous psychological phases. First, there is a free association phase where the mind wanders, and different images pop in and out of the mind. The next phase is focused thought, a transcendental state where you feel you are "in" the run itself, blending with the surroundings. Part of this ecstatic feeling could be induced by the release of brain chemi-cals (endorphins) after the first half hour of running. After about 45 minutes the mind becomes rather clear and ideas that just pop into it may have an amazing relevance to our life.

Visualization is a form of mental visioning that creates an inner picture of something we would like to achieve, have, or be in the outer world. There was a famous experiment done a few years ago with two groups of basketball players that demonstrated the effectiveness of visualization. Five players spent 5 to 10 minutes a day for two weeks visualizing making successful free throws *without practicing on the court.* The other five players practiced every day and did not visualize. At the end of two weeks, both groups were tested, and the group which did not practice on the court but *only visualized* themselves executing a perfect free throw had a much higher accuracy rate.

When I was a competitive skier, I used to visualize racing down the hill executing each turn with ease and elegance. In my mind, I would always finish the race with a winning time. I rehearsed the race over and over in my mind; as far as my brain was concerned, I had already won. Once in the race, my brain took over and my body followed its instructions. I raced with ease and elegance, made each turn on time, and finished the race standing up—with a very good time.

For professional athletes with a finely honed physical skill, the next step to excellence is honing the mind. Focused visioning and focused thought helps to establish the link between the mind and the body. It is believed that future events are planned and "created" in the frontal lobe of the brain. Visioning, meditation, and affirmation all help to stimulate the frontal lobe. The frontal lobe is very active, especially at night. While you're sleeping, the frontal lobe is always thinking and planning your future. This is another reason why you need to get enough sleep.

Affirmations are repetitive, positive statements you can make silently in the mind, out loud, or on paper. Affirmations are statements of an ideal or a goal you wish to achieve. Basically, the mind creates our outer world. Therefore, if you wish to change a physical aspect of your world, you must provide the inner foundation for that creation. First, decide what area in your life you are most interested in changing, and then make a positive statement about it the way you'd like it to be. For example, you might want to be healthier, more alive and vigorous: "I am healthy, and feeling healthier every single day." "My good health is boundless. I feel terrific!"

It's important, when you're working with the subconscious that you don't use negative forms of affirmations such as "I am no longer sick" or "My knee doesn't hurt any more." The subconscious cannot differentiate between positive and negative very well. It simply works on images, impressions and symbols. Always state the ideal in *present tense* and with *positive words,* as if you already possessed the thing you desire.

One thing I have noticed is that sometimes when I make an affirm-ation, for example, "I am getting healthier everyday," I hear a little voice inside that says "But that's not true. You're aging, you're not as young as you used to be." or some other negating statement. These are the negative beliefs that I am still holding. In making affirmations, I believe that it's important to recognize that these beliefs do exist, and ask yourself if you are willing to let these negative attitudes go. Sometimes, this kind of inner dialogue can clear up a long-standing block when you have been doing affirmations with no seeming results.

Repetition is important with affirmations, yet repetition without feeling and passion is worthless. Write your goals on post-it notes and stick them in the bathroom where you see them everyday. Put one in your car. Take an expectant attitude about the imminent arrival of what you wish. Be passionately involved in this process.

I suggest that you be careful of who you tell about your affirma-tions. It's not useful to have other people's negative assumptions, be-liefs, or sarcasm detracting or lessening your intention. Share your process only with those you are intimate with, and who you trust. The language of the subconscious is symbolic—be very aware of what you "feed" your inner self.

Both visualization and affirmations are what Emmet Fox, an ear-ly Unity Church teacher, called the "mental equivalent." He describes how to go about creating positive changes:

So the key to life is to build in the mental equivalents of what you want and to expunge the equivalents of what you do not want. How do you do it? You build in the mental equivalents by thinking quietly, constantly, and persistently of the kind of thing you want, and by thinking that has two qualities: *clarity* or definiteness, and *interest.* If you want to build anything into your life—if you want to bring health, right activity, your true place, inspiration ... form a mental equivalent of the thing which you want by thinking about it a great deal, by thinking clearly and with interest. Remember *clarity* and *in-terest;* these are the two poles.[21]

Footnotes:

1. Lazaris, *Lazaris Interviews, Book I,* (Beverly Hills, CA, Con-cept Synergy Publishing), 1988.
2. *Ibid.*
3. Roger Dalet, M.D., *How to Give Yourself Relief from Pain: by the Simple Pressure of a Finger,* (New York, Stein and Day), 1980.

4. Whit Reaves, Accupuncturist and O.M.D., Boulder, CO.
5. Conversation with Torbjorn (Tobe) Hanson, Applied Kinesiol ogy Practioner, Sports Performance, Danville, CA.
6. Heller Work: The Body of Knowledge, Mt. Shasta, CA.
7. Conversation with Dr. Harvey Lampell, reflexologist, Oakland, CA.
8. Conversation with Dorothy Weicker, Rolfer, Berkeley, CA.
9. Conversation with Julia Ireland, Rolfer, Sausalito, CA.
10. Rosen Institute, Berkeley, CA.
11. Michael Van Straten, N.D., D.O., *The Complete Natural Health Consultant: A Practical Handbook of Alternative Health Treatments,* (New York, Prentice-Hall Press), 1987.
12. Milton Trager, M.D., and Cathy Guadagno, Ph.D. *Trager Mentastics,* (Station Hill Press).
13. Conv. with Mark Bauman, Tragerworker, Redwood City, CA.
14. Paul Dong and Aristide Esser, *Chi-Gong: the Ancient Chinese Way to Health,* (New York, Paragon House), 1990.
15. Conversation with Mark Bersin, Feldenkrais practitioner, San Francisco, CA.
16. Dora Kunz and E. Peper, "Fields and Their Clinical Implications." in Kunz, *Spiritual Aspects of the Healing Arts.*
17. Delores Krieger, Ph.D., *The Therapeutic Touch: How to Use Your Hands to Help or to Heal,* (Englewood Cliffs, N.J., Prentice-Hall), 1979.
18. Janet Macrae, *Therapeutic Touch: A Practical Guide,* (New York, Alfred A. Knopf), 1988.
19. Van Straten, *op. cit.*
20. Michael C. Moore and Lynda J. Moore, *The Complete Handbook of Holistic Health,* (Englewood Cliff, N.J., Prentice-Hall), 1983.
21. Emmet Fox, *The Mental Equivalent,* Unity School of Christianity, Unity Village, Missouri, 64065

Further Reading:

John Feltman, Ed. of Prevention Magazine, *Hands on Healing,* Emmaus, P.A., Rodale Press, 1989.
Richard Gerber, M.D., *Vibrational Medicine,* Santa Fe, NM, Bear and Company, 1988.
Brian Inglis and Ruth West, *The Alternative Health Guide,* New York, Alfred A. Knopf, 1983.
Michael Murphy and Rhea A. White, *The Psychic Side of Sports,* Reading MA, Addison-Wesley Publishing Company, 1978.

Chapter 7

BASIC FIRST AID

If accidents happen and you are to blame
Take steps to avoid repetition of same.
                    Dorothy Sayers, *In the Teeth of the Evidence*

First Aid for Leg, Ankle, Foot and Heel Injuries

First aid treatment for most sports injuries is summed up by the short-hand term, **RICE—rest, ice, compression, and elevation.** After completing first aid, call your doctor or a sports medicine specialist for further treatment.

Figs. 7-1a and b, "Where does it hurt?" may help you find more information about your injury after first aid has been completed.

What to do for all Lower Leg Injuries:

- Rest. Avoid all pain-causing activity after an injury.
- Ice. For any injury, apply a refrigerated towel or an ice pack (make one by putting ice in a plastic bag) wrapped in a towel. To prevent ice burn, don't put ice or frozen packages of food directly on your skin. Ice your injury 20 minutes on the hour, or until the swelling and pain subside. Do this three or four times a day. Ice is helpful for controlling bleeding and numbing pain. For ankle sprains, after the ankle is numb, rotate *gently* in order to stimulate the lymphatic system to flush out tissue debris from bleeding and swelling. NOTE: For most people, ice treatment reduces pain and swelling. However, if ice *increases* the pain, try a heating pad (set to *low,* never high). Whenever heat seems to make an injury feel better, homeopathic *Bellis* may be a more effective first remedy than *Arnica* which is usually the first remedy given in trauma.

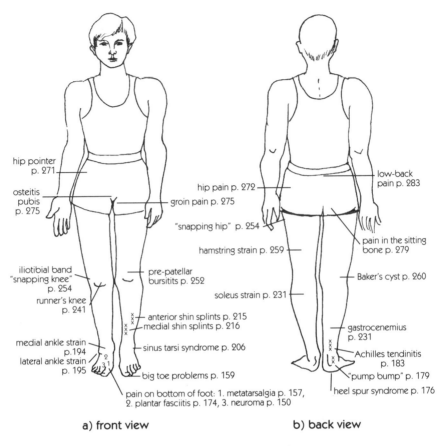

hip pointer
p. 271

osteitis
pubis
p. 275

hip pain p. 272

groin pain p. 275

"snapping hip" p. 254

hamstring strain p. 259

low-back
pain p. 283

pain in the sitting
bone p. 279

iliotibial band
"snapping knee"
p. 254

runner's knee
p. 241

pre-patellar
bursitits p. 252

soleus strain p. 231

Baker's cyst p. 260

anterior shin splints p. 215
medial shin splints p. 216

gastrocenemius
p. 231

medial ankle strain
p.194

lateral ankle strain
p. 195

sinus tarsi syndrome p. 206

big toe problems p. 159

Achilles tendinitis
p. 183

"pump bump" p. 179

heel spur syndrome p. 176

pain on bottom of foot: 1. metatarsalgia p. 157,
2. plantar fasciitis p. 174, 3. neuroma p. 150

a) front view

b) back view

7-1. Where Does it Hurt?

- If ice alone is not effective in reducing pain or swelling, try using alternate hot and cold applications (contrast baths). Immerse the injured part in ice cold water for 10 minutes. Then immerse in very hot water for 10 minutes. Alternating hot and cold tends to flush out the waste products of inflammation and helps recharge damaged cells to enhance healing.
- Elevation. Keep your foot higher than your hip or heart. Prop the leg on a pillow or soft chair. To minimize swelling, don't sit or stand with your foot on the floor. Keep the leg on pillows even in bed if you can sleep in this position.
- Compression or pressure. Sprains become swollen in the beginning to restrict movement and prevent further damage from mo-

tion. For ankle injuries, apply an ace bandage, extending from your toes to just below your knee. If the ankle is very swollen, use an inflatable air splint.

Non-elastic bandages are not advisable (unless you know how to wrap them) because the ankle may continue to swell, and a too-tight bandage will cut off the circulation. Check your circulation every 15 minutes by squeezing your big toe and watching the redness return. If the toe remains white, loosen the bandages right away.

The Walker and Runner's Medicine Chest

Homeopathic First Aid Remedies

Below are listed important first aid remedies to have on hand. See page 383 for full names and sources of these substances.

Apis	*Hypericum*
Arnica	*Ledum*
Arnica ointment or oil	*Lymphomyosot* (by BHI-Heel)
Belladonna	*Nat Carb*
Bellis	*Nat Sulph*
Bryonia	*Rhus Tox*
Calendula Oil	*Ruta Grav*
Calendula tincture	*Sulphuric Acid*
Cantharis	*Symphytum* ointment or oil
Carbolic Acid	*Traumeel* (by BHI-Heel)
Causticum	*Traumeel* ointment
Glonoine	*Urtica urens*
Hepar Sulph	

Doses and Potencies

A rule of thumb in homeopathy is that *the more acute the problem, the higher the potency you should use.* However, in first aid, use whatever potency you have on hand (6, 12, 15, or 30).

In a *severe* injury, you may use *Arnica* or another remedy every 15 to 30 minutes, until medical help arrives or there is marked improvement. In most cases, use the remedies every 4 hours until better.

Shock

Physical or emotional shock to system from accident, fall or injury:

Arnica: The first remedy to use in any trauma. Use any potency on hand or prescription-strength 200c or 1M every hour for 4 hours until noticeably better (up to 24 hours). In severe cases, *Arnica* may be used every 15 minutes. It should be taken as soon as possible after a traumatic or exhaustive event, *especially* by those people who may act confused or refuse to be touched. Typically, an injured person in shock may say that nothing is wrong—"I'm ok." Or "I'm fine, just leave me alone," while staggering around. *Arnica* is helpful in *all* forms of shock to the system such as: running a marathon, fatigue, jet lag, or weakness from infection (flu). Take it for head injuries or if you continue to feel poorly following a head injury.

Pain, Bruising and Swelling

Select one of the following remedies. Take in doses of 6, 12, 30 or 200 once every 4 hours for 24 hours:

Arnica: This is the first remedy to use for any injury. Symptoms to look for are: feels very sore, achy or bruised; with shock symptoms (dazed, cold, fainting, confused); bleeding; can't stand being touched; better lying down with head low, feet up; generally feels better warm; may feel better using cold compress on injury; for *severe* pain or injury, take every 15 minutes until the discomfort subsides.

Sulphuric Acid if: *Arnica* was given first and did not produce results within 1 to 4 hours; the injury is black and blue and very sore; feeling very hurried with rushing around accomplishing nothing (aimless hurriedness); feels cold and chilly, and doesn't want cold packs or ice.

Bellis if: *Arnica* was given first and did not produce results in 1 to 4 hours; there is bruising with deep, intense pain; injury feels much worse with cold and much better with heat; cannot bear to be touched.

Traumeel (a combinational remedy made by BHI): This remedy contains *Arnica, Calendula, Symphytum, Bellis,* and a few other ingredients which is synergistically formulated for trauma, strains, sprains, bruises, pain, inflammation and swelling. It's used in a pill form internally or externally in a cream for acute problems. Take every hour; after 24 hours, take one three times a day until better.

Hypericum: Take orally for pain if the injury is to nerves or parts rich with nerves; *Hypericum* is the *Arnica* of the nerves; for fingers or toes smashed in a door; sharp, nerve pain; for a fall on the tailbone.

Bryonia if: There is a slow onset of injury (such as a sprained ankle that swells after two to four hours); if you cannot move (or bear to move) the injured part; cannot bear to have injury touched; pressure makes injury feel better; very irritable; better if left alone; injured area is red hot; injury feels better with ice pack; along with above indicators, you also tend to gulp down cold fluids.

Ledum if: There is a slow onset of injury (such as a sprained ankle that gets worse in a few hours after the incident); injury feels cool to the touch; injury feels better with a cold pack; injured part is black and blue; for a black eye or bruise; for a bruise that doesn't go away.

Ruta Grav: For bruised shins, sprained ankles, and bursitis; for stiffness in joints that gets better with motion, but if too much activity joints feel worse; feels worse in the cold and damp; better warm.

Rhus Tox: For plantar fasciitis; tendinitis; stiffness that hurts when you first move; if motion makes stiffness better; if feels like a "rusty gate"; feels worse in the cold and is much better warm.

To Cleanse Wounds:

Calendula tincture: After cleaning a wound with hydrogen peroxide and betadine, you may use a solution of *Calendula tincture* diluted in water until it doesn't sting the skin. Soak sterile gauze in solution and apply directly to wound, covering with saran wrap. Change the dressing every 2 to 6 hours (moisten gauze with solution first so you don't pull off skin). Continue to expose to air so scab can form at night.

Calendula oil, ointment or cream is also very soothing.

For Painful Wounds:

Compresses can be made by soaking with tinctures of some remedies. Add a few drops of tincture to clean water to make a lotion for soaking compresses. Use moist compresses as described for *Calendula.*

Arnica: Don't use topically on open wounds. It may cause pain.

Hypericum: Take orally for pain. *Hypericum* is the *Arnica* of the nerves. For fingers or toes smashed in a door; sharp, nerve pain; can also be used topically in a tincture or lotion (tincture mixed with clean water).

Hepar Sulph: For painful abrasions or "raspberries"; take orally or make a tincture.

Ledum: Use a tincture; if the injured part is cool and feels better when cool.

Urtica urens tincture: For first-degree burns; for sunburn; for stinging pain.

Healing Ointment

To keep ointment in place on an injury during healing, cover with gauze and then apply a piece of saran wrap. Change about four times a day. If gauze sticks to the wound, moisten with peroxide to ease the removal.

Symphytum ointment: Promotes healing of abrasions and scrapes.

Arnica ointment or oil: Helps with inflammation and soreness of muscles; not for use on open or raw wounds.

Traumeel ointment same as above.

Calendula oil: Retards growth of bacteria; excellent for all wounds and lacerations; apply tincture to dressing; change dressing four times a day.

For Bee Stings

Take one of the remedies below:

Apis—6, 12, or 30 (use as high a potency as you can) once every hour until better if: bite is red hot and swollen; burning heat; bite or wound feels better with cold pack and aggravated by heat or warm applications; no thirst; there is a sudden, severe onset of allergic reaction.

Carbolic acid if: Shock reaction with terrible swelling and pain; for severe reaction to a sting that happens within 5 minutes.

Ledum—any dose available once every hour until better. For bee stings where the skin feels cool, and injury feels better with a cold pack.

Beyond First Aid for Head Injury

If someone has had a serious trauma, particularly if struck on the head, give *Arnica* immediately. The person is usually dazed or confused. Observe his state carefully; note if the personality seems to change. A fall or blow may also injure internal organs as indicated by increased pulse rate, pale skin, and increasing shock. If one pupil is dilated more than the other, go to an emergency room immediately.

Even though the patient may be responding to the homeopathic remedy, he should see a doctor or go to an emergency room as the remedy may wear off, causing him to go into shock. The injured person should be observed by a professional, and have someone nearby to call if the problem returns.

For Headache Following an Injury

Arnica: After head injury.

Nat Sulph if: *Arnica* doesn't work; for chronic headaches since head injury; may also be asthmatic; all symptoms are worse with damp.

Swelling after Injury

Lymphomyosot in either liquid or pills: 10 drops or one pill every hour for the first 6 to 8 hours, then three times a day until better; for edema or lymphatic obstruction; take every hour for a severe injury; then, after 6 doses, take it three times a day.

Arnica for swelling.

Puncture Wounds

Check tetanus vaccination; tetanus toxoid should be repeated every ten years. Go to an emergency room, if you haven't had a tetanus shot in the last ten years. Always allow a puncture wound to bleed freely to flush out dirt and germs. Clean with hydrogen peroxide, then take:

Ledum—highest dose available once every hour until better: for puncture wounds, take *Ledum* immediately; for bites or wounds that feels cool; better with cold pack.

Sunstroke, Heat Exhaustion

Signs of heat exhaustion: A muscle cramp in the leg or backside may be the first sign of a heat problem. Other signs are nausea, vomiting, dizziness and fainting. Continuing to run with any of these symptoms may lead to a stroke as the body's regulators are no longer able to cope. If the core temperature rises more than 2 C, permanent physical or mental damage can occur. Expert medical help must immediately be given in cases of heat exhaustion or stroke.

First aid for heat exhaustion:
- drink water or fluids immediately
- lie down
- cover with blankets if cold and clammy
- call paramedics or doctor
- take a dose of homeopathic *Arnica* every fifteen minutes; or *Glonium* or *Nat Carb*

>*Nat Carb:* Best remedy for sunstroke and heat exhaustion; *always thirsty;* nervous exhaustion; over-sensitive to light and noise; worse extreme cold; the typical person is usually a quiet type.

>*Glonoine:* Any sun on the head feels worse; worse heat; *no thirst;* dry mouth; cold extremities; hot, flushed head; better open air.

>*Belladonna:* Hot head; cold feet or legs; sudden onset from exposure to the sun; violent response; dilated pupils.

Burns and Sunburn

>*Urtica Urens* for: First degree burn; use a topical tincture; also good for hives (it's milder than *Apis)*.

>*Causticum* for: Second degree burn.

>*Cantharis* for: Third degree burn, or acid burn.

>*Hypericum* tincture: As a dressing over burns for pain.

>*Calendula* tincture: As a dressing over burns to promote healing (skin growth).

Drowning

Perform the Heimlich maneuver if possible on the drowning victim to evacuate water from the lungs. Wipe out the person's mouth to clear the passageway and begin artificial respiration. If the heart has stopped beating, give cardiopulmonary resuscitation (CPR).

Keep giving aid until help arrives. As soon as possible, give the

---

What To Do For Minor Burns

1. Give *Arnica* immediately for shock.
2. Pour *Hypericum* lotion over the burn. Prepare from *Hypericum* tincture—one-half teaspoon to one cup of clean water.
3. Give *Cantharis* orally every 10 to 15 minutes as needed to relieve pain and promote healing. Repeat whenever pain returns.

---

person *Antimonium Tartaricum* every 10 to 15 minutes. Do not put tablets directly into the mouth of an unconscious person. Instead soften two tablets in one-quarter teaspoon of water and place under the tongue where the mucous membranes can absorb the remedy. If the membranes are very dry, moisten with a little water with your finger.

Conventional First Aid to Have on Hand

Aspirin
Antiseptic solutions: Betadine and hydrogen peroxide
Surgical tape
Gauze
Ace bandages

Homeopathic First Aid for Travel

If you plan to travel to a competitive event such as a marathon or game, consider taking homeopathic remedies along in case you encounter a problem where medical attention may not be readily available. I suggest the following basic kit of remedies below. Add other ones if you have tendencies for chronic reactions to indigestion, diarrhea, cramps, anxiety, premenstrual tension, cystitis, headaches, or other common ailments. Ready-made travel kits are available by mail order or at your local homeopathic pharmacy.

Aconite for colds, flu, panic; fear of flying.
Apis for bee stings, puncture wounds or allergic reactions.
Arnica for shock, trauma; pain; bruising; sudden onset; jet lag.
Arsenicum Alb. and *Veratrum Alb.* for *turista* and diarrhea.
Belladonna for acute sunstroke.

135

Calendula tincture for scrapes and wounds.

Ferrum Phosphoricum for indefinite flu-like symptoms.

Glonoine for sunstroke with headache, or *Nat Carb* for chronic sunstroke.

Ipecac for nausea or vomiting.

Rhus Tox for muscle soreness and stiffness; sprains and strains; tendinitis; plantar fasciitis.

Nux Vomica for constipation; for overeating or over-consumption of alcohol.

Cocculus for travel sickness.

Cantharis for cystitis with terrible burning.

Staphysagria for cuts and lacerations; cystitis with cramping and burning.

Bryonia for headaches.

Gelsemium for headaches; jet lag; flu; fatigue.

Lycopodium for gas and stomach problems.

Taping Instructions

Taping and strapping is a valuable form of external support for an injured toe, foot, ankle, or knee. Taping can be used as a flexible cast to limit motion and to protect a healing area. Even though a taping job may lose 70 percent of its strength after 20 minutes of vigorous activity, it's still a good idea to wear the tape. Professional athletes are usually required to keep an injury taped, and may be fined if they practice or play without it.

Knowing how to tape and what to tape requires skill and experience. Taping can be used to support a weak arch (Fig. 7-2 and 7-3), to provide stability for a pronating foot, and to provide support for weakened muscles, tendons and ligaments. Taping can also protect vulnerable joints.

In addition to providing strength and support, taping also increases the sense of balance (proprioception). The skin under the tape conveys information to the brain more quickly—increasing the ability to respond to uneven terrain or sudden changes of direction. Tape on an injured part tends to heighten awareness of the injury—increasing the sense of protection to that area.

The classic foot taping to support the arch of the foot is called "low-dye" taping (named after Dr. Ralph Dye). Fig. 7-3 shows the three steps in taping the foot around the outside to stabilize a weak

7-2. Classic Low-dye Strapping
Used for: plantar fasciitis (pain on bottom of foot), heel-spur syndrome, flexible flat foot, pain in forefoot due to excessive rearfoot motion.

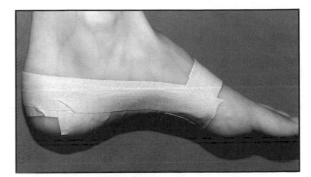

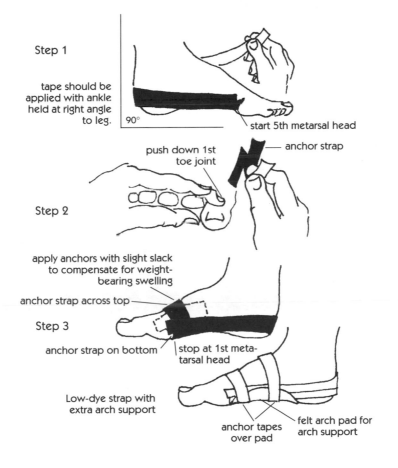

Step 1

tape should be applied with ankle held at right angle to leg.

90°

start 5th metarsal head

push down 1st toe joint

anchor strap

Step 2

apply anchors with slight slack to compensate for weight-bearing swelling

anchor strap across top

Step 3

anchor strap on bottom

stop at 1st meta-tarsal head

Low-dye strap with extra arch support

anchor tapes over pad

felt arch pad for arch support

7-3. How to Wrap a Low-dye Strap

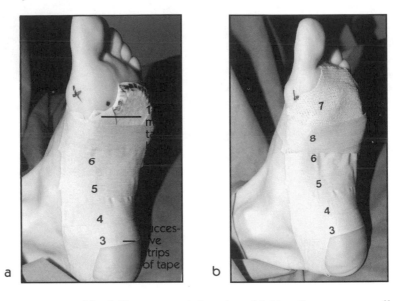

7-4. a) Metatarsal Pad. Shows a metatarsal pad taking the pressure off the 1st and 5th metatarsal heads with a low-dye strap for arch support.
b) Shows completed taping over metatarsal pad.

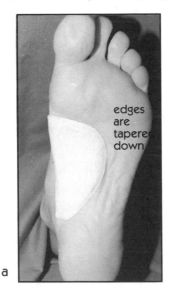 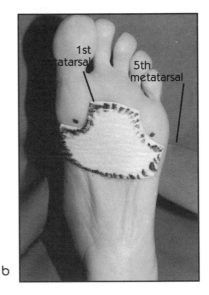

7-5. a) Arch Pad. Shows how arch pad goes on before low-dye strapping for increased arch support.
b) Metatarsal pad on the middle of foot helps keep pressure off 1st and 5th bones of foot

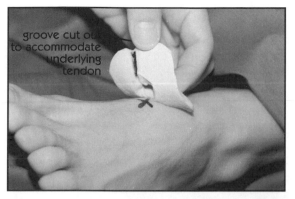

c) Shows a doughnut pad cut to fit over a "skier's bump."

or flat foot. Use ½" strips of tape length-wise and across the arch of the foot. If more arch support is needed, ¼" arch pads can be used for more support (see Figs. 7-3 and 7-5a).

Low-dye strapping is particularly help-ful for pain on the bottom of the foot (plantar fasciitis) or for heel spur syn-drome. For a painful heel spur on the bot-tom of the foot, add a foam pad or piece of felt with a hole cut out to accommo-date the spur and redistribute weight a-way from the painful point (see Fig. 7-5d) Low-dye taping can also be helpful for shin-splint syndrome when you're running fast on a track, as the extra support de-creases the foot's tendency to roll inward too far (excessive pronation).

Toe injuries can be taped to prevent motion which may interfere with healing. A piece of tape can be woven between the toes, using adjacent toes as natural

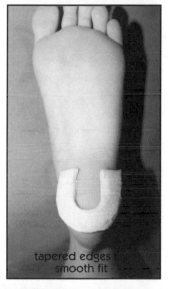

d) Shows a horseshoe pad cut out of 1/4" felt to take the pressure off the bottom of the heel (heel spur syndrome).

splints to prevent motion (see Fig. 7-6a, b, and c). A fracture or strain of the big toe also benefits from taping; however, I suggest you let your podiatrist show you how to tape the toe the first time.

For metatarsalgia (pain on the ball of the foot), felt pads may be cut to fit between the bones of the big and little toes (1st and 5th metatarsals) to redistribute weight evenly across the bottom of the

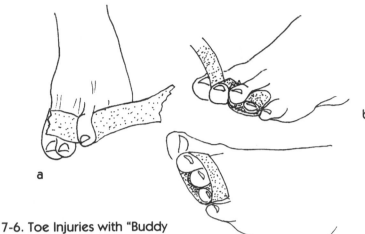

7-6. Toe Injuries with "Buddy Taping." Sprains, bruises, dislocations and fractures may be protected by "buddy taping" the affected toe to the next digit.

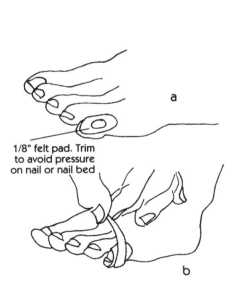

1/8" felt pad. Trim to avoid pressure on nail or nail bed

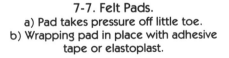

7-7. Felt Pads.
a) Pad takes pressure off little toe.
b) Wrapping pad in place with adhesive tape or elastoplast.

foot (see Fig. 7-4a, b and 7-5b). For bumps on the foot or heel, doughnut pads can be cut from felt and applied over the bump (see Fig. 7-5c). Note: When cutting a piece of felt or foam to fit over a bump, taper the edges down to fit more closely to the skin; they will be less likely to be pulled off and will fit in a shoe more easily. Make the size of the hole about ⅛" bigger than the bump.

Small corn pads (with no corn medicine on them) can be bought at the drugstore to place over hard corns to relieve pressure on the toe. Corn pads can be taped on (see Fig. 7-7a,b).

140

Fig. 7-8 shows a classic ankle strapping sometimes called a "basket strap."

Support and protection is also achieved by using padding. For example, you often see football players with foam taped to elbows or wrists during a game. Felt (with or without adhesive backing) or various thicknesses of foam are the usual types of padding used with taping. Adhesive moleskin is very useful since it adapts to shaping so well and is quickly applied. A great variety of products arc used to accommodate an injury or painful area including lamb's wool, moldable podiatry compound, tube gauze with silicone gel, and Spenco Second Skin.

By the way, adhesive tape stays fresh if kept in the refrigerator. It deteriorates in hot placcs (like the trunk of your car). Before applying tape, it's very important to wash the skin with soap and water and wipe with rubbing alcohol. This cleanses the skin of dirt and body oil. Taping around the circumference (e.g., around the top and bottom of the foot) should not be pulled tight. Keeping a bit of slack in the tape allows for the natural

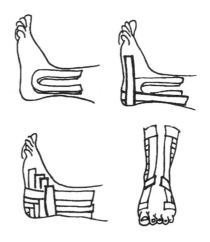

7-8. Ankle Strapping.

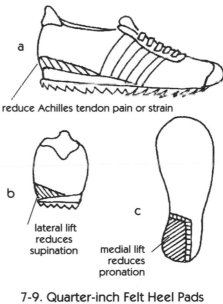

a

reduce Achilles tendon pain or strain

b

lateral lift
reduces
supination

c

medial lift
reduces
pronation

7-9. Quarter-inch Felt Heel Pads
Inside Shoe Used to:
a) reduce tension on Achilles tendon
b) reduce supination
c) reduce pronation

141

swelling that happens in weight-bearing. If you are taping over a bony prominence like the outside ankle bone, use some padding on the area to prevent injuring the underlying skin, nerves or tendons by cutting or compressing them.

Felt can be inserted into the shoe as a wedge to help correct over-pronation or excessive supination (see Figs. 7-9b, c). A ¼" heel pad put in the heel of a running shoe will also ease tension on a short, tight Achilles tendon (see Fig. 7-9a).

Taping and padding is a skill that takes experience to get right. However, you may try to tape and pad any minor strains, painful bumps, bunions, or irritated spots yourself. If your own taping and padding doesn't give you the relief you need, see a podiatrist or certified athletic trainer who can teach you how to do your own taping. Remember, if taping helps an arch problem or a tendency to over-pronate or supinate, then you can be sure that a permanent orthotic will also help.

Chapter 8

FOOT INJURIES

Something has licked my heel
like a surgeon
And I have a problem with
My right foot and my life.
    —James Dickey, Snakebite (1967)

Structure and Function

Your magnificent foot has twenty-eight bones, three arches, various muscles and ligaments, and a tendon named after Achilles, the greatest of Greek warriors. Your feet take you virtually anywhere. When your feet hurt, all is definitely not right with the world. Figure 8-1 shows the bones of the foot.

Your foot functions both as an adaptable and rigid structure as it moves in walking and running. *Arches* support you in an upright position, as well as disperse shock when you land on your feet (Fig. 8-2). The arch starting from your heel and stretching to your big toe, in the inside of the foot, is the *medial* arch (the arch you usually buy an arch support for when you have "flat" feet). On the outside of your foot is the *lateral arch,* stretching from the heel to the little toe, lying flatter, closer to the ground than the medial. In the ball of your foot is the *transverse* arch. Arch and heel injuries are usually caused by the same factors—too much motion (pronation or rolling inward) and too much impact shock.

Ligaments bind the foot bones together, and two are most important. The plantar ligament extends from the heel bone to the bases of the midfoot and the metatarsal bones. It helps to support the midfoot and lateral arch. The spring ligament, extending from the heel to the navicular, is very important because it helps to support the whole inside

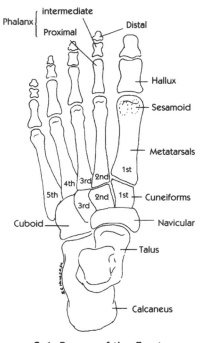

8-1. Bones of the Foot
(same as Fig. 2-2a)

arch. *Muscles* lie under and over the foot and extend down to the foot from the calf in order to move the foot and toes. The *plantar fascia,* a strong band of tissue, underlies your foot all the way from the heel to the base of the toes.

Stress Fractures of Foot Bones

There is a saying in sports medicine: "If you think it's a stress fracture, it's a stress fracture until proven otherwise." Stress fractures are microscopic cracks in the bones caused by the buildup of small amounts of stress that never get a chance to heal. Imagine bending a coat hanger back and forth. Repeated bending weakens the wire, eventually breaking it.

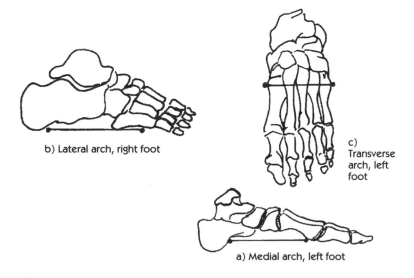

b) Lateral arch, right foot

c) Transverse arch, left foot

a) Medial arch, left foot

8-2. Arches of the Foot

A bone in your leg or foot, similarly weakened by repeated stress, is liable to bend and snap just like the coat hanger. As with invisible metal fatigue, stress fractures set the stage for a complete break, but may not even show up on an x-ray until weeks later. The only sure diagnosis will be a bone scan.

A stress fracture is almost always preventable. Think about it. You are the one who decides to climb the mountain, run the race, cycle through the desert. The body does not, on its own, arise in the morning and pound out a 12-mile run relentlessly five days a week. There has to be a decision by you to train, or, in the case of stress fractures, over-train. Achievements in athletics are so often equated in our minds with Discipline—and lots of it. So, we push the body. Self-discipline certainly is an asset as long as it includes rest and varied activity, so that the body can adjust to the demands we make. Fatigued muscles (such as tired legs at the end of a race) simply are not able to absorb shock. Fatigue creates the fertile ground for stress fractures to occur.

Since stress fractures result from over-use, pain may begin after an *increase* in your activities. The pain of a stress fracture usually begins with a slight tenderness around a bone. On the heel, a stress fracture hurts when pressed on either side of the heel. With repeated exercise, especially on hard surfaces, the pain increases. One way to differentiate a stress fracture from a strain or sprain is to put a tuning fork over the area of the suspected stress fracture. The tuning fork will cause the bone to vibrate producing pain. Another trick is to use Ultrasound which causes heat to come to the bone. If Ultrasound causes pain in the bone after a half hour, then you know you have a stress fracture. If Ultrasound seems to improve the injury, you probably have a sprain, strain or tendinitis. If your injury is a strain or sprain, there will be no pain from Ultrasound.

If you continue to run or exercise through the pain of a stress fracture, you risk breaking the bone completely. Bone injuries take four to six weeks to heal. See a doctor—preferably a sports medicine specialist—at the onset of the pain so that you can be treated with a cast, if necessary, or homeopathic medicines and physical therapy.

Healing stress fractures of the foot

Rest from high-impact activity such as running, aerobics, football, etc. Switch to a low-impact aerobic activity, such as swimming and cycling, and conditioning exercises such as yoga.

Correct any biomechanical abnormalities (e.g. foot imbalances, excessive pronation or supination, leg length discrepancies) with orthoses or rehabilitation therapy.

Select one of the following homeopathic Stage One remedies (during the first 24 hours), for pain, bruising swelling. Take in potencies 6, 12, 15 or 30 four times a day until better.

Arnica if bruising pain; better warm, but cold pack may numb injury and lessen pain and swelling; very sensitive to touch; worse with motion.

Bellis if more pain and deeper bruising than with *Arnica*; heating pad feels better than a cold pack; no tolerance whatsoever for cold.

Sulphuric Acid if *Arnica* doesn't work within six hours; *Bryonia* if you cannot move the injured foot or bear to have it touched, but pressure makes it feel better; better from cold pack.

Ledum if the foot feels cool to the touch (can be warm) and feels better with cold pack;

Lymphomyosot if very swollen; ten drops twice a day.

Traumeel, a combination remedy for initial pain and trauma after straining the foot.

Stage Two remedies (take 48 hours to a week after initial diagnosis). Take in potencies of 6, 12, 15, 30 or 200 once a day for three to four days or until better,

Rhus Tox if worse initial motion—stiff and sore first thing in the morning or after rest; better with continued movement; better with massage, motion, or yoga stretching; worse with cold pack; better with warmth; restlessness, continually trying to get comfortable; sore from lifting something heavy or exercising the day before.

Ruta Grav if better with rest, yet restless with an urge to move to get comfortable; stiff, sore, bruised and achy; better with heat; feel moody, fretful or despairing about the injury; weak, tired and cranky after lots of activity or movement.

Bryonia if slow onset of injury; can't bear to move the injured foot or to have it touched; pressure makes it feel better. Very irritable; injury is red hot; better with ice pack.

Ledum if slow onset of injury; feels cool to the touch (although may also be warm); better with a cold pack; injured part is black and blue.

Lymphomyosot 10 drops three times a day, or one pill three times a day, if very swollen (10 drops an hour until swelling subsides; then go to 10 drops three times a day.

Stage Three remedies (reparative phase—after two weeks, until healed):

> *Symphytum,* 30 four times a day for two weeks; or a single dose of 1M for bone healing. Then either
>
> *Calcarea Fluorica,* single 1M dose, after *Symphytum* or:
>
> *Calcarea Phosphorica,* single 1M dose for injury to ligaments and bones (see p. 223 for details).

During recovery from a stress fracture the doctor may put you in a soft or hard cast (or pad the injured area) if there is pain on walking. Choose a *firm-soled* shoe if not in a cast to prevent toe-off or pressure on metatarsal heads. Don't run for six weeks. Keep in shape on a stationary bicycle, a Nautilus machine or by swimming. For physical therapy, use electrical stimulation which *may* speed up bone healing and *will* decrease pain. Don't use Ultrasound therapy as this increases the blood flow to the area that's already inflamed and causes pain.

On the advice of your doctor, you can resume running after six weeks. Start with 5 minutes of running and 5 minutes of walking. Try three sets—a 30-minute workout. In a couple of days, increase to 10 minutes running, 10 minutes walking, three sets. After a week or so, increase the alternating sequence to 15 minutes until you build up gradually to your former pace.

Run on grass or soft surfaces. Check the cushioning of your shoes. Make sure your shoes are not compressed in the midsole.

Stop immediately if pain recurs.

Pain on Top of Foot (Stress Fracture of the Metatarsal)

The metatarsal (generally, the second or third metatarsal) is the most likely bone in the foot to get a stress fracture (Fig. 8-1). Pain, redness or swelling on the top of the foot, especially with excruciating pain when the bone is pressed, is a good indicator of this injury. There will be a small crack in the bone about an inch behind the joint where the toe meets the ball of the foot. X-rays may not show a crack in the bone for three to six weeks, but a bone scan will. X-rays, because they show the *healing* of a stress fracture only, generally lag behind what's actually present in bone by at least three weeks.

To treat a stress fracture of the metatarsal, see your doctor. Follow homeopathic treatment in the previous section for all stress fractures, and be sure to walk in *firm-soled* shoes, if you are not in a cast.

Pain Under the Bone Attached to the Big Toe (Sesamoid Stress Fractures)

If you have begun doing more activities on the ball of your foot lately, (e.g., increasing mileage, hill work, speed work or high-impact jumping sports), then you may have damaged the two little pea-like bones under your first metatarsal head. Even dancing or shopping in high-heeled shoes can damage these small bones.

If you feel an exquisite pain when you press hard on the joint under the big toe, then you have either bruised the bones, broken them, or have a fluid-filled sac there (bursa).

Functionally, sesamoid bones (see Fig. 8-3) work the same way as the knee-cap (patella) works. Both the patella and sesamoids increase the mechanical efficiency of the joints. They are not vestigial, useless little bones as is thought by doctors not familiar with the bio-mechanics of the foot. The main function of the metatarsal joint can be ruined if sesamoids are removed. Therefore it is very important to get the opinion of a second doctor if

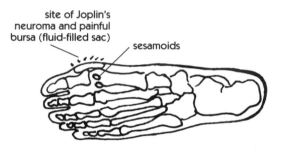

site of Joplin's neuroma and painful bursa (fluid-filled sac)

sesamoids

8-3. Sesamoid bones on bottom of foot are injured by too much running (or pressure) on ball of foot. Pain may also come from inflamed nerve or fluid-filled sac (bursa).

you're considering surgical removal of the sesamoids. For all sesamoid problems, the treatment will be the same.

If you think you have a sesamoid stress fracture, don't take medicine or get injections until you have a correct diagnosis with a bone scan or MRI (magnetic resonance imaging). Rest from all painful activity. Follow above treatment recommendations for general stress fractures. Do not allow the area to be injected with cortisone as this can mask the injury when using the foot, incurring more damage and slowing healing. If your sesamoids will not heal properly, you may have to resort to surgery, including bone graft, and/or partial or complete removal of the sesamoid. Again, surgery is only a last resort, as sesamoids should never be removed without good reason and a second opinion.

In the future, you can prevent the sesamoid problems by not running long distances on the ball of the foot, especially if your foot is bony, and the sesamoids already stick out too far on the bottom of the foot. It helps to wear shoes that are wide enough to distribute your weight more evenly on the ball of the foot.

Once you start running again, make a U-shaped pad out of felt, foam rubber, Spenco or Viscolas to apply right behind the first metatarsal head. Tape this to the foot and feel the comfort! Use two pads if necessary. Eventually, you can glue the pads into your running shoes and your regular shoes.

You can also have a rocker bar put onto the sole of your running shoe by an orthopedic shoe shop to relieve pressure on the sesamoids (Fig. 8-4). Have your shoemaker put a hard piece of 1/8" thick Neoprene on the *sole* right behind the widest part of shoe. The rubber piece should go clear across the sole, and taper at the front and back to create a smooth transition to the sole. This "rocker bar" helps your foot rock forward, taking the pressure off the ball of the foot and the big toe.

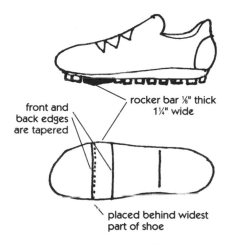

Women should not wear high heels if they have sesamoid pain. If the pain doesn't go away, you may need an orthotic.

8-4. A rocker bar of hard rubber applied to sole of shoe relieves pressure on sesamoids and ball of foot.

Case History of a False Sesamoid Problem

Holly, a twenty-seven-year-old pro golfer was on the women's golf tour when she started having pain and numbness under the ball of her big toe. Before she came to see me, she had been to several doctors and had had two surgeries for what had been diagnosed as tibial sesamoiditis. In the first surgery, the doctors removed her tibial sesamoid bone, but the pain had continued. In the second surgery, she was operated on for tarsal tunnel syndrome (a problem in the ankle which was thought to be causing the pain in the ball of the foot). Still the pain continued.

When she came to see me, I evaluated her and decided she had a bursa (painful fluid-filled sac) and Joplin's neuroma (inflamed nerve in the ball of the foot). See Fig. 8-5. First, I tried injection therapy into the painful area with homeopathic remedies. When these injections brought no relief, I injected again, adding cortisone. Nothing worked.

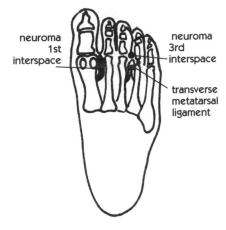

8-5. Sites of Inflamed Nerves Between Toe Bones (interdigital neuromas).

I then operated and found that she, indeed, did have a huge bursa, as I had suspected, which was so gristly that the injections had not been able to disperse the tissue. There was also a large, inflamed Joplin's neuroma. Taking out the bursa and the neuroma completely cured her.

Holly's case illustrates a very common mistake made by well-meaning doctors who tell countless patients that their sesamoids have to come out when there may be another problem, such as a bursa or Joplin's neuroma. In this case, the doctors weren't looking for a bursa; they assumed it was the sesamoid, and so they focused on the bone. To be fair, not much has been written in medical journals on Joplin's neuroma and bursas in the ball of the foot.

Another cause of pain in the ball of the foot besides inflamed bursas and neuromas is tendinitis in the small flexor tendon attaching to the foot bones. Tendinitis can be treated with homeopathic injections. Therefore, if your doctor tells you that you must have your sesamoids removed, *get a second opinion before having surgery.*

Pain in Mid-Foot (Stress Fracture of the Navicular)

See Fig. 8-1 to locate the site of this pain in the navicular bone. Refer to general treatment for stress fractures.

Injuries To Soft Tissues— Including Sprains and Strains

Pain on Top of the Foot in Front of the Instep (Midtarsal Joint Sprain)

You've just stepped into a pot-hole and twisted your ankle, or, jumping to dunk your basketball through the hoop, you've come down on another player's foot, twisting your ankle. Actually, you might think you sprained your ankle, but it's probably your foot that is really hurt (Fig. 8-6). Almost immediately there is swelling and pain, especially when you walk on an irregular surface. Many of you will keep right on running or playing. Don't do it! The first 24 hours is the crucial time to begin treating this serious injury. If you want to get back to your sport as soon as possible, you must not aggravate this injury with further stress.

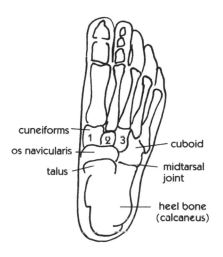

cuneiforms
os navicularis
talus
cuboid
midtarsal joint
heel bone (calcaneus)

8-6. Site of Pain in Front of the Instep (midtarsal joint sprain).

Call the doctor and rest from all painful activity. Apply an ice pack wrapped in towel, a refrigerated towel, or even a bag of frozen peas wrapped in a towel for 10 minutes three or four times a day. You can also use alternate hot and cold applications (contrast baths).

Elevate your foot higher than your hip or heart. Prop the leg on a pillow or soft chair. To minimize swelling, don't sit or stand with your foot on the floor. Keep the foot on pillows even in bed if you can sleep that way. Restrict movement. Apply an Ace bandage, extending from beneath toes to just below your knee. If the ankle is very swollen, use an inflatable splint. Elastic bandages allow swelling, which is more desirable than non-elastic. Your ankle may continue to swell, and too-tight bandages will cut off the circulation. Check your circulation every 15 minutes by squeezing your big toe and watching the redness return. If the toe remains white, loosen the bandages right away.

Use Stage One homeopathic remedies. For pain, bruising and swelling select one of the following remedies:

Arnica, Sulphuric Acid, Bellis, Bryonia, Ledum, or *Lymphomyosot* if very swollen. Ten drops three times a day, or one pill three times a day. To assist drainage, massage and immerse foot in contrast baths (alternate hot and icy cold). See details of remedies and doses in preceding section on stress fractures.

Your physician may inject homeopathic remedies into acupuncture points, joints, and ligaments to enhance and speed up healing. He or she may choose among *Traumeel* for trauma, *Zeel* (by BHI) for joint problems, *Rhus Tox* for pain with initial motion, and stiffness that improves with movement, *Ruta Grav* for stiffness and fatigue after movement, and *Lymphomyosot* for swelling.

Injections of insoluble cortisone are not advised as they can cause degeneration of tissue.

Hop or use a crutch—don't put weight on the foot. Don't try to drive; you won't be able to use the foot on the pedals. You may not be able to resume walking for three days up to two weeks, depending on the severity of the injury.

During your recovery from midtarsal joint sprain take Stage Two homeopathic remedies (24 hours to four to five days after injury). Select one:

Rhus Tox if you are worse on initial motion; stiff and sore first thing in the morning or after rest; better with continued movement; better with massage, motion, or yoga stretching; worse with cold pack; better with warmth; restlessness, continually trying to get comfortable; sore from lifting something heavy or exercising the day before. On the other hand,

Ruta Grav may be selected if the symptom complex resembles feeling better with rest; stiff, sore, bruised and achy; better with heat; feel moody, fretful or despairing about the injury; weak, tired and cranky after lots of activity or movement.

After taking one of these remedies follow with Stage Three remedies (reparative phase—from two weeks after injury until healed). First take *Symphytum* for initiating healing: take potency of 30 four times a day for two weeks or a single 1M dose (by prescription). Follow with: (see page 223 for details).

Calcarea Fluorica, one 1M dose following *Symphytum,* or

Calcarea Phosphorica, a single 1M once; for injury to ligaments and bones.

Whenever a ligament is torn, the balance organs (proprioceptors) are injured. Start flexing the foot up and down as soon as you can. An effective exercise to work all the joints, for instance, is to describe the alphabet (from A to Z) with the tip of the toes. Another good exercise is to pick up a towel or some marbles with your toes.

When you can bear weight on your foot, start to do balance exercises, and do them as part of your routine for at least six months. Any time you have hurt your foot or ankle, practice walking backwards and forwards, and to the right and left. Practice standing on both feet with your eyes closed, then on the injured foot with your eyes closed to re-establish communication with the nerves that provide balance.

On the advice of your doctor, you can resume running after six weeks. Start with 5 minutes of running and 5 minutes of walking. Try three sets—a 30-minute workout. In a couple of days, increase to 10 minutes running, 10 minutes walking, three sets. After a week or so, increase the alternating sequence to 15 minutes until you build up gradually to your former pace.

Run on grass or soft surfaces. Check the cushioning of your shoes. Make sure your shoes are not compressed in the midsole.

Stop immediately if pain recurs.

If the foot continues to swell in the evening, keep your leg elevated as often as possible during the day. Otherwise, stretch the leg out as you sit, moving the leg and foot frequently, pressing against the floor and flexing. This movement will increase circulation and drain the swelling.

Contrast baths help reduce swelling. Immerse the foot, alternately, in a pail each of hot water and icy cold water for 30 seconds at a time, unless you have a circulatory problem or if your skin is sore. Dip the foot until the skin becomes red. Contrast baths are helpful before starting simple foot exercises for therapy. Continued swelling, pain, or repeated sprains mean that you have a ruptured ligament and need to see your doctor. You may need an injection in or around the ligament to break up scar tissue.

If you repeatedly twist your ankle, have a shoemaker glue a piece of ¼" inch thick Neoprene or leather to the outer side of your running shoe (see Figure 8-7) to

8-7. Ankle Support:
to increase stability of shoe to decrease risk of ankle sprain have shoemaker apply 1/4" thick neoprene to outside of running shoes.

prevent twisting. This, however, could cause pronation problems, so be careful.

Pain on the Bottom of the Foot (Ligament Strain)

This injury may be the result of a sudden twist during a jump, or the result of running over and around rocks or holes in your path. Cutting-in maneuvers, such as twisting in soccer or basketball, can also strain ligaments. You may feel a sudden, slight tearing feeling. These strains also occur from repeated over-stretching, or after wearing ill-fitting shoes, especially shoes that are too flexible. Ligament pain can be quite intense, and may last for a period of months. Resting from painful activity is imperative. You may need an x-ray to rule out stress fracture.

For a ligament strain on the bottom of the foot, follow the same basic first-aid treatment in the section on midtarsal joint sprain and see your podiatrist. To prevent re-injury, use supportive strapping for three to four weeks. To waterproof for showering, wax the strapping or use plastic bags taped around your foot. See Chapter 7 on taping and strapping. Put underfoot supports in your shoes. Ask your doctor for specifics.

Do physical therapy three times a week, using an ice whirlpool with electro-galvanic stimulation. Begin exercise therapy (see Chapter 5 for exercises) on the advice of your doctor.

For homeopathic treatments, see above section on Stage One, Two, and Three homeopathic remedies.

Numbness or Pain from Instep to Toes (Tarsal Tunnel Syndrome)

During a run, your foot may swell. If you have tied your shoelaces very tightly, the pressure creates a numbing effect which is called tarsal tunnel syndrome. Another cause of numbness or pain may be an enlarged metatarsal bone that is under repeated pressure. The body responds to the pressure by creating a protective padding filled with fluid called a bursal sac (Fig. 8-8).

What to do for tarsal tunnel syndrome:

Tie shoes to allow for expansion, and if you have to, buy looser shoes. Change your lacing pattern.

To ease the pressure from the shoe, make a doughnut pad out of Spenco or felt to put on the sore spot on the instep.

One of the following homeopathic remedies given by your physician by injection may help:

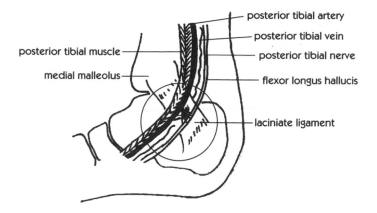

posterior tibial artery

posterior tibial vein

posterior tibial muscle

posterior tibial nerve

medial malleolus

flexor longus hallucis

laciniate ligament

8-8. Tarsal Tunnel Syndrome—a compression of nerves and vessels underneath the inner (medial) ankle bone.

Ruta Grav to reduce the jelly-like fluid of a bursal sac;
Rhus Tox if there is tendinitis; *Hypericum* if there is nerve inflammation (neuritis).

Pain on Top of Mid-foot (Extensor Tendinitis)

It is not uncommon to have inflammation along with pain on the top of the midfoot (extensor tendon). The lubricating sheaths which enclose the tendons cause the pain when the tendon is working. There may be a feeling of "grating" or "crackling." Check to make sure that the top of your shoe is not rubbing, or that your shoe laces are not too tightly tied.

Don't try to run through this pain. With rest, you may heal within two weeks. If your running shoes are unevenly worn down, you may need to be evaluated by a podiatrist. Foot orthotics could help with this problem. Try tying your shoes differently to change the pressure on the foot. Put a sponge rubber or Spenco pad under the tongue of your shoe.

Refrain from any foot exercises until pain subsides, and massage the top of the foot.

Select one of the following homeopathic remedies:
Arnica if sore, bruised, achy; ice feels good on pain.
Sulphuric Acid if *Arnica* has no effect in 6 hours.
Bellis if very deep bruising; very sore; if *Arnica* has no effect; *Rhus Tox* if leg hurts on initial motion; feels better with continued motion; much better with warm application; *Ruta Grav* if stiff and achy; worse with too much motion.

155

Pain on Outside of Foot between Ankle and Little Toe (Peroneal-Cuboid Joint Sprain)

You have damaged your cuboid joint by running along a banked or irregular surface. The cuboid joint, on the outside of the foot (see Fig. 8-6), is often sprained when the ankle joint is sprained. This injury happens if your foot turns inward too much when you run (functional high arch). Unfortunately, if you were wearing an arch support, this would have made matters worse. In the case of a functional high arch, your doctor would not have been able to diagnose your high arch unless you were running (for instance, on a treadmill in his office). If he did not observe your foot while running, it is likely that you were given an arch support which exacerbates the problem. A functional high arch requires an orthotic which holds the heel inverted, yet allows for a dropped first metatarsal. The Brooks kinetic wedge shoe is sometimes useful for this condition as are various foot orthotic modifications.

To treat this condition, rest from all painful activity after the injury. Ice for 10 minutes three or four times a day. When the injured part is numb from the ice, *gently* rotate foot in order to stimulate the lymphatic system to flush out tissue debris from bleeding and swelling.

Also try alternate hot and cold applications (contrast baths).

Keep your foot higher than your hip or heart. Prop the leg on a pillow or soft chair. To minimize swelling, don't sit or stand with your foot on the floor. Keep the leg on pillows even in bed if you can sleep that way.

Sprains become swollen in the beginning to restrict movement and prevent further damage. An external device to limit movement is the Ace bandage. Apply an Ace bandage, extending from beneath toes to just below your knee. If the foot is very swollen, use an inflatable air splint. Non-elastic bandages are not advisable (unless you know how to wrap them) because your foot may continue to swell, and a too-tight bandage will cut off the circulation. Check your circulation every 15 minutes by squeezing your big toe and watching the redness return. If the toe remains white, loosen the bandages right away.

During recovery from peroneal-cuboid joint strain, take the following homeopathic remedies in potencies of 6, 12, 15, or 30 four times a day:

Ruta Grav for pain and stiffness; take for two weeks or until pain and stiffness are gone. Then take:

Zinc (homeopathic) four times a day to strengthen ligaments, or *Calcarea Phosphorica,* single 1M dose after two weeks.

Case History of a Peroneal Strain with a Cuboid Misplacement

Paul Gartner is a forty-two-year-old car lot manager who is on his feet all day, walking miles around the lot. He came to me with a very painful heel spur syndrome for which I gave him *Rhus Tox* both orally and by injection. In addition, I made foot orthotics for his shoes, and recommended physiotherapy. Even with all this treatment, he didn't get much better.

After examining him again, I found that he was favoring the inside of his foot—which was sore—by walking on the outside of his foot. By walking like this, he had pushed the cuboid bone out of place. At first, when I tried to manipulate the cuboid back to the correct position, the tendon was in spasm and the cuboid wouldn't move. To relax the tendon, I gave him a trigger-point injection and then was able to put the cuboid back into place. I taped the foot to keep the cuboid in place, readjusted his orthotics, and he left with no pain at all. This story demonstrates how compensating for one problem can create another.

Pain Under the Ball of the Foot *Other Than* Sesamoiditis (Metatarsalgia)

Non-specific pain in the forefoot between the metatarsal heads is either a Morton's neuroma, or metatarsalgia. Metatarsalgia is an aching of the metatarsal bones or the joints where these long bones meet the toes. Morton's neuroma is a burning cramping pain between the metatarsal heads on the bottom of the foot. Metatarsalgia may be from an inflamed fluid-filled sac (bursitis) or from degenerated cartilage (arthritis). Morton's neuroma often has a fluctuating knife-like pain between two metatarsal heads. The nerve becomes impinged on the metatarsal heads and a large benign tumor is formed.

If you have pain on the ball of your foot, consider the following possibilities: bursitis, Morton's neuroma, sesamoiditis, Joplin's neuroma, or stress fracture of the metatarsal head.

What to do for various forms of metatarsalgia:

Bursitis. An inflammation with a fluid-filled sac (bursitis) on the metatarsal head can cause pain and puffiness.
  • Your physician can treat you with an injection of *Ruta Grav*, or cortisone. Anti-inflammatory medications may be helpful.

Morton's or Joplin's Neuroma. This is inflammation of a nerve with a benign nerve tumor between the metatarsal heads (Morton's neuroma), or at the bottom of the great toe where it meets the ball of the foot (Joplin's neuroma). These neuromas result from wearing tight fitting thin soled shoes, high heels, or tight sporting shoes such as ice skates or biking shoes.

- Treatment for burning shooting nerve pain going into toes, inject with *Hypericum* or *Ruta Grav.* Cortisone injections are a last resort, before surgery.
- In severe cases surgery may be necessary. Try orthotics and physical therapy first.

Maltracking of the Sesamoids. The little bones under the big toe (sesamoids) get pushed out of their grooves from anatomical deviations, such as bunions or displacement of the big toe (Hallus Valgus). When the sesamoids are outside of their normal tracks, these little bones grind away at the cartilage in the joint causing a great deal of damage as you walk. This leads to arthritis and is a serious ailment.

- Treat first with foot orthotics and good shoes—no pointed shoes or high-heels!
- Realign the big toe by taping away from the sesamoids.
- Physical therapy—ask your doctor.
- Rest from painful activities.
- Put a rocker bar on the sole of the shoe to relieve pressure. See Fig. 8-4.

Homeopathic oral remedies for maltracking of the sesamoids are either *Ruta Grav, Rhus Tox* or *Rhododendron,* followed by a single dose of *Calcarea Fluorica.*

Choose *Ruta Grav* if better with rest; tired and cranky with too much activity or movement; stiff, sore, bruised and achy; better with heat; worse with cold.

Choose *Rhus Tox* for stiffness; worse sitting; restlessness; if it feels better after moving around; worse with initial motion; much worse cold; better heat; if problem comes after becoming overheated and cooling off too suddenly.

Choose *Rhododendron* if pain is worse before a storm, but gets better after a storm.

Sesamoid Tendinitis. Pain in the ball of the foot can come from a problem with a tendon attaching to the sesamoid. Your physician may inject homeopathic remedies to treat inflamed tendons that attach to the sesamoids:

Rhus Tox if the tendon is stiff; *Ruta Grav* if the tendon is sore; *Zeel* or *Traumeel* if there is gristle.

Bunions: A bunion, through displacement of other parts of the foot (such as the sesamoids), can be a cause of pain under the ball of

158

the foot. In the case of bunions, if conservative (i.e., non-surgical) therapy fails, it is preferable to treat the bunion surgically in order to save the sesamoids.

Arthritis, a degeneration of cartilage over time, is another cause of pain under the ball of the foot which is the result of not taking care of some of the problems listed above. Have a lab test done to rule out a medical degeneration of cartilage (osteoarthritis). Refer to Chapter 17 for details of remedies for arthritis.

Pain and Swelling Where the Big Toe Meets the Foot or Within the Big Toe Itself (Turf Toe)

This injury is caused by over-bending the big toe upwards or downwards, or by tearing the ligaments in the toe joint. Over-stretching often occurs when playing sports on artificial turf. If not treated, turf toe can cause major problems in the joint such as arthritis.

To treat turf toe use an ice pack or hot compresses, whichever feels better. Rest the toe from painful activity. For pain, bruising and swelling take:

Arnica: potency of 6, 12, 15, 30; two to four pills every 4 hours for 24 hours. Injury usually feels better with a cold pack.

Bellis or *Traumeel,* if warm applications feel better; same dose.

Tape the big toe to stop motion. As long as you play on artificial turf, use a firm-soled shoe and fit your football shoe with a very firm plate on the bottom so your big toe will not bend.

During recovery from turf toe, take homeopathic remedies:

Ruta Grav; any potency four times a day for one week, then:

Calcarea Fluorica single dose 1M.

Swelling Where the Second Toe Meets the Ball of the Foot (Second Metatarsal Phalangeal Joint Sprain)

This sprain occurs when you run very fast and toe-off forcefully. During toe-off, the second metatarsal (usually the longest toe bone) joint is taking the most stress. Besides injury at toe-off, this pain may be caused by other forms of metatarsalgia listed below. Another name for this sprain is non-specific capsulitis (Fig. 8-9). The following conditions may be present.

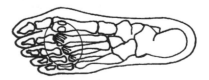

8-9. Inflamed Metatarsal Heads

1. **Bursitis**—pain with pressure, but not with motion under

under the second metatarsal head; this could mean a stone bruise.

2. **Neuroma**—burning and shooting pain between the second and third metatarsal is a nerve inflammation (neuroma).
3. **Arthritis**—pain with motion in the joint.
4. **Callus**—pain with direct pressure.
5. **Wart**—pain with movement side to side.

If you also have swelling on the *top* of the foot along with pain on the bottom, watch out for a stress fracture of the metatarsal.

To treat metatarsal joint sprain, follow the treatment recommendations in section on mid-tarsal joint sprain earlier in this chapter. Don't let this pain continue without treatment. If left untreated, the toe may become permanently bent (trigger toe). Don't use cortisone in this area, as it can damage the tendons and contribute to hammer toes.

Sudden Pain at the Arch (Middle of the Foot)—Rupture

You may be middle-aged or elderly, and experience this sudden tearing sensation while doing exercises, running or race-walking. If it hurts near the middle of the arch, you probably ruptured the plantar fascia (a long band of tissue under the foot), or the muscle (the abductor) under the plantar fascia. Usually the arch collapses if the rupture is not treated.

Another very serious problem is the over-stretching or rupture of the posterior tibial tendon. This is the tendon which holds up the arch. If you cannot raise up on the ball of the foot without assistance, you may have a rupture. If not treated, the whole foot will collapse, requiring surgery or braces. *This is a medical emergency requiring immediate attention.*

If you rupture an arch, call the doctor. Stay off the foot and discontinue all painful activity after the injury. Ice. If ice alone is not effective, another possible treatment is to alternate hot and cold applications (contrast baths). Keep your foot higher than your hip or heart. Prop the leg on a pillow or soft chair. To minimize swelling, don't sit or stand with your foot on the floor. Keep the leg on pillows even in bed if you can sleep that way. Wrap an Ace bandage around foot until you can get to the doctor's office.

Take Stage One remedies (first 24 hours):

Arnica for shock to system; two to four pills for up to 6 hours.

For pain, bruising and swelling take one of the following remedies. Take two to four pills of any potency every 4 hours for 24 hours.

Arnica if pain is reduced with ice or cold pack; if bruised, sore and achy.

Traumeel for same conditions as *Arnica.*

Bellis if heating pad feels better than a cold pack.

Sulphuric Acid, two to four pills every 4 hours if *Arnica* doesn't work within 2 hours.

Bryonia if you cannot move injured foot or bear to have it touched, but *pressure* makes it feel better.

Ledum if your foot feels cool to the touch (although it may also be warm) and much better with a cold pack.

Lymphomyosot if very swollen. Take 10 drops twice a day.

During recovery from arch rupture, take Stage Two remedies a week after initial diagnosis—6, 12, 30 or 200 once a day for three to four days or until better. Select either:

Rhus Tox if worse on initial movement; better with continued movement; stiff and sore first thing in the morning or after rest; better with massage, motion, or yoga stretching; worse with cold pack; better with warmth; restlessness, continually trying to get comfortable.

Ruta Grav if better with rest; stiff, sore, bruised and achy; better with heat; feel moody, fretful or despairing about the injury; weak, tired and cranky after lots of activity or movement.

Toes, Toenails, and Heels
Black Toenail (Subungual Hematoma)

Black toenails are caused by too short shoes, where toenails jam against the end of the shoe—especially when running downhill. The toenails are black because of a blocked-up hemorrhage under the nail. Most likely there is excruciating pain with this condition. It is important to take care of black toenail because, if you wait a week or two, the nail will start to come off. If the nail starts to crumble, clip it away to keep the area smooth so it doesn't catch on your socks.

If the nail is only black at the base, release the pent-up blood, and start the healing process. The procedure for doing this is actually painless and sounds worse than it feels, believe me!

Heat a paper clip till it's red hot and touch it to the nail, being very careful not to go too deeply. This will melt the nail and let the blood come out. Watch out! The blood usually spurts out quite far. Next soak your foot in hot water.

If the nail is black all the way to the end of the toe, and you are not diabetic or do not have circulatory problems, you can:

161

Slit the nail. Sterilize a sharp razor blade by boiling it for 15 minutes. Cool the blade and then make a small cut in the skin right under the toenail. Make a slit about ⅛" long. Again, this is painless because the skin in blistered and separated from nerve endings.

If the hole plugs up, repeat again after a few days.

Or, you can go to a podiatrist and he or she will drill through the nail, and drain the blood.

Choose one of the following homeopathic remedies:

Arsenicum Alb is the number one remedy; *Arnica* for bleeding under nail; *Bellis* if very painful bleeding under nail; *Graphites* if thick, black, rough; contracted toes.

Thick Toenail

Nails can be damaged by being stepped on. For example, your nail can be crushed by a horse stepping on your foot or by a 49'er fan at a football game! To keep the nail ground down and smooth, you'll have to go to a podiatrist every few months. If the nail is very disfigured, have it removed. Recovery will take several months or one to two years as toenails grow slowly.

Since thick toenails are a condition affected by diet and general health, a constitutional remedy may be advisable.

Select one of the homeopathic remedies:

Silica for corrugated (wavy lines) toe nails; *Thuja* for dry or corrugated nails; *Graphites* for deformed toes; *Calcarea Salts* for thick yellow nails; *Arsenicum; Fluoric Acid;* or *Sabadilla*.

Discolored or Crumbled Nail

This condition usually comes from a fungal infection or a combination of fungus and trauma. Select one of the homeopathic remedies for crumbled nails:

Silica; Graphites if crumbled nail has deformed toes; *Calcarea Salts* or *Antimonium Crudum* if brittle nails; grow out of shape; worse cold bathing.

For fungus, soak your feet in half a cup of white vinegar in a pan of water. In the office, I put little holes in the nails with a laser, and then apply a topical anti-fungal medicine.

Ingrown Toenail

Cut your nails straight across so they don't become ingrown at the corners. If they're already ingrown, file down not the top, but the surface near the ingrown side.

Silica is the number one remedy for ingrown toenails. Other homeopathic remedies which may help are:

Silica if ingrown nails are ulcerated or painful.

Nitric Acid if also ulcerated or painful; bleed easily; there is raw flesh; *Hypericum* if really painful nails; *Arsenicum* or *Graphites* for very hard nails. *Bellis* or *Sulphur* if there is pus around the nails or hangnails; *Thuja* if brittle, ingrown nails; with brown spots on hands; perspire; growths like warts. *Hepar Sulph, Rhus Tox, Nat Mur* for hang nails; dry, cracking skin; numbness and stinging; *Fluoric Acid* if splinter pain under the nail.

Psorium if filthy smell; very cold; infection around nails.

Graphites if crippled toes; brittle, sore; *Tucrium Marum* if pain in toenails growing into flesh; drainage from nail grooves; itching skin; worse in bed; *Lachesis* if unhealthy, red, raw sore flesh; worse with tight bandage; worse heat, better cold.

Corns on the Top and Sides of Toes

Hammer toes, those bent and clutched toes that have been stuffed into too-short shoes develop corns on the joints from constant pressure and friction. A corn is a protective hardening of skin that is painful when irritated.

For corns on the top of toes, wrap moleskin over the corns for temporary relief, but if they're very painful and hurt in all your shoes, see a podiatrist. You may need surgery to straighten the toes.

Corns between Toes

These corns probably will need to be trimmed out by a podiatrist. Wear cotton or sponge rubber between your toes.

If you have a bone spur, you'll need minor surgery. These corns and spurs are usually caused by high-heel shoes.

Soft Corns between Toes

Generally a result of tight shoes, soft corns are softened by sweat— hence the name. I don't recommend using corn drops or trying to cut corns off yourself with a razor.

One of the following homeopathic remedies may be useful:

Silica if there is perspiration, smelliness, rawness; *Baryta Carbonicum* for very raw, athlete's foot-like cracks; *Nat Mur* for violent itching; or *Zinc*.

163

Cracks on Heels—Fissures

Deep cracks on the heels called fissures are often accompanied by a callus. Runners usually get these cracks on the heels in dry, cold weather as a result of too-dry skin. It's helpful to rub hand cream into the heels often. Homeopathic remedies which may help are:

Calendula lotion for dry skin in general.

Lycopodium if one foot is hot, one foot cold.

Petroleum for big, deep fissures; thick skin.

Graphites for cracks with oozing discharge; unhealthy skin;
Rhus Tox for cracks worse with cold; stiff feet.

Calluses and Keratomas (very thick callus)

A very thick callus may be trimmed and treated by a podiatrist. You can continue to smooth down the area yourself with a pumice after a bath or in a bath, when calluses soften. Sometimes the thickened area will go away by taking a homeopathic remedy, but, generally, the best method is to take a remedy, improve your diet, and have a podiatrist trim the callus and check for biomechanical imbalances that are causing uneven pressure on your soles.

Homeopathic remedies which may help are:

Antimonium Crudum for thickness on soles of feet, but only if the patient fits the specific characteristics for this remedy; (craving pickles is part of the symptom complex); has painful heels; horny calluses; brittle nails; worse heat of sun; irritable; or try *Graphites* if *very* thick skin and calluses; unhealthy skin with fissures; calluses on toes; *Silica* if hard firm scars; crippled nails; cold feet; *Arsenicum Alb* for dry, rough, scaly skin; worse scratching; burning pain; calluses on soles of feet; may be restless, anxious, fearful type of person; *Sulphur* if thick calluses with burning in soles; *Phosphorus* for a painful corn on the heel; *Rununculus Bulbosus* if worse with feet hanging down.

Bunions

A bunion is a protuberance of bone on the inner side of your foot, usually accompanied by a bent big toe (see Figure 8-10). The bunion pushes the sesamoids (small bones under the big toe) out of alignment, so the bottom of your foot hurts, too. A predisposition for bunions is inherited, but imbalances in the foot or wearing pointed-toe shoes make bunions worse. If you have a short first toe (Morton's foot) *and* a very mobile foot which flattens out a lot, you are more likely to develop bunions. Bunions hurt because of pressure from your shoe. A long first metatarsal (Egyptian foot) that is crammed into a small shoe can create a bunion on the big toe joint.

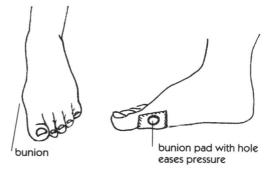

bunion

bunion pad with hole eases pressure

8-10. Bunions are bumps on the inner side of the foot which are aggravated by wearing pointed-toe shoes.

To treat bunions cut out the area of your shoe that's causing pressure on the bunion and put in elastic material. Cover the bunion with a doughnut pad to ease pressure. If there is a fluid-filled sac (bursa) over the bunion, your doctor might try homeopathic injections of:

Ruta Grav for sore, achy stiffness; or

Strontium Carbonicum for joint damage (arthritis) or *Zeel* for tender, damaged joints.

Oral homeopathic remedies which may help are (select one):

Silica for swelling around bunion or *Hypericum* for nerve-like pain or *Ruta Grav* for pain that is more like bursitis or *Arnica* if sore or feels deeply bruised.

Phosphorus if sore with burning, bursitis-like pain.

I don't encourage people to get injections of cortisone because it causes degeneration of the joint.

A bunion that is causing the big toe joint to be seriously misaligned could cause arthritis; therefore, have your bunion checked out, as an orthotic could help prevent major damage.

If you are a professional athlete and can function with the bunion, then wait until the end of your career to have surgery, especially if you are a dancer. Once surgery is done, your career as a dancer may be over. If, however, a bunion operation is necessary, simply have the bunion smoothed down; don't do a big procedure.

Stiff Big Toe (*Hallux Limitus* or *Hallux Rigidus*)

Hallux rigidus often results from an old injury that gradually stiffens the big toe joint. Runners (especially with a long first toe—Egyptian foot) may develop a toe with limited range of motion *(hallux limitus)* from the repetitive flexing of the toe. The joint may become painful when hopping, sprinting, landing from a jump, or from wearing ill-fitting shoes. If there is a gritty, sandpapery feeling when you move the joint, you may have arthritis and calcium deposits in the joint between the toe and the metatarsal. Whatever the reason for the stiffness, the answer is to get the toe elevated a bit off the ground so it's not getting hit every time you run.

One effective mechanical remedy for *hallux limitus* and *rigidus* is to apply a rocker bar of hard rubber under the shoe to relieve pressure (Fig. 8-4). Avoid wearing high-heel shoes (which concentrates pressure on the ball of the foot). Avoid buying running or sport shoes with thin cushioning in the forefoot and a wedged heel. If your stiff toe causes a lot of pain, you may have to resort to surgery to trim down the bones and relieve the pressure. Your doctor may also try homeopathic injections of *Ruta Grav,* or *Zeel* to free up the joint.

Oral homeopathic remedies include:

Ruta Grav if very stiff; *Strontium Carb* for arthritic joints; *Rhus Tox* for general stiffness; *Calcarea Fluorica* for bone spurs; *Hecla Lava* may help for bone spurs.

Don't use cortisone as it will contribute to the degeneration of the joint. Have surgery only if all else fails.

Hammer Toes

These toes are bent and claw-like from being scrunched up in shoes that are too small or high-heeled. Hammer toes are often bent within the toe, as well as where the toe meets the foot. Therefore, correcting hammer toes is often part of the treatment for pain in the ball of the foot (metatarsalgia). When the toe is bent, it pulls the fat pad forward, depriving the ball of the foot of its natural cushion. Obviously, wearing roomy shoes, sandals, and well-made shoes will help.

Hammer toes are treated easily with surgery. Felt or sponge rubber pads can be put across the top of the toes inside the shoe.

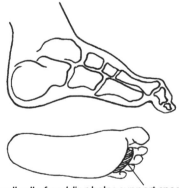

small roll of padding helps support space

8-11. Hammer Toes or "Claw-toes"

Or, you can put a small roll of padding underneath the toes to give them something to hold onto and fill in the space (Fig. 8-11). Going barefoot often helps the foot in general.

Skin Conditions

Troublesome skin conditions of the foot include blisters, warts and athlete's foot as well as dryness, excessive sweat, very smelly feet (brom hydrosis) and hot feet.

Blisters

Puncture the blister with a sterile needle. Express all the fluid, and then dab some betadine or hydrogen peroxide on it with cotton or a Q-tip. Cover with moleskin and tape (or a bandaid) until the moleskin or bandaid falls off.

Use *Calendula* lotion to bathe the clean blister. Use *Arnica* ointment only after blister is healed over and not open and raw.

Warts

Soak feet in a half-cup of white vinegar in a pan of water.

Don't use salicylic drops on warts because of the risk of burning your skin. A podiatrist can trim warts down and apply a mild acid to kill the fungus. If warts are resistant to all treatment, treat with either liquid nitrogen or a laser, which leaves virtually no scarring. Recurrence is rare as long as the surgeon removes all of the growth. High doses of vitamin A may help get rid of warts. Vitamin A is helpful for any kind of thickened skin, but since you can overdose on this vitamin *do not* take large doses without consulting your doctor.

Homeopathic remedies include:

Thuja for plantar warts and moles; if there is oily, sweet-smelling skin; can use topically with *Thuja* oil; *Antimonium Crudum* if horny warts on hands and soles or plantar warts; *Nitric Acid* if warts bleed on washing; *Spigillia* for warts on toes.

Athlete's Foot

Athlete's foot is an itchy, scaly malady caused by several different kinds of fungi. Specific medications are required, depending on where the condition is found on the foot.

Athlete's foot that occurs between the toes doesn't respond well to powders; instead, try conventional medicines such as Desenex Liquid,

---

The Frog-Blood Remedy

An age-old tale has it that warts are cured by putting the blood of a frog killed under the light of a full moon on the wart. Most assuredly, the wart will disappear if you take the trouble to go through this ritual.

Although caused by a virus, warts are also affected by psychological beliefs. I have tested the concept of auto-suggestion on some of my young patients. I tell children to eat one carrot (high in Vitamin A) a day to rid themselves of warts. When I question the ones who, on a subsequent office visit, still have their warts, they almost always admit that they didn't really eat a carrot every day. So, I tell them again to go home and eat a carrot every day. Very often, they return in a month or so with no sign of their warts.

Lotrimin and Enzactin Cream.

For athlete's foot on the bottom of the foot, use Tinactin. Talcum powder helps keep feet dry. In addition, soak your foot in a half-cup of white vinegar in a pan of water. Athlete's foot is contagious not only to other people, but to other parts of your body, so dry your feet with paper towels only and discard the towels. Wash bathmats and bathroom floors frequently.

Homeopathic remedies include:

Calendula soap or lotion is very good; oral Rhus Tox if itching, burning; better heat, worse cold; Sulphur if hot burning feet; athletes' foot between toes; worse heat, better cold; Psorinum if Sulphur doesn't work.

Dryness of Skin on the Foot

It's best to have a homeopathic workup in any chronic condition such as unusually dry skin. However, if you treat yourself, try topical:

Lanolin, Aloevera cream, or Arnica cream.

Excessive Sweat on the Feet (Hyper Hydrosis)

This is a condition which may be symptomatic of other problems, or simply a characteristic. Use homeopathic Zinc if always moving; restless; soles are very sensitive or cold.

Smelly Feet *(Brom Hydrosis)*

For smelly feet, wipe with vinegar and water. Also soak feet in a half-cup vinegar in a pan of water and put in some grass cuttings or liquid chlorophyll. Chlorophyll will help deodorize your feet. Change your socks regularly, and let your feet air out.

Homeopathic remedies include:

Silica, the main remedy: if icy cold, sweaty, smelly; yellow; offensive; *Graphites* if unhealthy feet; smells bad with or without sweat; eczema; *Rumex* for very sour-smelling sweat; *Staphysagria* for cold feet that smell like a rotten egg; *Pulsatilla* for warm feet with offensive odor or if worse if sweat is suppressed; tendency to get sick from putting feet in cold water.

Hot, Burning Feet

If your feet are so hot that you feel like sticking them outside the covers when you're in bed, here are some homeopathic remedies to consider:

Sulphur, Pulsatilla, Zinc for burning feet with restlessness; especially for older people. Check a *Materia Medica* for characteristics.

Happy feet are a blessing. In order to keep your feet pliable and flexible, walk barefoot once in a while at home, on the grass, or, best of all, on a beach covered with small pebbles. Walking barefoot stimulates the soles of the feet, energizing the points which correspond to your organs. Trading foot massages with a friend is a delightful and healthful exchange of energy.

Chapter 9

HEEL INJURIES

Time wounds all heels.
—Jane Ace, *The Fine Art of Hypochondria;
or, How Are You?*

There is a virtual epidemic of heel problems, especially stress fractures, in walkers. Many of my patients are women who have begun vigorous walking programs—often with inadequately cushioned shoes like flats or tennis shoes which bring on heel problems when worn on streets and sidewalks. I also see middle-aged runners showing heel spur syndrome or stress fractures of the heel. Our bodies rebel at the rigors of running or fast-walking on hard surfaces (chronic repetitive stress). While properly cushioned shoes are necessary, it is also important to walk or run on soft surfaces such as grass.

Another contributing factor to heel injury is tight muscles which don't absorb shock well. Bones become more easily damaged. It's important as we get older to do more flexibility exercises. As you know, "What you don't use, you lose." This is particularly true for older women who have not exercised regularly in early life. The risk of osteoporosis increases over time with lack of exercise and poor diet.

General Pain In the Heel

If you have pain in the heel that doesn't respond to conservative treatment—i.e., rest, applications of heat or cold, switching to non-impact activities, or wearing arch supports—have lab tests done to rule out arthritis, gout, or related conditions. If you have a history of gout, a test of your uric acid level may confirm the presence of the disease rather than an injury. X-rays should be done to check for heel spur or stress fracture. If stress fracture is suspected, but doesn't show up on x-

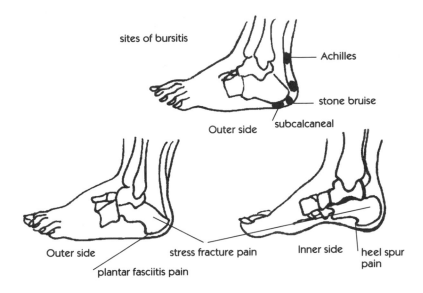

sites of bursitis

Achilles

stone bruise

Outer side subcalcaneal

Outer side   stress fracture pain   Inner side   heel spur pain

plantar fasciitis pain

9-1. Sites of Heel Pain.

ray, a bone scan is necessary. Remember, an x-ray does not show actual damage from a stress fracture for at least three weeks.

If the heel is red, hot and very sore, take your temperature. If the temperature is above normal, there's an infection, so see your doctor.

Stress Fractures of the Heel

A bone scan is the best way to differentiate a stress fracture from other causes of heel pain, such as heel spur syndrome, bursitis, or plantar fasciitis. Stress fracture pain is most intense on the sides of the heel rather than on the bottom (Fig. 9-1). There is considerable pain on arising in the morning and the pain gets worse throughout the day. Repeated pounding of the heel creates this over-use injury.

The only cure for stress fracture of the heel is rest. Physical therapy with ice whirlpool together with electrical stimulation decreases pain and may hasten healing. For initial pain and swelling, take:

Arnica, 30c (two) four times a day for the first 24 hours.

In two to three days, for pain, stiffness and soreness, take:

Ruta Grav in potencies of 6 or 12 (two pills) twice a day for two weeks or until better. Follow with *Symphytum,* potency 12 (two pills) twice a day. After two weeks take *Calc Phos* in potency 12 (two pills) twice a day until better if your body type is tall or lanky (occasionally stocky); if you are young and growing rapidly; tend to be a thirsty person.

Take *Calc Fluor,* a dose of 200 or 1M, to finish healing and prevent re-injury. Take if you tend to be warm and hurried; tend to be depressed, or are currently depressed; tend to have a big appetite.

You may use anti-inflammatory medicines which are non-steroidal (non-cortisone) like Naprosyn, Feldene, Advil, Motrin, but only on the advice of your doctor as they can cause stomach bleeding and irritation. Swallow with food. Avoid using these drugs if you are on medication for heart disease, ulcers, hypertension or kidney problems. Don't take them to mask pain so that you can continue to run. You may use NSAIDs with homeopathic remedies, but take them at least 20 minutes apart.

If you have much pain on walking, the doctor may give you a below-the-knee walking cast and crutches. After recovery (four to six weeks), an orthotic with a well-molded heel cup and extra padding (use Viscolas) is essential.

Ultrasound therapy aggravates a true stress fracture, whereas electrical therapy aids healing.

Pain in the Heel (Stone Bruise or Tennis Heel)

Your heel may feel sore as you push down on your heel or press it with your fingers. The heel has probably been bruised by repeated heavy footfalls or by landing on it in jumping sports. A fluid-filled sac (bursa) on the bottom of the foot develops from repeated impact, playing tennis or stepping on a stone. See Fig. 9-1.

To treat stone bruise or tennis heel, put an ice pack on the heel 20 minutes a day. You may also use heat if it feels better. Use hot compresses or a towel-covered heating pad (set to *low,* never high).

Discontinue activities that cause pain to the heel. Protect the heel with good shock absorptive inserts such as Viscolas or Sorbethane heels. Buy new shoes with good cushioning if the mid-soles of your shoes are worn out.

Substitute swimming, cycling, or working out on Nautilus equipment until better, for about four to six weeks.

Select one of the following homeopathic remedies. Take potencies of 6, 12, 15 or 30 (two pills) four times a day.

173

Silica or *Ruta Grav* if stiff; better with some motion, but worse with too much activity; if better with heat. If no results try *Benzoic Acid.* Follow after 2 weeks with *Symphytum.* After 2 more weeks take *Calc Phos,* a single 1M dose to finish the healing process.

Pain on the Bottom of the Heel (Plantar Fasciitis)

Here again there is pain on the bottom of the foot near the heel. The fascia, (tough, fibrous tissue), attaches at the heel bone and extends to the heads of the metatarsal bones (Figure 9-2). Too much tension or pulling of the plantar fascia causes microscopic bleeding. A strain in this area could be caused by a change of shoes or a change in your activity (new sport).

Your heel will probably hurt when walking, running, and upon standing after a period of sitting down. The damaged or inflamed plantar fascia frays like a rope. Once the fibers are frayed, a thick, inelastic scar forms. When the foot is rested (e.g., in the morning), this gristly tissue contracts and becomes very painful when first walking on it. Patients tell me they may hop around for 15 minutes before the tension eases. There is also pain when the toes are pulled toward the body in a stretch. Some patients describe the feeling as the sensation of a "rusty gate."

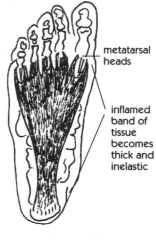

metatarsal heads

inflamed band of tissue becomes thick and inelastic

Bottom of foot

9-2. Plantar Fasciitis; pain could be a result of change in shoe or activity (new sport).

The most important measures for treating plantar fasciitis are to rest the foot, tape it, or insert orthotics into shoes. Taping is very important because the big toe must be kept from moving too much. Too much movement stretches and pulls on the the plantar fascia. Soft tissues generally take four weeks to heal.

Even though the pain of plantar fasciitis may subside after 15 minutes of warm-up, don't keep on running. See your doctor.

In the early stages, plantar fasciitis can be cured with Ultrasound therapy or electro-galvanic stimulation and a foot orthotic. Otherwise, the problem continues to worsen and may lead to surgery.

For pain, apply ice or heat, whichever feels better.

Select one of the following homeopathic remedies in potencies of 6, 12, or 30 (two) twice a day:

>*Rhus Tox* if very stiff after rest or in the morning; better with continued movement; restless; worse sitting.

>*Ruta Grav* if movement makes you tired and cranky; depressed; worse with stepping; *Phytolacca* if better sitting with foot up; worse with feet hanging down; if electric shock-like pain; better warm; better rest, worse motion.

>Take *Stellaria* if better or worse motion (hard to tell); shooting, darting pain; worse warm, better cool; *Rhododendron* if pain increases with an approaching storm;

>*Phosphorus* if pain is worse during storm; *Nat Carb* if there is a pulsating pain on the bottom of the foot;

>*Valerian* if worse sitting, better walking; (or *Rhus Tox*). *Causticum* if better on a rainy day; tends to be a rebellious type of patient.

For pain, you may take aspirin, unless you have medical complications such as ulcers, heart disease, hypertension or kidney problems. Don't take aspirin before running because it numbs the pain and allows you to run despite the injury.

Redistribute the weight in the foot by using an arch support, a heel pad, and by strapping your arch. Available over-the-counter supports are Viscolas, Spenco, Sorbothane, and Linco systems.

If you still have pain, replace the heel pad with a heel cup. You can buy heel cups in sporting goods shops.

Avoid exercise until pressure to the heel is no longer painful. Try race-walking *if* there is no pain.

If you still have pain despite the above self-treatments, have a podiatrist look at the entire weight distribution problem in your foot. Your physician may give trigger-point injection treatments of homeopathic *Rhus Tox* or *Ruta Grav.* If the area is very gristly, he or she may use *Zeel* to break up scar tissue. If it's very sore, *Traumeel* combined with *Rhus Tox* or *Ruta Grav* often helps. If results still aren't satisfactory, a short-acting cortisone, *Decadron,* can be added to the homeopathic remedies. The final step would be to add a long-acting cortisone to the foregoing mixture. If injected into the plantar fascia only, cortisone is usually not dangerous. However, cortisone injections into the fat pad of the heel are very dangerous since they may cause disruption

The Case of the Antidoted Paeonia Remedy

Sometimes one of my patients presents me with a vivid reminder of how allopathic (conventional) medicine can antidote (reverse) a homeopathic remedy. Barry, an advertising executive in his early forties, was running 4 to 5 miles a day when he came to see me for a heel spur. As part of his medical history, he told me that five years before he had had a rectal fissure which had been treated with homeopathic *Paeonia*. Since rectal fissures usually require surgery, I was quite impressed that it had completely gone away with the remedy.

To treat his heel spur, I injected *Rhus Tox*—to no avail. Next, I tried injecting *Ruta Grav.* Nothing. Then I put him on physiotherapy. Again, no improvement. I was forced to resort to a cortisone injection. The cortisone did work on the heel spur pain, but the rectal fissure came back—a very bad case. The reappearance of his former disease demonstrates how the cortisone had, after five years, reversed the cure of the *Paeonia* remedy. We repeated the dose of *Paeonia,* and his fissure went away.

of the anatomical arrangement of the fat pad, as well as softening or dissolving of the fat. If there is nerve injury (characterized by sharp pain), use *Hypericum.* Usually, three or four injections a week apart, will do the job. Once you see improvement, then take a single dose of *Calc Fluor* to finish the healing.

Generally, it's best to start with one remedy at a time so that you can determine the effects of each medicine. Injections of homeopathic and cortisone combinations are best used after trying single remedies.

Heel Spur on the Bottom of the Heel

A spur on the *bottom* of the heel occurs when the calf muscles are tight, creating excessive strain on the plantar fascia (the band of tissue on the bottom of the foot which is part of the Achilles tendon). With heel pain, it's important to stretch the calf muscles and to use physical therapy such as electrical stimulation or Ultrasound. See Fig. 9-1.

To treat heel spur on the bottom of the heel, ice for relief of pain. If ice doesn't make it feel better, use hot compresses or a towel-covered heating pad (set to *low,* never high).

See a doctor if the heel spur does not get better with rest. Even though you know you have a heel spur, rule out stress fracture, arthritis and gout with a medical diagnosis. Gout is a sudden pain which occurs at night with considerable heat and redness, and may appear to be a stress fracture.

If the pain is severe, homeopathic injections given by your doctor may give quick relief. Otherwise, if the pain is mild or if you hate the idea of needles, take oral remedies. I recommend three or four injections of *Rhus Tox* one week apart as well as oral *Rhus Tox*. In two months time, take a 1M oral dose of *Calc Fluor* to prevent recurrence of the heel spur. Even though I have had success treating heel spurs with homeopathic remedies, I have yet to see, on x-ray, a bone spur that has actually dissolved. While other physicians claim to have found this, I'm still waiting to see a case where the spur has been *dissolved* by a remedy alone. Homeopathic remedies do, however, give relief of pain.

I recommend using one of the following remedies:

Hecla Lava or *Fluoric Acid* to reduce size of spur.

Rhododendron if heel pain is worse before a storm;

Ruta Grav if you're tired and cranky after exercise; feel despairing of getting relief; or are very stiff in the heel; *Pulsatilla* if you're a young woman; if sensitive type of personality; if the pain seems to come and go (changeable); *Radium Brom* if heel is stiff; better with cold; *Calc Carb* if stout with flabby muscle tone; sweat easily; easily chilled; *Calcarea Fluorica* if tend to be a warm and hurried type; tend to be depressed, or are currently depressed; tend to have a big appetite; *Calc Phos* if tall, lanky, or stocky; if young and growing rapidly; tend to be a thirsty person; tend to be anxious and constantly complaining; *Phytolacca* if there is a pulling on the bones of the plantar fascia (where tissue attaches to bone).

If inflammation and pain are severe, you may take an oral, non-steroidal anti-inflammatory pill unless you have problems with ulcers, kidneys or hypertension.

After a day or two of rest, stretch your muscles by leaning against a wall with your feet flat on the floor. Stretch 5 minutes at a time (see Chapter 15 for stretches). Only when conservative therapy has been tried for six to eight months with no luck, should surgery be considered for heel spurs or plantar fasciitis. Following these surgeries, you will be in a walking foot cast for about three weeks. You will be ready to run in three to eight months.

The Effects of Cortisone—A Steroid

Steroid injections (cortisone) should only be used if homeopathic medicines fail, as they may cause degeneration of tissue. *Cortisone weakens your immune system.* When necessary to control pain, use Decadron, a soluble, short-acting cortisone which remains in the body only 24 hours. If there is still no major improvement, add a long-acting cortisone to the Decadron to prolong the effect of cortisone up to three weeks. No more than three or four cortisone injections should be given within six months.

Sometimes when I ask patients if they are getting steroids, they say no. However, they will say they are getting cortisone shots. They are unaware that cortisone *is* a steroid. Steroids weaken the immune system, increasing susceptibility to illness.

Case History #1: Heel Spur

The benefits of using homeopathic medicines for heel spurs was clearly seen with my patient, Tom Evans, a semi-professional prize fighter who runs to keep in shape. I first saw Tom fifteen years ago when he had a painful heel spur. He had the classic tale of "hopping around in the morning, with pain on the bottom of the foot" that is a common symptom of plantar fasciitis and heel spur syndrome. Throwing punches and back-pedalling during boxing had become painful, and road running, impossible.

I had done all the conservative therapies mentioned above. X-rays confirmed my diagnosis, and I eventually did surgery on his foot. He recovered fairly well, although he still had some stiffness in the morning after heavy workouts. I didn't see him again until recently.

This time he came to me with the beginning of plantar fasciitis and heel spur on the other foot. X-rays again showed the beginning of the heel spur, and this time I re-built his orthotics and gave him three injections of *Rhus Tox* a week apart. I also gave him oral *Rhus Tox.*

He had a full recovery from his problem, and two months later I gave him one dose of *Calc Fluor* to prevent a recurrence. He has been running and boxing in good form for several months!

Case History #2: Heel Spur

David is a superb young athlete, training for the Olympic trials in the 1500 meter dash. An excellent runner, he's in his late twenties. He came to me for a heel spur with plantar fasciitis. I gave him homeopathics which didn't provide much relief. Next I gave him cortisone shots and orthotics. The pain didn't get much better, and was really interfering with his training. He wanted surgery.

I made a small incision on his foot, just big enough to insert my finger. I detached the fascia and smoothed down the bone spur. I gave him *Arnica* before and after surgery for general shock and trauma. He was in a small footcast for four weeks, and after six weeks he started to run again. In David's case, surgery was the best answer.

Spring Ligament Strain

Spring ligament strain hurts on the bottom of the heel in the direction of the sole rather than towards the heel. This pain could be the result of a change in accustomed activities which over-stretches the spring ligament.

To treat spring ligament strain, follow the same treatment as for plantar fascitiis in the preceding section. Provide a good arch support orthotic and refrain from repetitive stress. Tape the foot for support.

Spurs on the Back of the Heel—Pump Bump (Retrocalcaneal Exostosis)

Your foot may have a naturally enlarged bump on the back of the heel. The enlargement may also have emerged after being irritated by the back of your shoe. The medical name for this unsightly growth is retrocalcaneal exostosis (see Fig. 9-3). The popular name, "pump bump," comes from wearing "pumps" that cut into the Achilles tendon. The higher the arch, the easier it is for the back of the heel bone to rub on the counter of the shoe. Also, a weak or flat arch that rolls inward (pronates), may contribute to the friction at the heel.

Pump bump can be painful, and may even develop its own bursal sac (protective pillow filled with fluid). It causes discomfort in ski boots, ice skates or high-top hiking boots.

To treat pump bump with first aid, apply ice for 10 to 15 minutes, massaging the area. If ice doesn't make it feel better, use hot compresses or a towel-covered heating pad (set to *low,* never high). After 24 to 36 hours, replace ice treatment with moist heat for 15 to 20 minutes several times a day.

Avoid running. Wear a backless shoe. If the counter of your running shoe is extremely firm, and you have a naturally large bump on the heel, use a hammer to break up the counter so it won't irritate your foot. An alternate strategy is to use a piece of felt or sponge rubber to make a donut pad to surround the bump, taking the pressure off (Fig. 9-3). Control the pronation (rolling movement inward) of your foot with an arch support or orthotic.

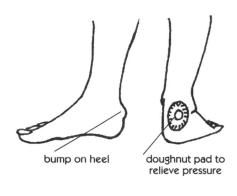

bump on heel   doughnut pad to
                      relieve pressure

9-3. "Pump Bump"
(Retrocalcaneal Exostosis)

Your physician may inject the inflamed bursa with homeopathic *Traumeel* or *Ruta Grav.*

Be aware that cortisone injections must be used with care by your doctor. If the needle misses the bump and hits the Achilles tendon, degeneration of tissue may occur. I recommend using Decadron first because it is a soluble, short-acting cortisone that only stays in the body for 24 hours. If your doctor gives you cortisone, decrease your activity for about three weeks to guard against any possible degeneration of the Achilles tendon.

Severe cases of pump bump can be treated surgically, removing the bony outgrowth, the bursa, and repairing the Achilles tendon if necessary. Unless there has been calcification at the point where the Achilles tendons attaches to the bone (because of excessive pulling), your recovery will be about four to eight weeks. Otherwise, it could be as long as twelve weeks. Stiffness due to scar tissue may take one to two years to go away completely, but responds well to stretching exercises. Take *Rhus Tox* pills (potency of 12) twice a day until better.

Pain in the Heel Cord Sheath (Achilles Tenosynovitis)

The sheath of the Achilles tendon is a loose, fatty tissue that elongates as the tendon itself elongates (like an accordion). The Achilles tendon connects the heel to the calf muscle. The tendon, with its rich blood supply, becomes easily inflamed when irritated. With irritation of the sheath, the fluid between the tendon and sheath expands, causing the tendon to swell within the confines of the tube. If the inflammation is left untreated, gritty deposits cause the tendon to stick to the sheath (adhesions). If enough inflammation builds up and eats into the tendon, the end result is a painful tendon problem.

One cause of friction may be wearing shoes with high backs or heel tabs. But, more commonly, the problem stems from an overuse injury resulting from biomechanical problems, excessive pronation (foot turns inward too much) or supination (foot turns outward too much), or too much shock being absorbed by the tendon.

Usually the Achilles tendon feels stiff first thing in the morning, and on starting exercise. The pain may ease during walking and running, but remains sore to the touch. There is usually pain 1 to 2 hours after running. Finally, the condition progresses to pain even with walking, and running is impossible.

For severe cases of tenosynovitis, I recommend having a magnetic resonance imaging test done (MRI) to determine the full extent of your injury. Ultrasound and xerogram tests are also helpful, but an x-ray usually is not.

Remove the cause of the friction by cutting down the tabs on the backs of your shoes or slitting the back with two vertical slits on either side of the heel.

If there is no spasm causing pain higher up the calf where the tendon joins the calf muscle (Fig. 9-4),[1] resume running and sports—provided you do thorough warm-up and cool-down exercises. Running uphill tends to be the most harmful activity for the Achilles tendon, so work first on stretching the calf muscles before resuming hill work. Use the Flex Wedge (stretching aid) to lengthen the Achilles tendon.

Avoid changing suddenly to wearing a racing shoe for a race. Wear shoes periodically before the race to condition your Achilles tendon. The lower heel on a racing shoe will cause more stress on the back of the heel. If you feel no pain during exercise, continue your sport.

Use physical therapy such as ice whirlpool and electro-galvanic stimulation. If pain continues, your physician may inject softening homeopathic mixtures to break up adhesions. I recommend a combination of ½cc of the softening enzyme *Wydase,* 1cc *Rhus Tox,* 1cc *Traumeel* and 1cc *Xylocaine* shaken hard 20 times (homeopathic succussion to potentize the solution). The injection should be given between the tendon and the sheath once a week for three or four weeks.

Select one of the following remedies (oral) to use for two weeks or until better:

> *Rhus Tox* if the heel is stiff after resting, but gets better with movement; if much better with heat; *Ruta Grav* if it's stiff; restless; better with motion but worse with too much activity (feel tired and cranky); you feel depressed about your injury; *Phytolacca* for pain and stiffness in Achilles tendon, especially where it attaches to the heel bone; pain is worse cold, damp; better warm; better rest, worse motion; worse with feet hanging down; better with feet elevated; *Stellaria* if better or worse motion (hard to tell); shooting, darting pain; worse warm, better cool.

Note: Any of the preceding three remedies may be used by your physician as an injection.

> Take *Calc Phos* in a potency of 6 or 12 twice a day until completely healed.

Try homeopathic remedies first, but you may also take conventional drugs for pain relief such as Advil, Naporsyn, or Feldene. Before taking, however, check with your doctor, as there is a risk of causing stomach ulcers with these powerful medicines. Swallow with food. Don't use if allergic to aspirin. These drugs can increase bleeding time if you have a cut, cause blood in the stools, and mask pain while running (increasing tissue damage). Take only for a short period of time.

Have deep tissue massage 10 minutes twice a day until better. Your physician will probably recommend physical therapy three times a week for three to six weeks.

Correct abnormal foot biomechanics with foot orthotics, better shoes, and temporary heel lifts made from Viscolas (excellent for dampening shock vibrations the same way your natural heel fat pad does). Surgery can repair the tendon sheath, but conservative therapy should be exhausted first.

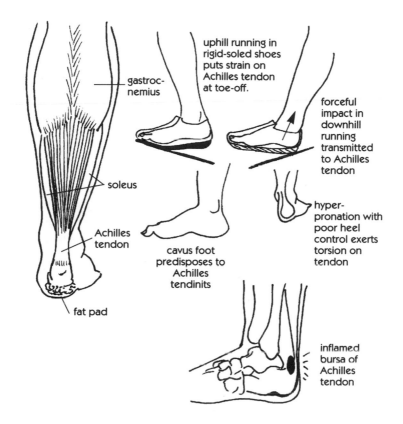

9-4. Achilles Tendinitis

Pain in the Heel Cord (Achilles Tendinitis)

Pain in the lower back of the leg, just above the heel, is Achilles tendinitis. Tendinitis means that the tendon is either degenerated or partially torn. See Fig. 9-4. There may or may not be inflammation of the
tendon sheath (tenosynovitis) at the same time.

The tendon is actually a cord inside a tube (sheath), and is not extremely elastic. When it over-stretches, it is very painful. Tendinitis
can result from sudden stretching—stepping off a curb or stepping in
a pothole. It may happen playing basketball or baseball, especially if
you're over the age of thirty-five or forty. As you get older, the blood
supply to the tendons decreases. If you're still exercising at age forty-
five with the same vigor as you did at age twenty-five, for example,

you can rather easily tear your Achilles tendon. Also, if your cholesterol is high, you're prone to more degeneration of the tendons. Poor circulation from arteriosclerosis or smoking decreases nutrition to the tendons, contributing to degeneration.

Achilles tendinitis means that the tendon could be degenerated, partially ruptured or completely ruptured. The tendon may rupture spontaneously after years of chronic pain. Sometimes, if the sheath is not involved, there is degeneration without pain. When the sheath is involved, there is always pain.

Case Histories of Achilles Tendinitis

Cynthia Smith, in her mid-thirties, jogged about 2 to 3 miles a day. One day, while running uphill, she overstretched her Achilles tendon. A few hours later, her heel was sore and inflamed. She dismissed the injury as a nuisance, without really treating it.

Her pain in the Achilles tendon went on for a period of two years, to the point where she had difficulty even walking comfortably, let alone running.

She came in to see me, and her x-rays showed ropy tissue in the heel. There was a sandpapery sensation (crepitation) when she moved her foot up and down. An MRI test confirmed that it was only the tendon sheath that was inflamed—the tendon itself was ok.

We tried physical therapy, injections with *Rhus Tox* and *Wydase,* and even orthotics. Nothing helped. She was depressed, despairing of any recovery. I felt surgery was next.

Fortunately, I happened to consult with a colleague, Dr. Tim Noakes, author of *The Lore of Running,* who had had a similar condition. He told me that he cured his tendinitis with deep massage— breaking up the adhesions between the tendon sheath and the tendon. He is an expert in sports medicine and a marathon runner and had not wanted to have surgery for his Achilles degeneration.

"Frankly, Steve," he told me, "it was painful. I even had the area iced before the massage to numb it, but I'm really happy with the results. It was worth it." After two months of massage therapy, he was able to run again, pain-free.

Cynthia was willing to try this treatment. Once the massage treatments were underway, I prescribed *Rhus Tox* and *Calc Phos.* She had treatments for two months, and was overjoyed that she was healed. I was amazed to find out that all the adhesions, lumps, bumps and sandpapery sensation were gone. Even though this was a lengthy process, she was able to avoid surgery and felt the massage—as painful as it was—was worth it.

Another patient, who had had a painful Achilles tendinitis for two years before I saw him, was Dr. John Richmon, Chief of Neurology at Oakland Kaiser Hospital. He told me that he had tried everything— stretching, exercises, icing, physical therapy with ultrasound, heel pad—and nothing had worked.

I injected *Rhus Tox* into his heel and did some loosening of the adhesions in the Achilles sheath. At first, his heel got much worse—he felt more pain and he limped more. When he called to report this un-expected symptom, I explained that he was getting what's called an "aggravation" of symptoms which sometimes happens with homeo-pathic medicine. I suggested he treat the heel with hot water jet soaks.

After about six weeks, I got a call from him. "Steve, I just called to tell you the pain has gone! I'm totally free of the pain for the first time in over two years. I don't even have that early morning 'catch' in my walking that used to plague me. I'm really grateful that this remedy worked." He's now back to running.

A third case of Achilles tendinitis concerns Dr. Paul Alway, an anesthesiologist at Alameda Hospital in Alameda, California. Dr. Al-way, in his early forties, had been training for marathons, running about 6 miles a day. He had run the Napa, California marathon and in-jured his Achilles. The pain started out as an aching during running. Then it progressed to aching an hour after running while he was mere-ly walking around. He kept decreasing his mileage, and finally he couldn't run at all. He was very upset.

I tried injecting *Rhus Tox*. There was some improvement, but it didn't last. We tried physical therapy, orthotics and rest, but nothing worked. I finally did surgery on him, and found the tendon sheath swollen and thickened. The sheath was all stuck down (adhered) to the tendon. I released the sheath, and the tendon itself was fine.

In preparation for the surgery, I gave him a dose of homeopathic *Arnica*. After surgery, I gave him *Rhus Tox* to help with the pain and stiffness. After two more weeks, I gave him a single 1M dose of *Calc Phos* to finish his healing. He is now happily back to running.

The first and most important preventive measure for Achilles ten-dinitis is stretching the Achilles tendon and calf muscle. The second is lifting the heel to reduce the tension on the tendon. Since the cause of Achilles tendinitis is almost the same as mid-calf pain, refer to the section on prevention measures for mid-calf pain in Chapter 11. The

Flex Wedge is excellent for stretching tendons and muscles.

To treat Achilles pain apply a refrigerated towel for 15 minutes to reduce swelling and inflammation.

Stop running for a few days or even two weeks. You'll be glad you waited if you run and then get a tendon spasm! Substitute non-pain producing activities such as swimming and cycling (put the seat high to stretch the leg). Don't start stretching exercises until pain is gone.

Select one of the following homeopathic remedies. Take potencies of 6, 12, or 30 four times a day until better.

Arnica for soreness; take for first two or three days;

Bellis if *Arnica* is not effective; very deep, achy pain; *Sulphuric Acid* if there is deep bruising and intense pain;

After two or three days, take:

Ruta Grav if stiff and sore; better with motion, but too much activity makes you tired and cranky; or *Rhus Tox* if stiff with initial motion, but continued motion makes tendon better; if always restlessly moving foot and leg to try to get comfortable; if it feels much better with heat; or

Phytolacca for pain and stiffness in Achilles tendon, especially where it attaches to the heel bone; pain is worse cold, damp; better warm; better rest, worse motion; worse with feet hanging down; better with feet elevated; or *Stellaria* if better or worse motion (hard to tell); shooting, darting pain; worse warm, better cool.

After a week, follow with *Calc Phos* in a potency of 6 or 12 twice a day until healed. You can also take a single 1M dose.

Have deep tissue massage with topical *Arnica* or *Traumeel* 10 minutes a day until better.

If pain persists, have a magnetic resonance imaging test (MRI) or xerogram done to rule out a tear or degeneration. Diagnostic Ultrasound can also be used.

Surgery, if needed, releases the damaged sheath and removes torn pieces. During surgery, healthy tissue can be placed in the tendon area to promote healing. The tendon is covered with healthy cells borrowed from surrounding (mostly fat) tissue. It's important to remove damaged tissue which, otherwise, would produce further abnormal tissue during healing. The new cells are influenced by existing tissue.

Your tendon may have ruptured from chronic overuse or a sudden acute stress. In the first case, you may have had accumulated stress that lead to hard, inelastic, gristle-like scar tissue. Since the tendon has lost its flexibility, it eventually ruptures.

Secondly, you may have had a sudden, severe pain in the heel cord, perhaps just after starting strenuous activity. Your muscles were either cold and tight or fatigued at the end of a run.

To determine if your tendon is completely torn, lie on your stomach and have someone squeeze the calf muscle gently. If the tendon is partially intact, the foot will move downwards. If the tear is complete, the foot will remain still. **Either way, go to the doctor immediately.** A complete tear requires surgical repair or casting. Tendons in an adult cannot heal without surgery; tendons of growing children can, under medical supervision.

Whatever the cause of Achilles tendon rupture, there are three main options for repair:

1. Open surgery. Surgery is usually the best treatment because the tendon can be completely repaired, and will become stronger after healing than with other treatments. During open surgery, healthy fat is placed around the tendon so that cells can begin the healing process. Otherwise, the injured tendon, full of scar tissue, does not have any healthy cells capable of healing the tendon. An advantage of open surgery is that you can be sure the tendon has been completely repaired. The doctor can take care of tissue degeneration, and reinforce the tendon with a graft of either natural or synthetic material. The disadvantage of open surgery is that you must have general anesthesia, you're in a hospital, and your leg will be in a cast for six to eight weeks. You may have adhesions and prolonged stiffness.

2. Closed surgery. This is called percutaneous (through the skin) surgery, similar to arthroscopy. The advantages are that it's done as out-patient surgery under local anesthesia. You are put in a below-the-knee walking cast for four weeks, and go into rehabilitation after four to six weeks. You have less chance of infection. A disadvantage of closed surgery is that the doctor is limited in what he or she can see in order to remove abnormal tissue. With closed surgery, there is slightly more risk of re-rupture than with the open surgery method, but less chance for re-rupture than with the third method—casting. I prefer percutaneous surgery or open surgery, both of which are usually more effective in the long run than the casting method.

3. Casting. In this method, your doctor casts the foot in a plantar-flexed position (toes pointing downwards) to keep the tendon shortened. In the cast and on crutches for ten weeks, you will have quite a bit of weakness in the leg when you get out of the cast—therefore the

---

First Aid For Achilles Ruptures

- *Arnica* for shock and trauma. Take a dose while waiting for doctor; repeat every 15 to 30 minutes in severe cases.
- Ice. Apply cold pack or refrigerated towel for 15 minute intervals till you see the doctor.
- Elevation. Keep injured leg supported on a pillow.
- Compression. Wrap an Ace bandage around the tendon while waiting to see the doctor. Check circulation every 15 minutes by squeezing your big toe. If the toe does not regain it's red color and remains white, loosen the bandages immediately.

---

higher risk of re-rupture as compared to surgery. The best candidates for the casting method are people who are high risk for surgery.

During recovery from serious Achilles rupture or degeneration, usually a cast is worn for comfort while healing. Work with a sports physical therapist who can monitor your progress on a computerized Cybex machine.

After the cast, you may go to a removable splint to enable you to gently move the heel to stimulate healing and clearing of congestion. The next step would be an Ace wrap—then a shoe with a ¼" lift and backless clogs.

Calc Phos is a helpful homeopathic constitutional remedy. Ask your doctor for dosage; take until completely healed.

A 10-minute daily massage is beneficial after healing is well-established. If swelling persists, apply ice as necessary.

As soon as the doctor allows, start putting your heel down to the ground to increase flexibility. Don't force the movement or cause pain. As soon as you can do this, do passive stretching exercises for the calf (see Chapter 15). Do about six stretching exercises every hour, if possible.

Wear heeled shoes or thick pads in the heel of your regular shoes. Try to walk normally and avoid limping. Do strengthening exercises for the calf. Start and finish with passive stretching for the calf (Chapter 15).

Substitute swimming or cycling (with the seat raised so that your tendon is not over-stretched). Progress to dynamic strengthening. When you can do those, resume your sport or running. To prevent recurrence of injury, do a daily session of stretching and include these in your warm-up and cool-down. If you have a cramp in your calves at night, drink plenty of water and don't add salt to your food. Take homeopathic *Cuprum* or *Mag Phos*. Don't let the tabs on the back of your shoes rub on your Achilles tendon.

Even a partial rupture will require eight to twelve weeks to heal. After rehabilitation, you can probably resume sport in about six months. Begin to build up your running *very slowly*. When no pain is felt, alternate running 5 minutes and walking 5 minutes for three sets (a 30-minute workout). In the next couple of days, run 10 minutes, walk 10 minutes. Then, a week later, increase the alternating sequence to 15 minutes each. When you can run 45 minutes easily, begin the cyclic (progressive) training schedule described in Chapter 3. *Never* restart your program where you left off. Give yourself rest days in between running days. Run, if at all possible, on grass or soft surfaces. Check the cushioning of your shoes. Make sure your shoes are not compressed in the midsole.

Footnote:

1. Fig. 9-4 Achilles Tendinitis adapted from drawing by F. Netter, M.D.

Chapter 10

 # ANKLE INJURIES

... he proceeded to leap—'fly' might be more appropriate—from one rock to another with arms stretched wide, often landing but a few inches from the slippery edge. ... Or he would stand motionless at the extreme limit of a massive rock, wheel about suddenly and make a great leap to the other side of the rushing water, never showing the slightest concern about the obvious danger that he might lose his balance and fall into space.

—Michael Murphy, *The Psychic Side of Sports*

Structure and Function of the Ankle

The quote above comes from a description by Peter Furst, an anthropologist who witnessed the Huichol Indian shaman, Ramon Medina Silva, demonstrate the meaning of balance. Such a dazzling display of unity of intention (mind) and body is an inspiring reminder of what lies within our human capacities.

Balance, the central factor of good health, is intimately connected with the ankle joint. Ankle ligaments house the balance mechanisms that monitor the position of your joints. This in-built awareness (proprioception) corrects you automatically when you over-balance—like a gyroscope on a ship. After a sprain or any injury to the ankle, you must regain your sense of balance.

The ankle joint is a simple hinge, but its structure is fairly complex. It is composed of the lower ends of the two shin bones, the tibia and fibula, which form a dome over the talus bone. The talus, in turn, sits over the heel-bone (calcaneus). See Fig. 10-1. Jutting out on either side of the ankle are the ends of the leg bones (malleoli). When you bump the inside of your ankle on the corner of the bed frame and wince with pain—that's the medial malleoli taking the brunt. The outer ankle bone (lateral malleolus) is the "crazy bone"—it hurts like crazy when you bump it, too. It is very easily fractured with a bad ankle sprain.

Protecting the inner side of the ankle is the tough medial ligament (deltoid). The deltoid's main function is to hold your foot to your leg by joining all the pieces—it joins the shin bone (tibia) to the foot (at the navicular bone); the navicular to the side of the heel (calcaneus) and to the back of the talus.

On the outer side, the lateral ligament joins the fibular malleolus to the talus and calcaneus. There are three outside ligaments (collateral ligaments) which are not as strong as the inside (deltoid) ligament.

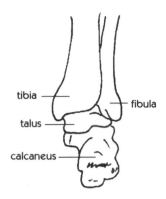

10-1. Shin Bones Sit Atop Heel Bones (back view).

Both the inner and outer ligaments hold the foot to the leg and provide stability.

Another important ligament (tibiofibular ligament) connects the two shin bones (Fig 10-2). There are other tendons as well that strengthen the ankle joint. The front is the least protected part of your ankle.

The ankle joint motion is hinge-like, meaning that the talus is a rounded surface, over which the shin-bone and fibula rock backwards and forwards. Sideways movement is prevented by the bone design and the ligaments. Pulling your foot up towards your shin is called *dorsiflexion* (see Fig. 10-3) and is accomplished by the muscles in the front of the leg (anterior tibial muscles) and the toe extensors. Pointing your toe down is called *plan-*

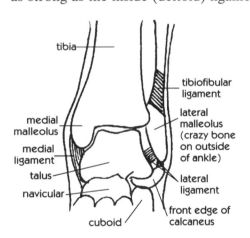

10-2. Left Ankle (front view)

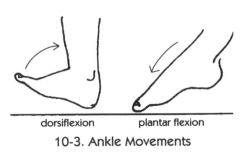

dorsiflexion   plantar flexion

10-3. Ankle Movements

tarflexion (Fig. 10-3), and is accomplished by the calf muscles and the toe flexors.

Ankles, besides giving you the ability to adapt to uneven surfaces, also produce propulsion and absorb shock. If you have a stiff ankle from injury or from over-taping for a sport, your shin bones can be damaged by unabsorbed shock, as can your foot or even low back.

Ankle Strains and Sprains

"I think I sprained my ankle!" is a commonly heard cry by someone who has twisted his or her ankle. When your ankle is hurting, it doesn't make much difference to you whether it's technically a strain or a sprain. However, once you're sitting in your chair with your leg up and an ice pack on the ankle, you may be wondering whether you should call the doctor. My advice is, yes, call the doctor, read the first aid treatment and recommendations below, and then read the following information on differences between strains and sprains.

Ankle strains

A strain is an injury between *muscle and tendon or tendon and bone*. It often occurs in conjunction with a sprain. A sprain is a potentially more severe injury which wrenches the ankle, tearing a *ligament connected to a bone*. If you have more than a very minor twist to the ankle, you should see your doctor as quickly as possible. It's possible that you have torn off a piece of bone (an avulsion fracture). The reason your doctor x-rays the ankle is not to see if it's sprained, but to see if there is a fracture (crack or break) in the bone. There are three grades of ankle strain:

1. Over-stretching of the tendon or muscle;
2. Partial tear of a tendon or muscle;
3. Complete tear of the tendon or muscle. This grade will require a cast or surgery.

Ankle sprains

There are two types of ankle sprains (and strains), depending on whether you twist the ankle inwards (inversion) or outwards (eversion).

Inversion. Inversion is the most common ankle injury because of the joint's natural tendency for turning inwards. An inversion sprain usually happens when your foot is in a dropped-down position (plantar-flexed) because the ankle is like a loose bag of bones in that position. For ex-

193

ample, you foot will be pointing downward as you step off a curb. Inversion sprains tear the outside (lateral) ligaments of your ankle. The most likely cause of twisting your ankle is stepping unexpectedly on an object like a rock, a pine-cone, a toy, or someone else's foot (Fig. 10-4). The twist tears the front lateral ligament (anterior) more easily because it's weaker. It is especially vulnerable when wearing a high-heeled shoe. There is also a tendency, with an inversion sprain, to injure your Achilles tendon or fifth metatarsal base (the outside of your foot). See Fig. 10-5 for inversion ankle injuries.

Eversion. The second type of ankle injury is an outward turning of the ankle (eversion sprain). It usually occurs on slippery or icy surfaces, as in high-speed sports like skiing (Fig. 10-6a). It can also happen in contact sports (being tackled), golfing, or simply stepping off a curb. If you have flat feet, you may have more of a tendency for an eversion sprain. The accident tears the inner (deltoid) ligament. See Fig. 10-6b, c, d, and e for different types of eversion ankle injuries.

Oddly enough, a slight sprain in the ankle (for in-

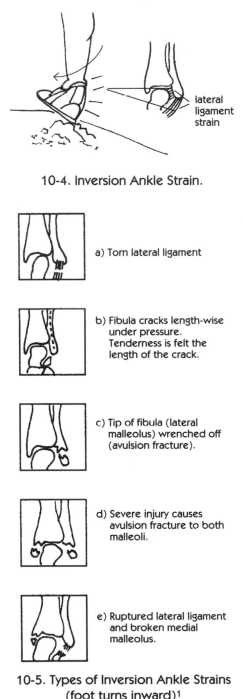

10-4. Inversion Ankle Strain.

a) Torn lateral ligament

b) Fibula cracks length-wise under pressure. Tenderness is felt the length of the crack.

c) Tip of fibula (lateral malleolus) wrenched off (avulsion fracture).

d) Severe injury causes avulsion fracture to both malleoli.

e) Ruptured lateral ligament and broken medial malleolus.

10-5. Types of Inversion Ankle Strains (foot turns inward)[1]

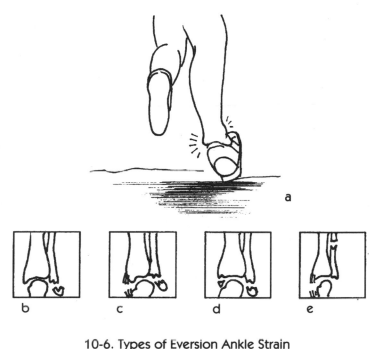

10-6. Types of Eversion Ankle Strain
a) Slipping on slick surface.
b) Fracture of fibular malleolus.
c) Fracture of fibular malleolus with rupture of medial ligament.
d) Fracture of both malleoli.
e) Fracture of fibula, rupture of medial ligament,
and separation of tibia and fibula.[2]

stance, a lateral ligament sprain) can be extremely painful, whereas a more serious ligament tear or bone fracture, may not be as immediately evident. A bad sprain is usually given poor medical attention. Patients have reported well-meaning, but dismissive, emergency room doctors saying, "Oh, well, there's no fracture." You're left to fend for yourself with an ace wrap, aspirin and crutches. Yet a bad sprain can be worse than a simple fracture; if not treated properly, it can take months or even years to fully recover.

Seventy-percent of ankle sprains which are treated conservatively—without surgery—will heal fine. Thirty-percent of ankle sprains with repeated injury will eventually require surgery. There are three grades of ankle sprains:

1. Over-stretching, but no tear, of the ligament. You won't need crutches, and will feel better in a day or two.

2. Partial tear of a ligament. It might be swollen and tender, but you'll feel better in a week.

3. Complete tear of the lateral ligament. You've probably torn the anterior (front) outside (lateral) ligament, and will need a cast and or surgery (Fig. 10-5a). With repeated sprains, you may very well tear the second (middle) and third (posterior) lateral ligament as well as the first, and then you're in real trouble. After three bad sprains, consider surgery to repair the ligaments. Repeated sprains can cause ankle arthritis!

Basic first aid for ankle strains and sprains

First aid treatment for injuries to the legs, ankles and feet is summed up by the short-hand term, R I C E:

Rest (staying off the injured part)
Ice (or heat or a combination of both)
Compression (ace bandages)
Elevation (keeping leg up to reduce swelling)

Ice your injury 20 minutes on the hour, or until the swelling and pain subside. Do this three or four times a day. Treating with ice helps control bleeding (bruising) and numbs pain. When the ankle is numb, you can start *gentle* motion in order to stimulate the lymphatic system to flush out the waste products in the tissues that come with bleeding and swelling. For most people, ice treatment reduces pain and swelling. However, if ice *increases* the pain, then try a heating pad (set to *low,* never high). If your injury feels better with a heating pad or hot compresses, then try homeopathic *Bellis* initially instead of *Arnica.*

If ice alone is not effective, try alternate hot and cold applications (contrast baths). Dip your ankle in a pan of hot water for 5 minutes, then switch to a pan of ice water. Keep both waters very hot and very cold as you alternate for about 30 minutes.

Keep your foot higher than your hip or heart. Prop the leg on a pillow or soft chair. To minimize swelling, don't sit or stand with your foot on the floor. Keep the leg on pillows even in bed if you can sleep that way.

The body's natural reaction to a sprain or strain is to restrict movement by "splinting." Splinting means the tendons contract and prevent motion. This protects you from further damage. Motion is also restricted by swelling. Swelling is the result of tissue damage with inflammation. Inflammation is important for healing. It sets in motion enzyme and chemical reactions which help the body rid itself of toxins.

Too much inflammation or too much splinting, however, is counter-productive.

An extrinsic way to restrict movement is to apply an ace bandage, extending from your toes to just below your knee. If the ankle is very swollen, use an inflatable air splint. Non-elastic bandages are not advisable (unless you know how to wrap them) because your ankle may continue to swell, and a too-tight bandage will cut off the circulation. Check your circulation every 15 minutes by squeezing your big toe and watching the redness return. If the toe remains white, loosen the bandages right away.

After completing first aid, call your doctor or a sports medicine specialist.

For homeopathic treatment select one remedy below that covers most of your symptoms. If a remedy is not effective within 2 hours, select another one. Use whatever dose you have in your medicine kit (usually 6, 12, 15 or 30). Higher doses of 200 or 1M are available only with a prescription from a health care provider. Generally, the low potencies are given once or twice daily in these cases. *Discontinue taking a remedy as soon as you feel better.* Remedies can be contaminated by touching them. Drop pills into your mouth directly from the cap of the bottle. However, do not swallow the pills; instead, put the pills under the tongue and allow them to be absorbed by your mucous membranes. Homeopathic medicines can be taken in conjunction with conventional medicines such as non-steroidal inflammatory drugs or antibiotics.

Stage One remedies (first 24 hours) for injuries for shock of injury:

> *Arnica:* take any dose on hand or prescription-strength 200C or 1M an hour every 4 hours for 24 hours or until better.

For pain, bruising and swelling, select one of the following remedies (in potencies 6, 12, 15, 30). Take four times a day until better.

> *Arnica:* once every 4 hours for 24 hours if a cold pack on the injury feels better than heat (even though you may prefer to be kept warm); if you're extremely sensitive to pain (like the princess in the fairy story who could feel a pea under nine layers of mattresses!); sore, lame, bruised; if it feels dislocated or sprained.

> Use *Sulphuric Acid* if *Arnica* helped some, but not as much as expected; if the injury is black and blue and very sore; if you are aimlessly restless ("I'm late, I'm late," but you're not going anywhere—like the Mad Hatter); if worse with excessive heat or

197

cold; when better warm or lying on affected side. For severe cases take one to two doses an hour apart; milder cases twice a day until better.

Bellis if there is bruising with deep, intense pain; if the injured part feels much worse with a cold pack and much better with heat. Use *Bellis* when you cannot tolerate ice at all.

Use *Bryonia* if you cannot move the injured foot; if you cannot bear to have it touched; if pressure makes it feel better; when better lying on painful side; if there is redness or a hot feeling; if it feels worse with warmth, better cool.

Ledum if it feels cool to the touch; can be hot and inflamed (e.g., with gout); if it feels better with a cold pack; if you have easily-sprained ankles.

Phytolacca if better rest; worse motion; if worse with feet hanging down; better with feet elevated; if worse cold or damp. This remedy has an affinity for Achilles tendon, ankle joint and rear foot.

Use *Stellaria* if difficult to tell if better or worse with motion; if you tend to be worse with warm; when better cool; for stitching, migratory pain.

Use *Lymphomyosot:* ten drops three times a day, or one pill three times a day, if very swollen. Combine with massage and contrast baths to aid drainage.

For inflammation you may take the following conventional medicines:

Aspirin is still the number one medicine to reduce inflammation unless you have ulcers, a heart or kidney problem or are on an anti-coagulant medicine. Check with your doctor before taking aspirin and take with food. Stop if there is any blood in the stool, nausea, vomiting, or ringing in the ear. The usual dose is one to two aspirins every four to five hours.

Non-steroidal anti-inflammatory drugs (NSAIDs) such as the most common over-the-counter ones, Advil and Motrin, are also taken for inflammation and pain. Use the same precautions as for aspirin.

If you still have pain and swelling in the morning after elevation and ice pack treatments, call your doctor even if you don't think anything's broken. You may need x-rays. Other treatments by a physician for ankle strains and sprains:

• Injection therapy can be given by a physician immediately after a trauma, during recovery and after surgery. He or she can inject homeopathic remedies into acupuncture points, joints, and ligaments to enhance and speed up healing. Injecting ligaments causes a mild inflammatory response (aggravation) that promotes healing. Injection medicines should be combined with ½cc Wydase, a natural softening and spreading enzyme (hyaluronidase) and 1cc Xylocaine, an anesthetic. Homeopathic choices for injections are:

Traumeel for trauma and inflammation. This is a combination remedy (has several homeopathic remedies together) and promotes healing. *Traumeel* drops are for internal consumption, while *Traumeel* cream is for external use.

Zeel promotes healing of joint problems.

Rhus Tox if worse initial motion; for stiffness all the time; if much better warm.

Ruta Grav for stiffness which gets better after movement; if restless with too much rest; also pain or fatigue with too much activity.

Phytolacca for Achilles tendon; for stiffness of Achilles to the attachment to the heel; for weak and stiff ankles; if better with feet elevated.

Stellaria for stiff, painful joints; if better or worse motion; if better cool or cold; worse warm; good for sinus tarsi, subtalar or ankle joints.

Lymphomyosot for swelling.

Your physical therapist will decide the best course of treatment. With injury, the electrical charge in the cells of the injured area actually reverses. The cells, in order to heal, must be recharged and awakened. Submersion in an ice whirlpool, together with electrical stimulation, works very well to re-charge and awaken the cells, especially if done in the first 24 to 48 hours.

In my office, we have found good results using Ultrasound, another form of physical therapy, to speed up healing. We also use interferential therapy with a computerized Dynatron machine. The Dynatron machine combines two different wavelengths of electrical energy and stimulates the tissue where the two wavelengths meet to form an interference pattern.

Contrast baths also clear congestion and recharge the battery of the cells which stimulates healing. Acupuncture or acupressure is another method to recharge the batteries in the cells and promote drainage.

Accuscope combines acupressure with electrical stimulation (using micro-current or homeopathic stimulation) and is very good for injuries. It is a gentle, subtle form of stimulation as compared to electro-galvanic stimulation.

Therapeutic massage wakes up tissue, increases circulation and releases or prevents soft tissues from sticking (adhering) to bones, tendons or ligaments. This is performed only after healing has taken place.

The goal of rehabilitation exercises should be four-fold: to promote strength, balance, flexibility, and endurance. Your physical therapist will advise on exercises or see Chapter 15. The main type of exercises will be peroneal strengthening; stork stand for balance; and range of motion (describing the alphabet from A to Z with the end of the big toe).

Manipulation is important in some ankle injuries where the joint has to be moved back into place, as is mobilization, a gentle movement performed by osteopaths, podiatrists, physical therapists, chiropractors, and conventional doctors.

During recovery use Stage Two remedies (24 hours to four or five days). After initial pain and swelling have been reduced, consider the following remedies. Take potencies of 6, 12, 30 or 200 once a day for three to four days or until better. Choose one:

Rhus Tox if it is stiff and sore in the morning or after rest—worse initial motion; if it feels better from movement, and you tend to be *restless;* if it's better with massage; if it's worse with cold pack; much, much better with warmth.

Ruta Grav if it's better with rest; if motion feels better but too much activity or movement makes you feel cranky and tired; if stiff, sore, bruised and achy; if better with heat; if you feel moody and fretful about the injury ("Will I ever get better?"); if there are torn ligaments.

Ledum if joint feels cool to touch (may also be warm); if better cool applications; *Phytolacca* if better with rest; worse with motion; if worse with feet hanging down; better with feet elevated; if it feels worse with cold, damp. This remedy has an affinity for Achilles tendon, ankle joint and rear foot. Use *Stellaria* if it's difficult to tell if better or worse with motion; if you tend to be worse when warm; better cool; for stitching, migratory pain. Select

Bryonia if red and inflamed; worse with any motion; if you cannot move the injured foot or bear to have it touched; if better with pressure or tight wrap; if better with cold pack; better with rest; better lying on affected side.

Rhododendron if worse before a storm; worse cold, wet; worse rest; if better with motion, but worse too much motion.

Use Stage Three remedies to strengthen and prevent re-injury. This is the reparative phase—i.e., two weeks after the injury, when the affected part is feeling better. Take the following:

Calcarea Phosphoricum. If you can, have your homeopath give you a prescription for a single 1M dose. Otherwise, go to a homeopathic pharmacy and get doses of 12 or 30 and take twice a day for two weeks.

If the ankle continues to swell at the end of the day during recovery, keep your leg elevated as often as possible during the day. If you can't do that, stretch it out as you sit, and frequently move your leg and foot, pressing against the floor and flexing. This will keep the circulation going and drain the swelling.

Also try contrast baths (dipping into a pail of hot water and a pail of cold water with ice) unless you have a circulatory problem or if your skin is sore. Dip the foot in hot water for 30 seconds, then cold, alternating for about 10 minutes, or until you see your skin becoming red. The baths will help you in starting some of your simple foot exercises for therapy.

Guidelines for recovery from ankle injuries

To stay in shape:

- Substitute swimming, cycling, and non-impact aerobic activity to rest your injury for up to four to six weeks.
- Flexibility and balance. Many injuries damage the balance organisms (proprioceptors) in your ligaments; therefore, it is imperative that you re-establish your proprioception. The following exercises will help you take care of this vital necessity.
- Foot flexion. As soon as pain permits (within hours), start doing up-and-down flexes of the injured foot. A technique for exercising all the joints is to describe the alphabet (from A to Z) with the end of your foot. You can also practice picking up a towel or some marbles with your toes.
- Backwards and sideways walking. When you can bear weight on your foot, you must start to do some balance exercises, and do them as part of your routine for at least six months. Any time you have hurt your foot or ankle, practice walking backwards

and forwards, and to the right and left. If you play any team sport, you need to practice running backwards, as you sometimes do in games.

- Stork test. First practice standing on both feet, eyes closed, with arms outstretched. When you can stand on the injured leg alone with your eyes closed and arms outstretched for one minute, you have succeeded in re-establishing your balance.

Useful equipment during recovery

- Mini-trampoline for bouncing.
- Exercise bike for alternative, non-impact aerobic activity.
- Treadmill to assist in walking and running and in biomechanical diagnosis.
- Balance board for restoring injured balance mechanisms in ligaments (proprioceptors).
- Ankle rehabilitation machine for comparing an injured part to an non-injured part. A Cybex machine is a state-of-the-art computerized diagnostic machine which is very helpful for testing and monitoring muscle strength and dynamic muscle imbalances. These machines are used by sports medicine specialists.

External aids for supporting feet and legs

Wear one of the following supports for two to three months while you are healing, or if there is *any* chance of re-injury. If you re-tear an injury, you may have to have surgery, so don't take a chance.

- Tape. Taping can be done by your trainer, physical therapist or doctor. Tape is a necessity for professional athletes. Bandages enhance your proprioception and increase your strength by at least 15 percent.
- Ankle braces. Braces may lace up or have metal supports.
- High-top running shoes. High-tops increase proprioception and give ankle stability.
- Casts. Scandinavian studies have shown, believe it or not, that there is no difference in the final result whether or not you are put in a cast in an ankle injury. The primary reason for wearing a cast or a brace is for comfort, unless, of course, you have torn all three ligaments. In that case, a cast will hold you together and is essential. Other studies show that *removable* cast braces do help. They allow for stability and gentle, protected motion. The foot is held up and the tendons and muscles are protected from

healing in an over-stretched position. I prefer a posterior splint that can be easily removed for bathing and physical therapy. It's worn for three to four weeks while the ligaments heal. You might also try an air cast or air splint.

Resuming your running

Begin to build up your running *very slowly*. When no pain is felt, run 5 minutes and walk 5 for three sets (a 30 minute workout). In the next couple of days, run 10 minutes, walk 10 minutes. Then, a week later, increase the alternating sequence to 15 minutes. When you can run 45 minutes easily, then you can begin the cyclic (progressive) training schedule described in Chapter 4. *Never* restart your program where you left off. Give yourself rest days in between running days.

Run, if at all possible, on grass or soft surfaces. Check the cushioning of your shoes. Make sure your shoes are not compressed in the midsole. Stop immediately if pain recurs. To restore balance, run in figure-8's, gradually decreasing the size of the loops. For this exercise, you need to be fairly well healed from any injury.

Alternative therapies following healing

Once healing has taken place, you may consider various alternative therapies which can offer increased energy and balance to your whole system. Refer to Chapter 6 for descriptions of the various bodywork therapies and movement practices which will help your physical and mental functioning.

Repeated strains and sprains

A tear in the ligaments (connecting tissues between bones) not properly treated may leave you with chronic instability and weakness of the ankle which causes you to twist your ankles frequently. Thorough attention at the beginning of an injury can help lessen later complications. Walking or running on uneven ground is especially dangerous for you. Repeated injuries damage a joint and cause arthritis. Loose bone chips, remnants of earlier damage, can also be the cause of pain following the recovery of a sprain. If you have chronic instability or twisting, wear a brace during activities or change your sport.

If you continue to twist your ankle, have a shoemaker glue a piece of firm rubber, ¼" thick to the outer side of your running shoe to prevent twisting (see Figure 8-7). This, however could cause pronation problems, so be careful.

Wearing a brace, taping, or high-top shoes *may* prevent further re-injury.

Surgical repair may be needed for chronic ankle sprains. There is little difference between repairing an ankle ligament immediately or waiting for a couple of weeks. I usually delay a surgery decision in order to give the ligament a chance to heal on its own. However, if you have three consecutive ankle sprains, then surgery is probably indicated. If you're young and healthy and want to continue in sports, get your ankle surgically repaired.

Emotional states contribute to ankle strain and repeated ankle injuries. The ankle area corresponds to the sexual and pleasure center in the Indian Ayurvedic system which is based on the seven energy centers of the body called chakras. When you step off a curb and sprain your ankle, or when you twist your ankle on the tennis court or on your hiking vacation, you may be expressing an unconscious feeling of guilt about having fun or pleasure. For example, an injury to your ankle could be an expression of guilt or anger over a sexual relationship. It could also mean that you feel guilty playing tennis when you should be working or studying. Repeated injury may be investigated and understood by hypnotherapy or, possibly, psychotherapy.

Case History: Ankle Sprain with Associated Tendon Strain

Sheldon Roberts, a twenty-eight-year-old distance runner, awoke before dawn one fall day, and rather reluctantly jogged down his driveway in the cold morning air. Not particularly alert this morning, he stumbled into a pothole just as the sun was rising, hindering his vision. For two days, he tried to walk it off (he was actually hopping around and had to borrow a pair of crutches) before deciding to come in to see me. He limped into my office on his crutches, his ankle very swollen and black and blue. The pain was deep, intense and throbbing, and he couldn't stand for me to touch the area.

He had damaged the tendons along the outside of the ankle (peroneals), and had pulled the Achilles tendon. Fortunately, he had no fractures. He had ruptured two, if not three, of the lateral ligaments which meant that he had a grade-three strain.

His initial symptoms clearly indicated the homeopathic remedy *Bryonia*. These symptoms were: 1) he couldn't stand to have his ankle touched; 2) his ankle was red, hot and swollen in addition to being deeply bruised; 3) an ice pack made his ankle feel better; and 4) the pressure of an ace bandage gave some relief. I immediately gave him

Bryonia which produced *remarkable* improvement in about a half-hour. He was amazed at the lessening of pain and swelling.

In addition, a physical therapist in my office put Sheldon's ankle in an ice whirlpool with electro-galvanic stimulation which further reduced the pain and inflammation. With the swelling down, we gave him an open-in-front fiberglass cast (posterior splint). I prescribed *Bryonia* (potency 12) once an hour for the first day depending on the amount of pain or swelling.

Since his posterior cast was removable, he was able to return to the office daily for electro-galvanic stimulation, which speeded the healing. The removable cast also allowed him to shower. At the end of one week, after physical therapy, the ankle was very stiff and hurt at the beginning of motion. It felt much better with heat, and there was considerable swelling at the end of the day. The peroneal and Achilles tendons were inflamed and sore. I injected the ankle joint and tendon with *Rhus Tox* and *Lymphomyosot.* It worked like magic—the swelling and stiffness went away. I then put Sheldon on *Rhus Tox* (potency of 12—two pills) twice a day after an initial loading dose of 200C.

In two weeks, he was put into a canvas lace-up splint with metal on the sides to give more stability. We applied the splint in such a way that there would be no excessive stretching of the injured outside ankle ligament while he was immobilized. Elongation of those ligaments would have left him with ankle looseness and weakness even after he had healed.

After a month he was given a single 1M dose of *Calcarea Phosphorica* to guard against re-injury. Further rehabilitation was done with ankle exercises. Most important was re-establishing his sense of balance in the nerve endings in the ligaments. For example, in the beginning, with eyes closed, he could only balance on his foot for a few seconds before he fell to the side. This balance exercise is called the stork stand. It took about three weeks before he could balance for at least a minute on his previously injured side.

To increase range of motion, Sheldon practiced running in figure-8's as well as hopping back and forth and from side to side. He also used a bike to increase range of motion in the ankle, a tilt board for balancing, and did backward walking. Altogether, his healing took place over a period of four months, and demonstrates the necessary steps that must be taken to heal ankle strains and sprains. He wore the brace for three months whenever there was a chance of re-straining the ankle.

Summary of What To Do For a Mildly Twisted Ankle

- Stay off the foot, and keep it elevated during the day.
- Apply either ice pack (with towel) or heating pad, whichever feels better.
- Try alternating heat and cold applications.
- Support with an ace bandage.
- Take homeopathic *Arnica* during first 24 hours.
- Take *Rhus Tox* or *Ruta Grav* for stiffness during the next few days.
- Take *Calc Phos* or *Calc Fluor* in two weeks.
- Resume walking or running only if there is no pain or swelling.
- Check shoes for arch support, rearfoot control, and shock absorbency.

Sinus Tarsi Syndrome

Sinus tarsi syndrome, commonly associated with foot or ankle sprains, can cause major discomfort, but is often not diagnosed or treated. The sinus tarsi is the joint on the outside of the foot just below the ankle joint (see Figure 10-7). It's one finger below and in front of the outside ankle bone. When the ankle joint is sprained, the ligaments in the sinus tarsi are also sprained. When these ligaments heal, they form a rubbery mass which causes pain when the foot moves from side to side. There is also swelling just below the outside ankle bone.

You may have sprained your ankle eight to twelve weeks before, but there may still be pain in this area. Another cause of sinus tarsi syndrome is from walking around with your foot toed-out (pronated) as an unconscious protective measure after twisting your ankle. In this case, the abnormal pronation to protect the foot invites damage to the sinus tarsi.

To treat sinus tarsi syndrome x-rays are necessary to rule out small

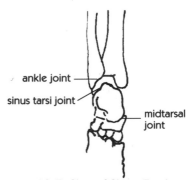

10-7. Site of Sinus Tarsi Syndrome and Midtarsal Joint Sprain (right ankle, front view)

fractures. Magnetic Resonance Imaging (MRI) is the best diagnostic method for sinus tarsi syndrome if x-rays are inconclusive.

Your physician can inject homeopathic remedies to help dissolve the rubbery, gristle-like mass in the sinus tarsi. Use the following remedies in combination with a local anesthetic such as 1cc of Xylocaine and ½cc Wydase, a natural enzyme (hyaluronidase) found in the body that lubricates joints and softens scar tissue. Inject one dose, one week apart, or more often, for a total of three to four injections.

> *Ruta Grav* (1cc). Add *Lympomyosot* 1cc to the mixture if there is substantial swelling. Use *Rhus Tox* (1cc) instead of *Ruta Grav* if it's very, very stiff and hurts at first, but gets better after you start moving it.

> Use *Silica* if there is a lot of scar tissue. Then take oral *Silica,* potency 12, twice a day for two weeks.

If there is no improvement after one or two homeopathic injections, your doctor may add a soluble cortisone—the kind that dissipates from the area within 24 hours—to the homeopathic mixture above. If there is still no improvement, then a mix of soluble *and* insoluble cortisone can be used, which will remain in the sinus tarsi for three weeks.

I prefer to use the cortisone treatment before resorting to surgery because there are no major tendons or joints in the sinus tarsi that would be at risk of cortisone degeneration. If the mass is very firm, simple surgery can be done.

Foot orthotics are necessary if you also pronate or supinate too much.

Sprain of the Midtarsal Joint

The midtarsal joint is just in front of the sinus tarsi and is the big joint where the midfoot joins the rearfoot (see Fig. 10-7). This joint allows side-to-side motion of the foot. Sprains in the midtarsal joint can occur by themselves, or in combination with an inversion ankle sprain. When this sprain occurs, often a piece of bone is torn off, calcifies in the ligaments, and gets caught in the joint when walking on uneven ground.

Even if there is no bone fracture, the ligaments may heal with so much scar tissue that the pain is often as bad as the pain of a fracture.

To treat midtarsal joint sprain, first call your doctor and do basic first aid—see preceding section on ankle strains. Use Stage One and Stage Two homeopathic remedies.

Your doctor will probably give you a walking cast for four to six weeks, and you will have to do physical therapy.

Take a single 1M dose of homeopathic *Calc Phos* for final stage of healing.

If the fracture heals and is still very stiff, your physician can inject with 1cc of Xylocaine and ½cc of Wydase in combination with 1cc of one of the following homeopathic remedies:

Zeel or *Traumeel*; *Rhus Tox* when the ankle is worse with initial motion; if worse after resting, but better with continued motion; if much worse with cold or wet; if much, much better when warm. Use *Ruta Grav* for stiffness; if worse with too much motion; if you feel tired and cranky; if better with warmth, but not as much better as *Rhus Tox*. Use *Phytolacca* for puffy, swollen feet; shifting, electric-like pain; if better with rest; worse with motion; worse with feet hanging down; better with feet elevated; worse when cold or damp. This remedy has an affinity for Achilles tendon, ankle joint and rear foot. Use *Stellaria* for bruised joints; swelling of joints; darting pain; soreness to touch; when better in evening; if better in cold air; worse when warm; when worse or better from motion. Use *Ledum* for easily sprained ankles; if ankle is cool to the touch (although it may be warm); if feet get so sore, you can barely step down; better soaking feet in ice water.

Bryonia for stitching or tearing pain; if much worse motion; much better rest; better lying on affected side; better cool; better with support.

If your fracture hasn't healed properly, you may need surgery to take out the small piece of bone that has pulled off. It's often a good idea to get an MRI or CAT scan before doing surgery to make sure all the damage is seen.

If you have not had a fracture, avoid walking on the injured ankle. Your doctor will probably recommend some physical therapy and that you keep your ankle taped.

If the ankle is still painful or stiff after three weeks, your doctor may inject with the above-mentioned remedies.

Bone Spurs in the Ankle

Bone spurs in the front or back of the ankle can be a source of pain when you move your ankle. For example, a bone spur on the back of the heel (posterior spur) is painful for jumpers, dancers, and basketball players when they raise up on the ball of the foot (plantarflexion). Bone spurs will hurt when running, standing on the ball of the foot, and wearing high-heels. The big toe will hurt, too, because of secondary damage to the flexor tendon. Pulling the foot towards the body (dorsiflexion) causes pain in the front of the ankle from an anterior (front) spur. See Fig. 10-8.

Spurs are formed from either tension on the bone or compression on the bone. With tension, the bone is pulled by a muscle, ligament or tendon. As the bone is being pulled, it begins to grow in the direction of the tension. With compression, the bone is pressured by a another bone. Tension or compression bone spurs are caused by trauma, such as sudden, severe stretching. This is usually within the Achilles tendon where it attaches to the heel bone. The *os trigonum* may also be fractured (pulled off). See Fig. 10-8.

Multiple ankle sprains eventually cause spurs. An ankle sprain tears a tissue, causing microscopic bleeding, which calcifies and becomes a bone spur. Therefore, to prevent formation of these spurs, it's necessary to flush out blood and inflammation products from tissue with physical therapy, movement or massage.

A foot that has been in an abnormally stretched position in a cast for a long time can form tension spurs. Usually, a foot hangs down while it's in a cast. This pulls on the bone, causing a tension spur. In addition, cartilage shrinks from immobility, producing an arthritic condition which leads to spurs. If possible, use a removable cast to allow gentle motion in the injured part, according to the tolerance of pain and the strength of your damaged tissue.

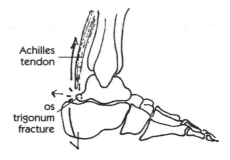

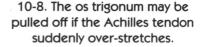

10-8. The os trigonum may be pulled off if the Achilles tendon suddenly over-stretches.

Outpatient Surgery to Remove Spurs

Jack came to me with pain in the ankle which I diagnosed as an anterior (front of ankle) impingement spur. A year before, he had fallen off his bicycle, fractured his leg badly and had to have surgery. He had been immobilized with a non-ambulatory cast for six weeks, with his foot mildly plantarflexed (pointing down). After that he had been in a walking cast for four weeks, followed by eight weeks of physical therapy. At the end of this lengthy recovery, he could walk all right, but he still had stiffness in the front of his ankle.

Now, a year later, his stiffness was worse, and x-rays revealed the anterior tension spur that had resulted from his time in the casts.

The solution for Jack was arthroscopy. I gave him *Aconite* to relax before the surgery and a local anesthesia to stop pain. There was a stand-by anesthesiologist in case Jack needed it. I made very small incisions in the heel, and the arthroscope, which has a tiny TV camera the size of a pencil eraser in it, allowed me to find and remove the bone spur. Jack watched it all on color TV! Five weeks later, he had no pain, and began gradually to resume walking and running.

Compression spurs are caused by bone hitting bone. This pressure causes excessive bone growth and calcium deposits. For example, if you're a lineman on a football team (with your foot always forced up against your ankle), you may develop a spur in the ankle—a condition called the "nutcracker syndrome."

Spurs grow and begin to limit the motion in the ankle joint, which is called impingement. A bone spur in the front of the ankle is called an anterior impingement; in the back of the ankle, it's a posterior impingement (*os trigonum* or posterior shelf). To treat bone spurs, first get an x-ray to determine if a bone spur is present. It may be that you suffered an injury six months to a year ago, but the numbness and pain only began recently with increased activity or mild re-injury.

Surgery is generally indicated for bone spurs. Arthroscopy is a non-traumatic out-patient procedure which works well if you can find a sports specialist who is trained in the use of the arthroscope. While arthroscopy is preferable because you may not need a general anesthetic and incisions are small, *some* bone spurs may only be operated on with traditional open surgery.

During healing select one of the following homeopathic remedies. Take four times a day in doses ranging from 6, 12, 15 or 30 until better:

Rhus Tox if worse initial motion; if there is stiffness that gets better with continued motion; if much, much better warmth.

Ruta Grav if there is initial stiffness in walking which gradually gets better with motion; if too much motion makes you feel tired and cranky; if better warm but not as much better as *Rhus Tox*.

Check for biomechanical imbalances with your podiatrist or sports specialist.

Fracture Within the Ankle Joint (Osteochondral Injury)

Sometimes small fractures of bone (osteo) or cartilage (chondral) are not seen in the initial diagnosis of ankle injury. They may show up six to eight months later on x-ray. Fractures may have a small bone chip floating in the ankle joint.

To treat a fracture within the ankle joint, a physician will remove bone chips with an arthroscope or by open surgery.

To enhance healing of the joint, select one of the following homeopathic remedies in potencies of 6, 12, 15 or 30 four times a day:

Arnica for the first 24 hours (post operative).

Ruta Grav following *Arnica*, once a day for two to fourteen days.

Lymphomyosot injection or drops can be used if there is substantial swelling. Take ten drops three times a day until the swelling subsides.

Traumeel ointment can be rubbed onto the incision.

Calcarea Phosphorica, a single 1M dose after two weeks to enhance recovery.

Calcarea Fluorica, one dose same as above.

Arthritis and Severe Ankle Joint Damage

Arthritis (inflammation of a joint) can occur many years after damage to the cartilage in the ankle joint. X-rays will show changes in the bones and loss of a smooth outline. Arthritis may occur gradually without any serious pain, or may cause stiffness, pain and swelling. See Chapter 17 on arthritis.

Footnotes:

1. Fig. 10-5. Types of Inversion Ankle Strains was adapted from a drawing from *Sports Injuries: A Self-help Guide,* V. Grisogono.

2. Fig. 10-6. Types of Eversion Ankle Strains, *ibid.*

Chapter 11

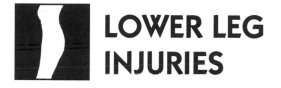

LOWER LEG INJURIES

... he runs with almost no effort, as a shadow flits and drifts and
darts. There is no gathering of muscle for an extra lunge. There is
only the effortless, ghostlike, weave and glide upon effortless legs ...
—Grantland Rice describing Red Grange on the football field.

Structure and Function of the Lower Leg

The two bones of the lower leg bear the regal latin names of tibia and
fibula. The tibia, the main weight-bearing bone, is the hard ridge you feel
in the front of the leg. It has little protective muscle or fat covering and
is vulnerable to trauma (especially in
field sports) and to overuse injuries
like stress fractures. Alongside the
tibia, at the outside of the leg, is the
thinner fibula which serves mainly as
a lever for muscle attachments. It only
moves in conjunction with the knee
and the ankle. See Fig. 11-1.

In the front of the leg, the anterior tibial muscles move the toes and
ankle upwards. The muscles which
turn the foot inward are behind the
tibia where the leg is fleshier. Those
which turn the foot outward, the peroneals, are behind the fibula.

In the back of the leg, the largest
muscle of the calf (gastrocnemius)
lies just behind the knee and runs
down the back of the leg. The other

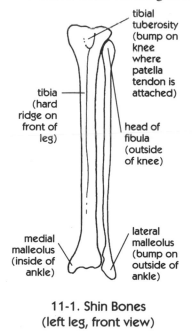

11-1. Shin Bones
(left leg, front view)

213

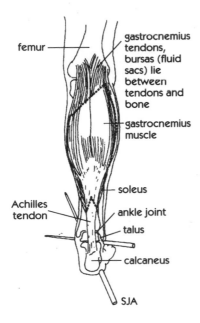

femur

gastrocnemius tendons, bursas (fluid sacs) lie between tendons and bone

gastrocnemius muscle

soleus

Achilles tendon

ankle joint

talus

calcaneus

SJA

11-2. Right Leg (back view)

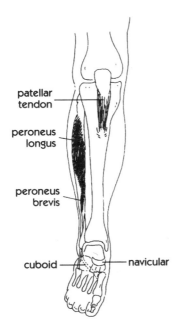

patellar tendon

peroneus longus

peroneus brevis

cuboid

navicular

11-3. Right Leg (front view)

major muscle, soleus, is attached to the back of the leg bone and lies just under gastrocnemius, feeding into the Achilles tendon. See Fig. 11-2. Gastrocnemius and soleus contract to pull the heel back and up when you point your toes down or stand on your toes. They allow you to walk, run, jump, and hop. They also help you to bend the knee against resistance, for example, when doing hamstring curls with weights. Soleus does not affect your knee.

There are several important tendons in the lower leg. There are the hamstring tendons—those hard cords you feel in the back of the knee—and adductors, which pull the thigh-bone inward. The patellar tendon at the end of the thigh muscle (quadriceps) straightens the knee, and is attached to the bump on the knee (tibial tuberosity). See Fig. 11-3. The Achilles tendon is very thick and very powerful (see Fig. 11-2). It is connected to the middle of the back of your heel and is separated from the upper part of the bone by a small sac of fluid (bursa) which allows friction-free movement.

Many of the foot movements involve co-ordinated action between different groups of tendons. Lower leg tendons are protected by an enclosing sac of synovial fluid to ensure free movement.

The lower leg can be injured in four main areas: the front (anterior), the back (posterior), and the inner (medial) and outer (lateral) sides.

General Pain in the Front of the Shin

Although most sports injuries are the result of the accumulation of long-term stress, sometimes a pain indicates a serious internal or medical problem. If shin pain develops gradually, the cause could be a circulatory disease, a referred back pain, or—in very rare cases—a bone tumor. More likely, however, the pain is caused by an overuse injury.

If you have general pain in the front (anterior) of the shin, keep a record of when and how the pain developed so that you can give your doctor an accurate account of its progression. Meanwhile, don't continue to run through the pain. Alternate days of walking and running. Avoid running fast.

Listen for a heavy foot slap when you run. The muscles in the front of the leg may be weak and need strengthening. Avoid running downhill, and don't overstride. Check your shoes for excessive wear in the back of the heel which indicates overstriding which is common with shin splints in the front of the leg. Also check your shoes for signs of pronation or the inward collapse common with posterior medial shin splints. Pronation may also happen with shin splints in the front of the leg.

Consult your sports medicine specialist for x-rays and lab tests to rule out a medical cause of the problem. Have a biomechanical diagnosis.

Shin Splints (Front and Inside of Lower Leg)

Shin splints, sometimes called tendinitis, means pain in the lower leg which worsens during exercise or running. Shin splint syndrome, whether on the front or on the inside of the leg, is a catchall term for pain in the muscles or tendons, the covering of the bone, or the bone itself.

There are two types of shin splint syndromes. The first and most common is called posterior medial shin splint syndrome which occurs on the inside of the leg. The second is called anterior shin splint syndrome and occurs in the front of the leg. Both are caused by virtually the same conditions.

The tendons or muscles in the shin may fray, much like an old rope. They often heal with gristle-like, inflexible scar tissue. The pain worsens when you run on hard surfaces, run too fast for the conditioning of your muscles, or run too far for the endurance level of your training. The faster you run, the more impact and shock your legs must absorb.

Particularly vulnerable are young women on college and high school track teams, who may not be, initially, in as good shape as the men. They may have slacked off during summer vacation and started running again too far too soon. Sometimes a coach will push a young athlete too hard. Young men and women may not want to admit to any pain when they are training, in an attempt to please their coaches, who have a tendency to become father figures to younger athletes.

Shin splints are very common in jumping sports such as high-impact aerobics and basketball, as well as in ballet and gymnastics. Overstriding and downhill running often produce shin splints.

Posterior medial shin splints

Shin splints on the inner side of the leg hurt when the heel hits the ground while walking fast or running. Posterior medial shin splints (Fig. 11-4) also hurt when the inner side of the calf is pressed about four fingers above the inside ankle bone. The pain may extend up the side of the leg about the width of a hand. Shin splints usually cover a broad area. If your pain is concentrated at only one point, you are more likely to have a stress fracture.

With posterior medial shin splints, you have strained the posterior tibial tendon that at-

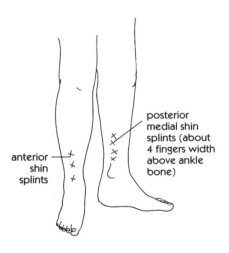

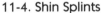

11-4. Shin Splints

taches to the arch of the foot. The main function of this tendon is to slow you down (as the foot hits the ground) and to control the amount of pronation (flattening) of your arch. The most common causes of medial shin splints are:
- Over-pronation (inward turning of the foot when running).
- Overstriding.
- Running on hard surfaces.
- Changing from a relatively softer running surface to a harder surface.
- Mileage increases.
- Seasonal training when competitive athletes go onto the track.

Case History of Posterior Medial Shin Splints

Joan Sutherland was a forty-two-year-old woman who was running 4 miles five days a week. When I saw her, she had been running for about a year and a half, and had just increased her mileage to five and six mile runs to prepare for a 10 K race (6.2 miles).

She complained of pain on the inside of the right leg about five fingers above the inner ankle bone. The pain covered a broad area about the width of three fingers.

"I have an aching pain when I first start to run," she said, "then it goes away. After about an hour of running it comes back as more of a sharp pain." She'd had the pain for about a month already, and it was getting to the point where she couldn't run at all. She had pain now even with walking. It was worse when the weather was cold and damp. She said it felt better with a heating pad.

I took x-rays which were negative for stress fracture. The tuning fork test did not cause a sharp pain which would have indicated a stress fracture. When I held her foot and asked her to push in, she had some pain which indicated an inflammation of the posterior tendon but no rupture.

Biomechanically she had excessive pronation with about five degrees of forefoot varus (moderately flat-footed and slightly knock-kneed). As I continued to examine her she told me, "I hope I'll still be able to run. It's become really important to me. I've never looked better, you know. I'm so much more trim from running. And the other thing is, I need to run to deal with the stress from my job."

My diagnosis was medial shin syndrome with posterior shin splints and periostitis (inflammation of the covering of the bone). I gave her a neoprene sleeve for support during the healing process. In addition, I gave her temporary orthotics for her shoes, and casted her for permanent ones since she was determined to keep running and would need them. I gave her the homeopathic remedy *Ruta Grav* since she had the indications for that remedy: she was worse with cold and damp, better when warm. She was also restless, but if she walked too much she hurt (a key symptom for *Ruta Grav*). *Ruta Grav* is also indicated for problems in the bone covering (periosteum).

During the recovery process, I put her on physical therapy with electro-galvanic stimulation. To keep in shape while healing, she rode an exercise bike and swam for about two weeks. About three weeks later, she was much better and was able to do a walk/jog program. At that time I gave her a single 1M dose of *Calc Phos*. After four weeks she started building up her running mileage, and was fine after that.

To treat shin splints on the inside of the lower leg, wrap the lower leg in an icy towel after running. If heat feels better, use a heating pad (wrapped in a towel to protect skin from burning). Elevate the leg on a chair with a pillow for temporary relief. Take *Arnica* for initial pain and swelling. If you don't have homeopathic remedies for pain and swelling, use aspirin, Advil or Tylenol. Check with your doctor if you are taking any other drugs for conditions such as stomach irritation, heart disease, high blood pressure or kidney problems. Always take these drugs with food. However, don't use these drugs to mask the pain in order to continue to run through the pain or do any other activity that may damage your leg or cause pain.

See your doctor as soon as you can. Take x-rays to rule out stress fracture or the possibility that a piece of bone was pulled off (avulsion fracture). To test further for stress fracture, do a tuning fork test or a bone-scan. A tuning fork will cause pain in one particular area if there is a stress fracture.

After diagnosis, take homeopathic remedy (potency 6, 12, 15, or 30 four times a day for two weeks):

Ruta Grav which is the number one remedy for shin splints.
After two weeks take *Calc Phos*—a single dose of 1M. This remedy is especially helpful for young, growing girls who have shin splints.

Massage leg for 10 minutes twice a day. Use a heating pad—set to *low,* never high, at bedtime or during evening.

Walk or run on grass or a soft surface. Substitute cycling and swimming for running. Do stretching exercises, such as wall pushups, to stretch the calf. Strengthen inner leg muscles (posterior tibial) by walking on the outside of the feet and walking on the toes. Don't resume full activity until completely healed—from two to four months.

Check with a podiatrist about orthotics. Most people with shin splints need orthotics for excessive pronation. Also check your shoes for sufficient shock-absorbing capacity. A compression bandage such as a neoprene sleeve helps hold the muscle closer to the bone. With shin splints the muscle tends to get pulled away from the bone. Some coaches and trainers tape the leg for support, and may tape the feet with the same effect as an orthotic.

Anterior shin splints

Anterior shin splints (see Fig. 11-4) often happen to athletes at the beginning of track season when they return to the track after having run outside on softer trails.

To treat shin splints in the front of the lower leg, refer to above section for posterior medial shin splints as treatment is virtually the same as for anterior shin splints.

Stretch the muscles in the *back* of the leg by using a Flex-wedge (exercise aid) or by doing wall push ups. Check to see that your toes are not bent and clutching like fingers (hammer toes). If you do have hammer toes, put a small roll of padding under your three middle toes to give them something to grab onto. Wrap gauze around the rolls to hold them in place or get ready-made ones, called crest pads, from your podiatrist.

Check shoes for cushioning and wear patterns. Put the shoes on the table and make sure the heels are perpendicular to the table surface. If the shoe is rolled in or out, you may have a problem; a heel lift may help.

Also check running posture. Weight should be over your hips— don't lean forward or overstride. Shorten your stride when walking and running and *slow down*. Shin splints are a common problem in walkers. If you are exercise walking and have pain in the front of the shin, you are walking too fast. Your muscles are not yet developed sufficiently for faster walking. Check your arch support or foot orthotic with the help of your podiatrist.

Chronic, severe shin splints that happen every track season may require surgery. Surgery consists of releasing the fascial sheaths around the muscle and stripping the muscle from the bone. This is a fairly uncomplicated procedure. You can expect to heal in five to six weeks.

Shin Splint Syndrome in a Professional Athlete

Susan Lakshaw, a twenty-five-year-old professional triathlete, came to me complaining of shin splints, pain in her knee, and pain over her hip. She was, understandably, concerned about the pain as she makes her living competing in sports events. Video analysis of her running on a treadmill showed she pronated too much (her foot rolled inward). She also had a long second toe (Morton's foot) and a weak arch.

I gave her foot orthotics, but she developed yet another problem—this time a pain in the midfoot (near the cuboid bone). After analysis I found that, during running, the foot orthotic was providing too much correction which went unnoticed while she was merely standing on the orthotic or running slowly. I modified the foot orthotic, and from then on she had no problem in her training. This case underscores the need to be evaluated *while running* for complete diagnosis.

During treatment, while I was solving her particular shin splint problem, Susan began using high-potency *Arnica* before and after races. She also used *Rhus Tox* for stiffness in the Achilles tendon, iliotibial band, and plantar fascia after exercising. Susan was quite thrilled to have the aid of these safe, natural remedies for her sports activities. She told me she felt much more "in charge" of her own recovery and continuing health.

Shin Pain from Tibial Stress Fractures

Stress fracture is always related to an increase or change in an activity involving repetitive movements and impact. You may be susceptible to this injury if your running style is biomechanically faulty—for example, if you turn your foot inward as you run. Also, if you run pulling your foot up hard, as you do when running uphill, stress is created from the muscles pulling against the bone. Running on a banked surface, as well, creates abnormal strains to the shin.

At no time should you ever make a sudden change in the amount of any repetitive exercise you do. You must allow your body time to adjust to any training changes. Never re-start a training schedule at the same level you stopped it. You must start again in slow stages. Since stress fractures are a result of increased work load on unprepared muscles and bone, it is necessary to strengthen and stretch anterior, posterior, medial, and lateral lower leg muscles to prevent injury (see Chapter 15 on exercises).

The pain of a stress fracture may start out as a mild ache after exercising. You might try to ignore it and keep running through it every day. However, you'll find that the pain gradually gets worse to the point that it hurts to walk, or even when you're in bed. If you rest a few days, the pain may ease up, allowing you to keep running, but it's better to stop running before the pain interferes with your daily activities.

Bone scans are the best way to identify the stress fracture. X-rays won't show actual stress fracture damage until three weeks later. The old saying is "If in doubt, treat it as a stress fracture."

If you think you have a stress fracture, your physician can do a simple test with a tuning fork. If the vibration creates a tenderness in

---

Early Warning of Stress Fracture

There is a phase just before a stress fracture called "stress reaction of bone," which shows up on a bone scan as tiny cracks. If you can catch the overuse injury at this stage, and stop running, you can prevent a stress fracture or a full-blown fracture.

Shin splints are the very first sign of stress reaction of bone, occurring on the front of the leg (anterior shin splints) or, occurring on the side (posterior medial shin splints). Listen to the early warning signs and reduce your exercise program.

---

one point, it's usually a stress fracture. If the pain is diffuse over a large area, it's not a stress fracture. A bone scan will show a stress fracture or an inflammation of the covering of the bone (periostitis).

To treat a stress fracture, rest the leg for at least four weeks by avoiding weight-bearing activities that cause pain. It takes six weeks for bone to heal. Don't run, jump or walk too far. Substitute cycling or swimming for high-impact running or exercise.

Homeopathic remedies (ask your doctor for correct dose) to enhance healing are (take in sequence indicated):

Ruta Grav. Take first for inflammation of the covering of the bone (periostitis). Then take *Symphytum* for two weeks; then either *Calc Fluor* or *Calc Phos* (see details of remedies in next section on contusions).

Trauma to the Shin

A hard blow to the shin can damage the covering of the tibia (periosteum) causing a big, tender bruise (periosteal hematoma). A very hard blow can damage or crack the shin bone. The skin may or may not be broken.

Basic first aid for shin trauma—bruise (contusion)

Use this first aid procedure for all lower leg injuries. Call the doctor as soon as first aid has been done.

- Rest from all painful activity after an injury.
- Ice. Apply a refrigerated towel, an ice pack (or a bag of frozen peas) wrapped in a towel. To prevent ice burn, do not put ice or frozen food directly on the skin. Ice your injury 20 minutes on the hour, or until the swelling and pain subside. Do this three

or four times a day. For most people, ice treatment reduces pain and swelling. However, if ice *increases* the pain, then try a heating pad (set to *low,* never high). In this case, your homeopathic remedy would be *Bellis* instead of *Arnica.*

- If ice alone is not effective, another possible treatment is to alternate hot and cold applications.
- Elevation. Keep your foot higher than your hip or heart. Prop the leg on a pillow or soft chair. To minimize swelling, don't sit or stand with your foot on the floor. Keep the leg on pillows even in bed if you can sleep comfortably.
- Be sure your tetanus vaccination is up-to-date if you've broken the skin.
- To clean out wounds: If your skin is broken, clean out with hydrogen peroxide or wipe off with rubbing alcohol. Then clean again with Betadine and apply *Calendula* solution or ointment. To keep ointment in place on injury, cover with a piece of gauze and then apply Saran Wrap. Other ointments for wounds are: *Arnica* ointment. This should *not* be used on open wounds as it tends to cause irritation; *Symphytum* ointment for an open wound or abrasion; *Traumeel* ointment; *Hamamelis* for bruising, or if the contusion has worsened an already existing condition of varicose veins; Neosporin, a conventional anti-bacterial ointment.
- For infection, see a doctor.

Stage One remedies (first 24 hours) for injuries:
- Shock of injury:

    Arnica—any dose on hand every 4 hours for 24 hours or until better.
- Pain, bruising and swelling. Take one of the following remedies in potencies of 6, 12, 15, 30 or higher every 4 hours for 24 hours or until better:

    Arnica if very sore, achy, bruised feeling; cold pack tends to feel better than warm on injury. Take *Sulphuric Acid* if *Arnica* was given first and did not produce results in 4 to 6 hours; if the injury is black and blue and very sore; if feeling hurried, rushing around accomplishing nothing (aimless hurriedness); cold and chilly; worse with cold packs or ice. Take *Bellis* if *Arnica* was given first and did not produce results in 4 to 6 hours if there is bruising with deep, intense pain; if worse with cold and much better with heat; cannot bear to be touched.

You may also take NSAIDs—Advil, Motrin, or other non-steroidal anti-inflammatory drugs, but not if you have ulcers, as these drugs affect the stomach lining.

During recovery from a contusion (bruise) or wound, don't resume your sport until bruising and swelling are gone. Use padding for protection from further injury. If you notice swelling over the shin after two or three days, don't rub the leg. Apply ice twice a day or more.

Take Stage Two homeopathic remedies after initial pain and swelling have been reduced (24 hours to four or five days), select one of the following remedies in doses of 6, 12, 15, 30 or 200 once a day for three to four days or until better.

Rhus Tox if worse with initial motion; if injury feels better with continued movement; much better warm. *Ruta Grav* if injury feels worse with rest, but weak, tired and cranky after too much movement.

Take Stage Three remedies two weeks after injury to enhance healing. These remedies are prescribed according to your individual constitution. To improve the accuracy of your selection, you may want to consult several of the *Materia Medica* listed in the Resource Guide at the end of the book.

Symphytum—one dose daily for two weeks, then go to one of the *Calcarea Salts*. If you are uncertain about which fits you best, take *Calc Phos*. Select one and take in a potency of 6 or 12 twice a day for a month:

Take *Calcarea Arsenicum* if prone to be fastidious; refined in nature; restless; if you tend to be always hurried; if overly concerned about your welfare—like to have someone go to the doctor with you; if you have a tendency to sip fluids in small amounts.

Take *Calcarea Carbonicum* if you are stout, hard-working but tire easily; have fair hair, blue eyes; if you sweat easily; are easily chilled; if you feel better with warmth; better lying on the injury; worse in the morning.

Take *Calcarea Fluorica* if you tend to be warm and hurried; easily depressed or have a fear of financial ruin while injured; have a big appetite.

Take *Calcarea Phosphorica* if you are tall, lanky or stocky; young and growing rapidly; if you tend to be a thirsty person; tend to be anxious and constantly complaining; may moan during sleep; sympathetic to others.

Take *Calcarea Silica* if you tend to be sickly; have frequent colds and sore throats; lack stamina; are frequently chilly; a yielding type.

Take *Calcarea Sulphuricum* if you tend to be large (can be slender); are a philosophical, absent-minded professor type; sweaty hands and feet; tend to be warm and prefer cooler weather.

- Injection therapy may help following trauma, during recovery and after surgery. Your physician may inject acupuncture points, joints, periosteum (bone covering), muscles or ligaments to enhance and speed up healing. Injection possibilities are:

    Traumeel for trauma.

    Zeel for joint problems.

    Rhus Tox for stiffness and achiness; if worse on initial motion; better with continued motion.

    Ruta Grav for stiffness; worse with too much motion; cranky.

    Lymphomyosot for swelling.

- Physical therapy—daily if possible; at least three times a week. Try ice whirlpool (first 24 to 48 hours), electrical stimulation and Ultrasound.

- Contrast baths (alternating very hot water and ice water) help to clear congestion and recharge the battery of the cells, stimulating healing.

- Your physician will give you air splints or suggest crutches if necessary.

- To stay in shape while healing from shin trauma, substitute swimming, cycling, and non-impact aerobic activity to rest your injury for up to four to six weeks. Continue flexibility exercises (see Chapter 15).

- Flexibility and balance. Balance organisms (proprioceptors) in your ligaments have been damaged. Therefore, to re-establish proprioception, do the following:

    1. Foot flexion. As soon as pain permits (within hours), start flexing the injured foot. Describe the alphabet (from A to Z) with the tip of your foot. You can also practice picking up a towel or some marbles with your toes.

    2. Backwards and sideways walking. When you can bear weight on your foot, start balance exercises, and do them as part of your routine for at least six months. Any time you have hurt your foot or ankle, practice walking backwards and forwards, and to the right and left. If you play any team sport, you need

to practice running backwards, as you sometimes do in games.
3. Stork test. First, practice standing on both feet, eyes closed, with arms outstretched. When you can stand on the injured leg alone with your eyes closed and arms outstretched for one minute, you have succeeded in re-establishing your balance.

Resuming sport

Your bruise should heal, if properly treated, within eight weeks. Begin to build up your running *very slowly*. When no pain is felt, run 5 minutes and walk 5 for three sets (a 30-minute workout). In the next couple of days, run 10 minutes, walk 10 minutes. Then, a week later, increase the alternating sequence to 15 minutes. When you can run 45 minutes easily, you may begin the cyclic (progressive) training schedule described in Chapter 3. *Never* restart your program where you left off. Give yourself rest days in between running days.

Run, if at all possible, on grass or soft surfaces. Do figure-8 running. Weave back and forth in figure-8's, gradually decreasing the size of the loops. Don't do this exercise, unless you are fairly well healed. Check the cushioning of your shoes.

Alternative treatments following healing of shin trauma:

* Have therapeutic massage to wake up tissue and increase circulation. Massage also releases or prevents soft tissues from sticking (adhering) to bones, tendons or ligaments.
* Hypnotherapy may help find possible emotional causes of repeated leg problems.
* Therapeutic yoga is very good for flexibility and balance.
* T'ai Chi or dance therapy helps with balance and flexibility.
* Alexander technique, Heller work, Feldenkrais and Trager work may be beneficial for integration and enhancing of healing.

Pain When Pulling up the Foot
(Anterior Tibial Tendinitis)

If you draw your foot up hard against resistance and feel pain over the large cord on top of the ankle (anterior tibialis tendon), you have anterior tibial tendinitis. The tendon may feel sore to the touch. Putting the heel down hard (e.g., in bowling) can be painful if the tendon is inflamed. This tendon on the front of your shin works hard to decelerate. It keeps your foot from slapping the ground when you walk or run. Fast race walking, especially on hard surfaces, can cause this pain.

To treat anterior tibial tendinitis, first see your doctor. Don't run or walk if it causes pain. Rule out bone spurs with an x-ray.

After the pain has gone, begin to gently stretch the affected tendon, and work out with swimming. Don't keep running or doing your sport until you have regained pain-free flexibility.

After diagnosis, take homeopathic remedies (potency 6, 12, 15, or 30 four times a day for two weeks):

> *Ruta Grav* for stiffness and soreness. After two weeks take *Calc Phos*—a single dose of 1M. This is especially helpful for young, growing athletes.

Make sure your shoes don't have tight laces. Have regular massages, and ask your physical therapist about hydro therapy.

Warm compresses or a heating pad may help relieve minor pain.

Swelling or Numbness Within Lower Leg (Acute or Chronic Compartment Syndrome)
Acute Compartment Syndrome

Sudden pain and tightness in the front leg, especially with numbness between the first and second toe, means serious trouble. Swelling in the leg compartment that houses the muscles can cut off circulation to the leg. You may feel a crunching sensation underneath the tendons in the front of the ankle or foot when moving the foot up and down.

This is a medical emergency. Call your doctor immediately and tell him or her to meet you at the emergency room, or go directly to an emergency room.

To treat acute compartment syndrome:
- Ice immediately. Keep packed in ice on the way to the emergency room.
- Elevate leg.
- Do not put weight on leg while going to doctor's office.
- Don't try to drive yourself.
- Take one of the following homeopathic remedies:

> *Arnica* immediately. Use whatever dose you have on hand, and take every hour for the first 24 hours; *Bellis* if heat usually makes pain feel better; or *Sulphuric Acid* if *Arnica* does not produce improvement in 2 hours; *Cuprum* for violent, hard cramping; *Mag Phos* for less severe cramping.

Chronic Compartment Syndrome

If numbness in the front leg starts gradually after a few minutes of running, and happens every time you run, you have chronic compartment syndrome.

To treat chronic compartment syndrome:
- Ice for temporary relief.
- See your doctor for advice regarding surgery.
- Use homeopathic remedies listed above for acute compartment syndrome.

Case History of Chronic Compartment Syndrome

Sally Robinson, twenty-four, enjoyed running with her husband. She had been running for about two years. As she increased her mileage, she noticed a cramping sensation or pain in the front of her leg with firm swelling over the whole front of the leg. In addition, she occasionally felt a tingling sensation between her first and second toes. The tingling went away when she dropped down to a fast walk, but with running, the tingling returned.

When I observed her running on the treadmill in my office, swelling began after five minutes. She had chronic compartment syndrome. I explained that her muscle was like a salami in a sheath. When she ran, the muscle swelling was trapped within the sheath of her leg compartment. The cure, in Sally's case, was a simple surgical procedure to release the tough covering over the anterior tibial muscle. After seven weeks in a non-rigid cast, she slowly resumed running, and has had no trouble since.

What To Do For "Charley Horses"

These cramps often happen in bed at night following a day of more-than-usual exercise. Sometimes women will have these pains after walking on high heels all day. The toes curl up rigidly, and the foot or calf muscle spasms. Cramps are sometimes so severe as to wake you out of a sound sleep. Take homeopathic *Mag Phos* or *Cuprum Metallicum* for relief. For chronic cramping or twitching at night, have a homeopath do a constitutional evaluation.

Alexander's "Charley Horses"

Alexander, a sixty-four-year-old veteran of the Normandy invasion in World War II, came to me complaining of terrible cramping in the calves. "These cramps just come on out of nowhere," he said, "and they're so bad I just have to stop in my tracks. I get doubled over with the pain it hurts so much." As he was telling me the story, it happened right there in the chair.

The cramp was so violent, it was as if there was a fist in the muscle. I immediately got some homeopathic *Cuprum* (copper). I had him open his mouth, and dropped in one dose. All the cramping stopped. He knew nothing of homeopathy and was completely surprised at this quick result. Later, he told his friends, "It was the damnedest thing that ever happened to me." He continued to take *Cuprum* whenever a spasm would hit, but he seldom gets them anymore.

Night Cramps in Seniors

I've heard many complaints by my senior patients about night cramps. Many of them have been taking a conventional medicine, quinine sulfate, for cramping. When I've prescribed homeopathic *Magnesium Phosphate,* almost every one of them has said it works much better. Most of them have stopped using the quinine sulfate.

One dramatic case of homeopathic remedies curing cramps was Helen Goodman, a sixty-year-old patient from Aptos, California who walks for exercise. She complained of twitching and cramping of the legs which awaken her every hour during the night. She had suffered from this malady for twenty years. Nothing had helped.

I evaluated her circulation and nervous system, which were fine. After taking a homeopathic history, I found that she had had a death in the family about twenty years ago. Also at this time, she had moved to Aptos from Sacramento. In listening to her, it seemed that she had suppressed a lot of grief throughout her life. Her twitching and cramping had begun at the time of the death and the move. Interestingly enough, during this period she also suffered severe migraines.

The indications for a homeopathic remedy based on her personal characteristics (emotional reactions, living habits, type of personality, and food preferences) were for *Nat Mur* (homeopathic sea salt). As it happens, *Nat Mur* fit her personal characteristics and is also indicated for muscle twitching. I gave her one dose of *Nat Mur.* The next day, her husband called me. "We can't believe it! We're thrilled. Her cramping and twitching have completely gone away." However, there was one problem. "She had a very bad migraine this morning, though. What do you think of that?" he asked.

I prescribed *Bryonia,* and after that the migraines disappeared, and neither headache nor twitching has returned over a period of ten months.

There are several homeopathic remedies that may work for leg twitching and restless legs. Take in a potency of 6 or 12 once a day until twitching stops:

Nat Mur if you have twitching in the lower leg upon falling asleep; *Mercurius* for twitching that migrates from place to place; *Arsenicum* for twitching that wakes you up; *Coffea* for twitching when over-excited from exhilaration and excessive joy; *Nux Vomica* for twitching and restlessness with incessant thoughts of business or professional concerns; *Pulsatilla* for twitching with restlessness and obsessive worry; *Calcarea Salts* for restlessness with repetitive thoughts; *Mag Carb, Arsenicum, Chamomilla, Colchicum,, Kali Carb, Lycopodium, Zinc, Sepia,* and *Stramonium.* To differentiate these remedies, it will be necessary to consult with a homeopath or look for the characteristics in a *Materia Medica.*

Pain Caused by Shin Strain (Anterior Tibial Muscle Strain)

A sudden pull (or chronic overuse) of the anterior tibial muscle (front shin muscle) causes this pain. The injury is a result of a dynamic imbalance between weaker muscles in the front of the lower leg and stronger muscles in the back of the leg. For example, if you trip while running forward, your toes are caught and pulled downward. Running or jumping on awkward surfaces, or forcibly pushing off on your toes can also injure the front leg muscles. Another possibility is landing heavily on the heel and pulling the toes up hard during running. See Fig. 11-5.

If the muscles are imbalanced (e.g., through poor training), a sudden pulling can partially tear the front tibial muscle. The tear fills up with

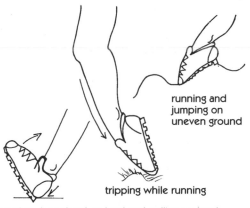

running and jumping on uneven ground

tripping while running

coming down hard on heel and pulling up hard

11-5. Anterior Tibial Muscle Strain

blood, and the blood becomes a gristle-like mass. This inflexible, rubbery mass in the muscle creates long-term stiffness and pain. Even when you do stretching exercises, the pain comes back after a period of inactivity. Injuries to muscles take a long time to heal.

To treat anterior tibial muscle strain, apply ice at least once a day for 10 to 20 minutes to reduce swelling and avoid development of compartment syndrome (numbness in the leg from muscle swelling).

Do a gentle foot press on the injured leg as follows:

- **If the strain is mild, and the pain is minimal,** kneel down, with the top of your foot underneath you flat on the floor. Gently sit back on your heels until you feel a pulling sensation. Hold to a count of ten. Do not force the movements, and do not bounce! Try to stretch the muscles at least six times, three times a day. Don't do this until your leg is fairly healed or free of pain.

Avoid painful activities. If your pain does not go away within a week, you may have the more serious problem of a stress fracture.

Try a deep massage (10 minutes twice a day until better) with *Traumeel* cream or *Arnica* ointment; if it's stiff, use *Rhus Tox.*

See a physical therapist for electrogalvanic stimulation over the involved area. He or she may suggest therapy three times a week for 10 minutes each time to stimulate the tissue. Your therapist can also try Ultrasound with electrogalvanic stimulation to disperse the scar tissue and encourage normal tissue to form instead.

Your physician may give you injections to break up scar tissue. I recommend a mixture of 1cc of Xylocaine (a local anesthetic); 1cc of Wydase (a softening enzyme); and one of the following homeopathic remedies:

Ruta Grav if stiff, sore, achy; fatigued from too much motion; *Rhus Tox* if stiff, sore; worse with initial motion; better after continued motion; tend to be restless;

Arnica if bruised; very sore, achy; cold pack eases pain; *Traumeel* for pain and swelling and trauma.

Take one of the following oral remedies (two doses of 12 or 30 twice a day until better):

Ruta Grav if it's stiff and sore, and you feel depressed about being injured; *Rhus Tox* if it's stiff and feels worse initially after resting, but gets better after moving around; worse with a cold pack, better with heat; you are restless; *Arnica* if leg is sore and feels bruised; *Bellis* if *Arnica* doesn't work; or *Sulphuric Acid* for deep bruising.

I do not recommend an injection of non-soluble cortisone because it may weaken surrounding healthy tissue. Cortisone deposits cause local irritation.

Do gentle exercise to strengthen the front shin muscles (anterior) and stretch the back calf muscles (posterior) twice a day for 10 minutes until better. This will correct the dynamic imbalance that has been created by overuse. For instance, when you run, you naturally strengthen the calf muscles as they repeatedly pull your foot up against gravity. The calf muscles are strengthened in the back and become proportionately tighter.

Pain on the Bump of the Knee (Tibial Tubercle)

You've just been squatting and lifting a very heavy weight and felt the knob of bone below your knee pull away from the shin (tibia). See Fig. 11-1. You may be, on the other hand, a long-distance runner who has accumulated stress in the lower leg by increasing your mileage, speed, or downhill running. Perhaps, in another instance, you were working out on the trampoline and did too many knee-drops—traumatizing the knee.

The pain is localized over the bone whenever you work your thigh muscles (quadriceps) under load—e.g., running, squatting, or kicking. You feel soreness if you press it or kneel on it. This damage to the tubercle, caused by repetitive tendon pulls, may be a stress fracture, bone bruise, bursitis or tendinitis. Since overuse caused the problem, rest will cure the problem. Various names for this condition are housemaid's knee, carpet-layer's knee or jumper's knee. If, of course there is a severe tearing or fraying in the tendon, then surgical repair is necessary.

For treatment of pain on the tibial tubercle, refer to Jumper's Knee in Chapter 12.

Pain in the Back of the Leg and Heel Cord (Pain in the Calf and Attachments to Leg)

Since this pain involves the Achilles tendon, please refer to the section on the Achilles tendon in Chapter 9 on the heel for full details.

Pain in the calf can be healed by stretching and strengthening exercises (see Chapter 15). Heat and soaking in a hot tub are usually helpful to release tight calf muscles.

For relief of pain or swelling use *Arnica,* 6, 12, 15, or 30 four times a day for two to three days or until better;

It will be necessary to strengthen muscles in the front of the leg. Use Flex wedges (special slanted wedges for stretching the lower leg and Achilles tendon).

Physical therapy or acupressure and deep tissue massage can be very helpful.

Pain on the Inner (Medial) Side of the Lower Leg

Refer to preceding section on shin splints for posterior medial shin splint syndrome.

Posterior Tibial Tendon Insufficiency

Posterior tibial tendon insufficiency is a form of posterior tibial tendinitis. Older people are susceptible because tendons are less strong and resilient as are people with too much pronation which biomechanically stresses and weakens the tendon. The posterior (back) tibial tendon may stretch, partially rupture or completely rupture spontaneously. This is a serious problem. Once the posterior tibial tendon has lost its strength or function, the arch quickly collapses. This is called a posterior tibial insufficient foot.

With this injury, you will not be able to raise up on the ball of the foot unassisted. *This is a medical emergency.* If the condition is not quickly corrected with a cast, brace, or surgery, arthritis may develop. You could become crippled within three to four months.

Alice Miller's Story

Alice, a fifty-seven-year-old woman, was 5'4" and weighed about 185 pounds. She had been walking about four miles a day every morning with a group of women. She was dieting and watching her weight, and enjoyed the firming and toning results of her walking program. One morning she stepped off a curb and noticed her arch started hurting.

After this incident, her foot became stiff each morning when she got up. It was hard for her to get around at first, but after walking around a while, the arch loosened up. However, the inside of her arch was swollen as well as painful, and the whole foot began to hurt. After waiting about a week, she came to see me because she couldn't walk anymore without great difficulty.

When I asked if she could raise up on the ball of her foot, she was unable do it on her injured foot without help. I concluded that she had partially ruptured her arch. An x-ray showed that her arch was already flattening significantly, and an MRI confirmed the partial rupture.

I put her in a removable cast for about four or five weeks, which allowed her to have physical therapy. After that I made her a special, strong orthotic. Since her discomfort continued, I finally had to repair the arch surgically after she healed.

To treat minor cases of posterior tibial tendon, wrap in an icy towel after running. Elevate the injured leg on a chair.

Take *Arnica* for initial pain and swelling or homeopathic *Sulphuric Acid* if *Arnica* doesn't help within 6 hours. If you don't have homeopathic remedies for pain and swelling, use aspirin, Advil or Tylenol. However, check with your doctor before taking if you are under any other medication for stomach irritation, heart disease, high blood pressure or kidney problems. Take with food, and don't use drugs to mask the pain in order to continue running or doing any other damaging activity.

Don't resume full activity until injury is completely healed—from two to four months. See a podiatrist for advice on orthotics. Most people with this problem will need orthotics.

Do wall pushups to strengthen and stretch the calf muscles.

Strengthen calf muscles by using an elastic band or old inner tube attached to a door knob. Sit in front of the door and pull the tubing towards the body. Pull and release ten times. Do three sets twice a day.

As in Alice's case, sometimes the tendon is damaged to the extent that surgical repair is necessary. In that case, surgery is preferable to continuing to use a damaged, non-healed tendon which can snap and fall completely apart.

Pain on the Outer (Lateral) Lower Leg (Peroneal Tendinitis)

This pain comes from walking fast or running on the crown of a road with a foot that is too turned-out (supinated). This causes pain in the peroneal tendon (Fig. 11-3). The peroneal tendon does most of the work in moving the foot towards the outside. Occasionally, this tendon is inflamed around the cuboid bone which may be out of place from a biomechanical stress. Peroneal tendons can become partially torn or ruptured in conjunction with bad sprains or strains and may need surgical repair. Fibular (the outside ankle bone) stress fractures are also sometimes associated with peroneal tendinitis.

To treat peroneal tendon pain, ice, rest, tape or bandage for support. A doctor may use manipulation to return the cuboid bone to its correct position. If there is a spasm and movement is not possible, a homeopathic injection may be necessary prior to manipulation. A cuboid pad or an orthotic helps keep the bone in place. If pain or swelling persists, have an x-ray or MRI to rule out tendon damage or stress fracture.

Select one of the homeopathic remedies below for pain, bruising and swelling. Take potencies of 6, 12, 15 or 30 once every 4 hours for 24 hours:

Arnica if very sore; bruised, achy; cold pack may numb the pain; *Sulphuric Acid* if *Arnica* helped some, but not as much as expected; *Bellis* every 4 hours for the next two to three days or until better, if *Arnica* was given first and did not produce results in 4 to 6 hours; there is bruising with deep, intense pain; worse with cold and much better with heat; cannot bear to be touched; *Bryonia* if you cannot move the injured foot or bear to have it touched; pressure makes it feel better; *Ledum* if injury feels cool to the touch (although it may be warm); better with a cold pack.

After initial pain and swelling have been reduced (24 hours to four or five days), take one of the following Stage Two remedies in potencies of 6, 12, 15, or 200 once a day for three to four days or until better:

Rhus Tox if it feels better with continued movement and warmth; *Ruta Grav* if it feels worse with rest or if there are torn ligaments; if it's better with motion; worse with too much motion; *Stellaria* if you can't decide if it feels better or worse with movement; *Phytolacca* if it feels worse with leg hanging down.

Take *Calc Phos*—a single 1M dose—after two weeks on either of the above remedies to enhance healing.

Pain in the Back of the Lower Leg

Pain in the Mid-Calf (Gastrocnemius or Soleus)

With this injury, you feel a small localized spot of pain in the back of the calf, especially after sprinting up stairs or after a sudden overstretching movement that may have torn the muscle or tendons. Another possible cause of pain in the calf muscles is uncommon stress during activities in which the knee is bent against strong resistance

234

(e.g., weight lifting with knee squats). This causes inflammation (bursitis) in a fluid-filled sac (bursa) under the tendon (Fig. 11-2).

The soleus muscle is usually the culprit in mid-calf pain. If you're a runner with short, bunchy, inflexible calf muscles (soleus and gastrocnemius), you will be less able to handle accumulated stress or a sudden pull in the leg. Soleus will tighten and become sore.

To prevent mid-calf injury to gastrocnemius and soleus muscles, do stretching exercises *as a weekly routine.* Wall pushups are effective for releasing the soleus. You can also push against the wall with flat feet, dip one knee slightly, and hold for five seconds. Repeat with other leg. A Flex Wedge is a great aid in leg exercises and stretches. It consists of two wedges with adjustable struts. When you stand on them, the leg is automatically stretched.

You can also insert a sponge rubber, Viscolas, Spenco or Sorbethane heel lift in running and regular shoes.

To treat mid-calf pain, apply refrigerated towel after running.

It may be helpful to use a heating pad at night (set to *low,* never high). Don't try to do stretching exercises until your pain has gone away. Rest if your leg continues to be painful. Don't run through this pain.

Select one of the following homeopathic medicines in potencies of 6, 12, or 30 four times a day for two days:

Arnica for soreness; *Bellis* if *Arnica* is not effective; *Sulphuric Acid* if there is deep bruising and intense pain.

After two days, select one of these remedies:

Ruta Grav if stiff and sore; *Rhus Tox* if stiff with initial motion, but continued motion makes it better.

Then take,

Cal Phos after *Rhus Tox* or *Ruta Grav* until fully recovered.

Have deep tissue massage 10 minutes a day until better with:

Topical *Arnica* or topical *Traumeel* cream.

Chapter 12

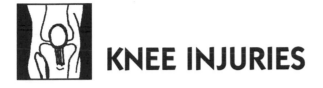 KNEE INJURIES

It went to pieces all at once—all at once and nothing first.
—Oliver Wendell Holmes.

The Structure and Function of the Knee

The knee is one of the largest joints in the body, and one of the biggest problems for runners and athletes. It is extremely vulnerable to traumatic injuries as well as to overuse injuries. About 30 percent of all running injuries occur to this joint.

The knee consists of three major components: thigh bone, shin bone and knee-cap. The bottom end of the thigh bone (femur) meets the top end of the shin bone (tibia), and is capped by the knee-cap (patella)—see Fig. 12-1a. At the end of the thigh bone are two rounded knuckles called condyles which match (although not perfectly) the receiving surface of the top of the shin bone.

The knee-cap (patella), a loose bone formed in the lower end of the quadriceps muscle group, sits atop the juncture of the thigh and shin bones. It slides over the thigh bone condyles during knee movements. Between the knee-cap and the thigh bone is a fluid-filled gap.

Another fluid-filled gap exists between the thigh and the shin bones. This gap actually consists of two compartments, one on the inner side and one on the outer side of the knee. The inner gap is called the medial meniscus; the outer gap is the lateral meniscus (Fig. 12-2). The two menisci are rubbery, elastic pads that buffer the junction of the two joint surfaces.

A special type of cartilage called articular is found only in bone ends that meet to form moving joints, and covers the bone surfaces in the knee. Articular cartilage is a functional part of the bone structure and is different from the knee cartilages (menisci). Articular cartilage

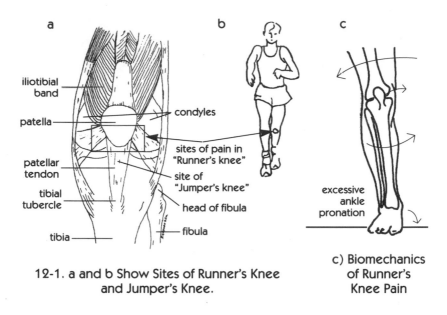

a

iliotibial band

patella

patellar tendon

tibial tubercle

tibia

b

condyles

sites of pain in "Runner's knee"

site of "Jumper's knee"

head of fibula

fibula

c

excessive ankle pronation

12-1. a and b Show Sites of Runner's Knee and Jumper's Knee.

c) Biomechanics of Runner's Knee Pain

is like teflon—once damaged, it doesn't repair itself. The cartilage will never be as good as it originally was, even with surgery. The joint capsule, the covering which encloses the joint, is lined with another kind of lubricating (synovial) membrane.

Ligaments and tendons play a big part in the control and stability of the knee. When you walk and run, the knee is stabilized by strong ligaments attached on either side. Ligaments in the back protect the knee, but do not function as major stabilizers. Within the knee joint, two strong ligaments (the cruciates), criss-cross each other to hold the joint together (Fig. 12-2). Once the cruciate ligaments are injured, the knee is unstable and will not support weight. The patellar tendon is the only tendon on the front of the knee; there are many more tendons on either side of the lower part of the knee. On the outer side of the knee lies a strong band called the iliotibial band, which links the outer hip muscles with the top of the shin bone, and which stands out as a firm long band when you straighten your knee (Fig. 12-3). This band gets a lot of use in repetitive movements; it is cushioned with fluid-filled sacs (bursas) which can become inflamed in over-use injuries.

The knee was built to operate with a backwards and forwards motion, exactly like a mechanical hinge. However, because it is part of the larger structure of the entire upper and lower leg, the knee not

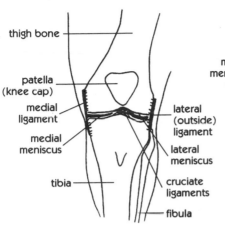

12-2. a) Left knee (front view)

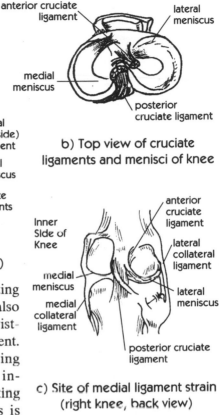

b) Top view of cruciate ligaments and menisci of knee

c) Site of medial ligament strain (right knee, back view)

only functions as a hinge permitting bending and straightening, but also allows the foot to rotate in a twisting movement when the knee is bent. For instance, when you are sitting down, you can turn your feet inwards and outwards without lifting your heels off the floor. This is achieved through rotation at the knee. If there are any biomechanical problems of misalignment, these complex movements may cause trouble over time.

The powerful hamstring muscles in the back of the thigh do the main work of bending the knee (Fig. 12-4). One of these muscles, the gastrocnemius, is working, for example, when you bend with resistance—as you do in weight lifting. The quadriceps muscles on the front of the thigh straighten your knee. These thigh muscles are prone to be weak-

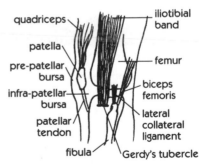

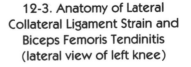

12-3. Anatomy of Lateral Collateral Ligament Strain and Biceps Femoris Tendinitis (lateral view of left knee)

er than the hamstrings because they don't resist gravity as much as your calf muscles do in pulling the leg back each time you walk or run.

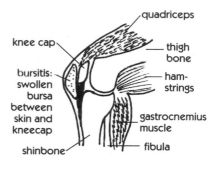

The knee joint is both very stable and very mobile. Its stability comes from the strong binding ligaments, as well as from the powerful thigh and hamstring muscles that control movement. On the other hand, the knee joint is mobile because the bones are not closely

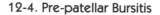

12-4. Pre-patellar Bursitis

bound. The knee, as stabilizer, helps us to stand, walk, and hop—absorbing shock when we jump. The knee, as mobile facilitator, also allows us to kneel, crouch or squat. We can perform many complex leg movements such as dancing, skiing, or staying atop a horse because of our knees.

If you have pain in your knee, determine if it occurs in the front (anterior) of the knee, outer side (lateral), inner side (medial), back (posterior), or within the joint itself. Check the list below to find the possible causes of knee pain.

1. Pain in the Front of the Knee:
    Runner's Knee
    Jumper's Knee
    Carpet-Layer's Knee (Pre-patellar Bursitis)
    Intra-articular Plica
2. Pain on the Outside (Lateral) of the Knee and Thigh:
    Iliotibial Band Syndrome
    Lateral Collateral Ligament Strain
    Tendinitis of Biceps Femoris
3. Pain on the Inner Side (Medial) of the Knee:
    Medial Ligament Strain
    Pes Anserinus Tendinitis
    Pes Anserinus Bursitis
4. Pain behind the Knee:
    Baker's Cyst
    Tendinitis of the Hamstrings, Calf, Gastrocnemius,
    Soleus, Popliteal
5. Pain within the Knee Joint
    Medial Meniscus Degeneration or Tearing

Lateral Meniscus Degeneration or Tearing
Cruciates Rupture
Chondromalacia
6. Pain From a Medical Condition
Arthritis
Gout
Infection

Injuries to the Front of the Knee

Knee-Cap (Patella) Pain—Runner's Knee

Runner's knee is the most common form of knee injury. Fancy names for this pain are patellar compression syndrome, mal-tracking of the patella, or chondralgia patella. They all mean pain on the front of the knee! Runner's knee happens to new runners, tennis players, basketball players, as well as to the veteran marathoner. It can even happen to exercise walkers.

You may feel this pain when you run—wondering what it is, wondering if it's going to get worse—probably deciding to run despite the ache. You may think you just didn't warm up enough, and you keep hoping it will disappear.

Runner's knee can also occur later in the day after a run. It may even crop up the next morning after a workout the day before. A characteristic symptom is that the knee gets stiff after being in one position too long, followed by a sharp pain upon standing erect. Squatting and kneeling, of course, make it worse, and the knees will probably feel worse running downhill or walking down stairs.

Runner's knee usually starts as an ache, becoming more severe over time. It's hard to define because it occurs intermittently and may not stem from a sudden injury (although direct injury is also a cause). There may be some swelling around the knee-cap, and a grinding sensation (crepitation) under the knee-cap.

If you have had a slow onset of pain in the knee, think about how you've been running or exercising. Have you been running on a banked surface? Have you increased mileage dramatically? Have you been running hills a lot or doing speed work? Have you changed shoes lately? Do you need to replace shoes? If the pain started almost as soon as you began running, it's probably a problem in the knee itself unless your alignment is really off.

If the pain started after you've been running a while, it's proba-

241

Self-Test For Runner's Knee

You can do your own examination if you suspect you have runner's knee. Have a friend help you. Sit down in a chair and stretch one leg out straight, supporting the foot on another chair in front of you. Now have your friend squeeze your extended leg just above the knee. As she squeezes, she should push the outside of the knee-cap towards the center of the knee with her other hand. As she pushes, tighten your thigh muscle. If you have pain when you do this, you've got runner's knee.

Runner's knee can be treated fairly simply as long as you work on correcting the weaknesses or imbalances that are pulling your knee out of alignment.

---

bly caused by a foot imbalance. Foot problems such as a weak arch or excessive pronation are the main cause of runner's knee because the abnormal strains pull the knee-cap off its tracks (mal-tracking of the patella). See Fig. 12-1c. The re-surfacing of an old knee injury is also likely to happen after you've been running awhile.

To determine what might be causing your knee pain, have a friend watch you while you run, checking for a pronation problem (rolling inwards of the leg, knee or foot). Also, review the check list on running form in Chapter 2. Remember, in running, the foot lands under a bent and flexed knee, which is more susceptible to instability. As long as your foot is pointing straight ahead and under the knee, the hinge joint will be working fine. However, if the foot toes in or out, the knee will be abnormally rotated. Abnormal rotation of the knee, which can be caused by other imbalances in the leg as well as the foot, causes the knee-cap to be pulled off the ends of the thigh bone knuckles (condyles). When the knee-cap does not ride smoothly over the condyles, or when it rides to the outside, you experience the pain of runner's knee.

If you have one leg shorter than the other (either actually shorter or functionally shorter), you tend to rotate the short leg to the outside (toe-out) as an unconscious way of increasing stability. This rotation causes the knee-cap to be less stable and to receive more force.

Particularly susceptible to runner's knee are people built with a wide pelvis. The wide pelvis rotates the thigh bones inwards, thus creating more rotation in the knee itself.

Case History of Runner's Knee

A perfect example of runner's knee caused by a wide pelvis is Susan Power, a thirty-eight-year-old runner and tennis player.

She is an executive in the real estate business, and a hard-driving Type A personality—characteristic of many of my running patients.

Her initial complaint included aching pain under both knee-caps with stiffness in her knees after periods of rest. She had pain after thirty minutes of sitting with her knees bent which got worse when she stood up. Also, going up and down stairs was painful, particularly after a long tennis match or after about 6 miles of running.

In addition to the knee pain, she had achiness in both arches of the feet. When I examined her, there was the characteristic grinding, sandpapery sensation (crepitation) in the knee joint.

Susan's wide pelvis created a slight knock-kneed effect, and when I video-taped her running on the treadmill, I saw that both feet rolled inwards when she ran (excessive pronation). Tight hamstrings and tight inner thigh muscles also caused the thighs to rotate inwards, creating a compensatory outward foot angle (pronation) that, of course, made the problem worse.

Susan's case is a good example of the many aspects of treatment of runner's knee:

- She was x-rayed to rule out arthritis or cartilage damage (chondromalacia).
- Orthoses. Two different pairs of temporary orthotics were made to correct the over-pronation of her feet. A running orthotic was made with rearfoot and forefoot control. For tennis, which requires that she be able to rotate and move from side to side, I made a flexible foot support with no rearfoot control.
- Shoes. For running, she needed new shoes since her old ones were much too run down. I recommended buying a running shoe that would fit her type of foot—one with a straight last which also controls excessive pronation and provides good rearfoot control.
- Exercises for strength. She was given exercises to strengthen her thigh muscles (quadriceps), especially the inner thigh muscles (vastus medialis).
- Exercises for balance. She was instructed to balance on one foot and bend her knee to an angle of thirty-five degrees, and then come up to a straight knee position twenty times, twice a day.

243

This is an *eccentric* quadriceps strengthening exercise which means that she was strengthening the muscle as it was elongating.

- Alternate sport. I recommended that she play tennis doubles with a good volley partner (to minimize running) rather than the more strenuous singles. Yoga would help stretch her muscles and open her to the quieter aspects of movement, and I suggested she take a class.

- Homeopathic remedies. She was first given homeopathic remedy *Ruta Grav* for soreness and stiffness, and two weeks later, *Rhus Tox* for stiffness after rest. To finish the healing process, I gave her a single 1M dose of *Calcarea Phosphorica* for bone and cartilage strengthening.

- Biofeedback. After a few weeks of strengthening the thigh muscles, she still tested weak in the muscle, so I used biofeedback electronic stimulation to get better results from her workout. To help her re-establish the mind-body connections in the thigh, she contracted her inner thigh muscles (vastus medialis) as she was having electro-stimulation.

- Running form. She was instructed on the treadmill to correct over-rotation and wobbling at the hips. I suggested Alexander work to help her with structural re-alignment.

- Running patterns. Later, she did some varied terrain running for flexibility.

- Health regained. Within two months, Susan told me she felt much better in her knee, with pain only when she overdid exercise. She was very pleased with the results of the exercises, physical therapy and foot supports. In particular, she told me she was thrilled to have a general increase in energy which she attributed directly to the homeopathic remedies.

What to do for runner's knee

As you can see, a "simple" pain in the knee can bring big challenges and major changes in your activities and sports program. The following are recommendations for a variety of treatments that will aid your full recovery from runner's knee:

- For temporary relief. Ice. Apply an ice pack wrapped in a towel for ten minutes. You can also use a refrigerated towel. Rest ten minutes, then repeat. Do this three or four times a day. For most people, ice treatment reduces pain and swelling. However, if ice increases the pain, then try a heating pad (set to *low,* never high).

In this case, your homeopathic remedy would be *Bellis* instead of *Arnica.* Or, alternate hot and cold applications (contrast baths).
• Pain and swelling. Select one of the following remedies according to your symptoms. Take two to four pills per hour for 24 hours:

Arnica for initial trauma and bruising pain; if better when warm; if very sensitive to touch; if worse with motion. A cold pack may numb injury and lessen pain and swelling.

Take *Bellis* if there is more pain and deeper bruising than with *Arnica;* if a heating pad feels better than a cold pack; if there is no tolerance whatsoever for cold.

Take *Bryonia* if red and inflamed; if worse with any motion; if better with rest; better cool; better pressure or tight wrap.

Colchicum if there is redness, pain, and swelling; if one joint only is affected; for shifting pain; if pain includes damage to tendons and ligaments; if weakness is always present; use for chronic forms of knee-pain; for knee-pain with gout; if worse with any motion.

Sulphuric Acid if *Arnica* doesn't work within six hours.

Traumeel for initial pain and trauma after straining knee.

Rhus Tox if your knee feels worse on initial movement, better with continued movement; if it is stiff and sore in the morning; much worse at night or after rest; if it's better with massage; if it's worse with cold pack, better with warmth; if you are very restless, always adjusting for comfort; if injured part is never at ease; always in motion; restless and exhausted; worse with too much walking; for weakness after a sprain; if there is pain in joints, bones, muscles, tendons and ligaments; for lameness; for sudden onset of discomfort after being exposed to cold, damp air while overheated or perspiring; for muscle twitching and nerve-like pain.

Ledum if the knee feels cool to the touch (may also be warm) and feels better with a coldpack; if worse in a warm bed; if better at the beginning of movement.

Benzoic Acid if there are cracking sounds (crepitation) and pain in the joint; for a swollen knee; if worse in open air or uncovered; for a gouty knee.

Pulsatilla if knee pain shifts and moves; if better when cool; if better with gentle initial motion.

Rhododendron if worse before a storm; if worse when cold and wet.

Calc Carb if knee pain is worse arising from a seat and climbing stairs; for stiffness and discomfort while sitting.

Causticum if pain is not relieved by motion (try if *Rhus Tox* doesn't work); when better in a warm bed; if much worse in cold air, but all right in damp weather.

Lymphomyosot if knee is very swollen, take ten drops twice a day.

- Rest from painful activities.
- Elevate the knee and keep the leg straight as much as you can.
- Apply an ace bandage for pressure, extending from your toes to just below your knee.
- If you still have pain and swelling in the morning after a few days, call your doctor as you may need x-rays.
- You can use anti-inflammatory medications (non-steroidal) such as Advil and Nuprin, as well as prescription drugs, including Feldene, Motrin, Ansaid, Clinoril, Indocin, Anaprox, Orudis, Dolobid, and Meclomen. However, check first with your doctor before taking any drugs.
- Homeopathic Remedies. After treating with *Arnica* during the first twenty-four hours, I recommend the following additional homeopathic remedies. Choose one to fit your symptoms and take 6, 12, 15, 30 or 200 once a day for three to four days or until better.

Rhus Tox (see details above).

Take *Ruta Grav* if knee is better with rest; if tired and cranky with too much activity or movement; if better with heat (but use *Rhus Tox* if much better with heat); worse with cold; if you feel moody, fretful and despairing about the injury; if pressure feels better; worse lying down; tends to be a more prolonged problem as compared to *Rhus Tox;* exhausted with too much motion.

For tight hamstrings:

Take *Bryonia* if worse with *any* motion or touch; if the knee is red, hot and swollen; with shiny red inflammation; if you are irritable; if your knee feels better with cold packs and pressure; if better cool; worse heat.

Take *Rhododendron* if there is achiness that hurts more before stormy weather; if better with warm wraps; if much better with continued motion; weakness and worse with rest; if pain moves from joint to joint.

One of the *Calcarea Salts* below should be taken *after* using one of the above remedies for about two weeks. Note: if two weeks time has already lapsed after your knee injury and you have not yet taken any homeopathic remedies, start first with one of the above remedies before progressing to the *Calcarea Salts.*

Take *Calc Carb* (use after *Ruta Grav*) if: worse rising from a seat; worse when cold and damp; arthritic-type complaints; if your knee feels better with heat; if your knee feels worse with cold; if your knee feels better sitting with the leg straight; if your knee feels worse going upstairs.

Take *Calc Fluor* (use after *Rhus Tox*) if: there are spurs in the joint and bony growths.

Take *Calc Phos* (use after *Rhododendron*) if worse with any change in weather.

Take *Hecla Lava* (use after one of the earlier remedies above) for bony growths.

- Homeopathic injections for runner's knee:

Your physician can use one of the three remedies below in combination with Wydase, a natural enzyme found in the body.

Ruta Grav—see typology above.

Traumeel—for pain and swelling.

Zeel—for pain, swelling, and dispersing of gristly tissue.

Rhus Tox—see characteristics above.

Rhododendron—see characteristics above.

Bryonia—see characteristics above.

Phytolacca—if joint is stiff and swollen; much better rest with leg elevated; better heat; much worse walking around;

Stellaria—sometimes better or sometimes worse motion; better cool, worse warm.

Calc Fluor—for spurs or exostoses (pump bumps).

Hecla Lava—for spurs or exostoses.

- Physiotherapy.
- Heel lifts. If your runner's knee is caused by having one leg physically shorter than the other, use a ¼" heel lift inside the shoe of the short leg.
- Orthoses. If you have a functional short leg syndrome (i.e., the leg is held abnormally when you run), you need to correct your feet with foot orthotics. Orthotics may be used in conjunction with exercises to correct for leg muscle imbalances that also contribute

What To Do If Runner's Knee Is Mileage-Related

You may have been feeling fine running or walking twenty miles a week, but when you increased by, say, another ten miles, you began to have achiness in the knees. If you continued your increase of mileage in spite of this warning ache, then you may begin to have real pain. This is the result of accumulated stress, and the knee joint becomes inflamed. To avoid further stress and allow healing to take place, decrease the amount of running or race walking by 25 percent. Run uphill, but avoid downhill as much as possible. Substitute another form of non-painful activity. Try cycling as long as you avoid hills; stay in lower gears and keep the seat up high (in order to straighten the knees as much as possible). Swim with fins to strengthen front thigh muscles, and keep knees fairly straight when doing the crawl. Don't swim the breaststroke because the whip kick stresses the knees. To strengthen inner thigh muscles, try squeezing a basketball tightly between your thighs.

Take one of the homeopathic remedies below. Take four times a day for two weeks or until better. For detailed characteristics see preceding descriptions. *Ruta Grav, Rhus Tox, and Rhodo* are all similar in that they are worse with cold and damp; better when warm; worse with rest; better with motion.

to functional short leg syndrome.

- Tracks. If you have knee problems, avoid running on indoor tracks where you circle thirty or forty times. This makes your foot turn inwards constantly, and even if you alternate directions, a problem could occur.
- Exercise and activity. If you are substituting indoor activities when you can't run outside, avoid stressful ones such as rope jumping which may cause too much stress to the forefoot (metatarsals) as well as the Achilles tendon. Swimming may be your best choice of aerobic activity. You can also use an exercise bike as long as the seat is raised to prevent stress to the knees. A stair-climber may work if you do most of your climbing in the ankle. Low-impact aerobics can be used providing there is no pain.
- Rehabilitative exercises. See Chapter 15.

Pain Immediately below the Knee—Jumper's Knee (Patellar Tendon Strain)

The patellar tendon is a mighty mite of a tendon, short but powerful. It extends from the lower end of the knee-cap to the top of the shin bone (the tibial tubercle). See Fig. 12-1. Because it is an important element in all movements of the knee, it is very susceptible to overuse injury through repetitive exercise, such as long-distance running, intensive hill-running, hopping, kicking or squatting. Sudden injury to the tendon can occur when a kick is blocked in football, stumbling while running, or during jumping or long jumping.

The tendon is particularly at risk when it is fatigued or not warmed up sufficiently. Faulty posture, imbalanced leg bones, or bad shoes will affect the angle of tension on this tendon, creating maltracking of the knee-cap.

Pain from a patellar tendon strain, caused either by sudden injury or by overuse, does not stop your knee from working. As a result, scar tissue forms in the tendon which limits its movement and increases pain. Continuing on this downward spiral of injury, the tendon then becomes bound down by adhesions which stick the tendon to the tissues around it. Bone spurs (calcifications) can occur in the tendon.

To treat patellar tendon strain, call a sports medicine specialist. Keep your knee straight as much as possible—no bending or squats! Use an ace wrap or a brace, and take Stage One homeopathic remedies (during the first 24 hours) which are the same as for runner's knee in preceding section.

During recovery avoid activities which cause pain over the tendon. Don't run on hilly ground, squat, hop, jump or swim the breaststroke. If you can run without pain on soft ground, or do one-quarter squats, or swim the crawl, then you can continue to exercise.

Stretch the quadriceps (see Chapter 15) within the limits of pain to restore flexibility and prevent the formation of adhesions. Stretch ten times, three times a day and before any exercise session.

Do static (isometric) quadriceps contractions at frequent intervals during the day, but don't do an excessive amount at one time. Make sure that you do one or two static quadriceps contractions at least three times daily, along with your stretching exercise.

After maintaining your quadriceps tone for a couple of weeks, go on to strengthen them on a leg press machine as your doctor allows. Don't bend your leg more than thirty degrees to the fully straightened position, and start with light weights. Start with three sets of ten, increasing slowly by one or two steps in each session. Once you have increased resistance by six increments from the original weight, you may press from a 90 degree bend.

If you are not able to use a leg press machine, practice knee bending movements as soon as you are free of pain (see Chapter 15).

Once healing is fairly well established, stretch the tendon. Kneel on a soft firm surface. Sit back gently onto your calves, holding the tendon on the stretch. Be very slow and gentle. Stop immediately if *any* pain is felt.

When you can do half-squats on the injured leg, you can begin to resume your normal activities *in easy stages*. If you play football, do some practice kicks by yourself before playing with others.

Sudden Tearing underneath the Knee (Patellar Tendon Rupture)

This injury happens when the bent knee is under heavy stress, as, for example, when you are doing full squat exercises in weight-lifting. Suddenly, you feel something give out. What has happened is a partial or complete tear of the patellar tendon. The tendon works hardest when the knee is fully bent and carrying the brunt of your body weight. Nevertheless, sometimes a surprisingly minimal amount of stress creates a major tear. This happens in cases where the tendon has been weakened by steroid injections.

In the worst case, the tendon may tear away completely from its bottom moorings in the shin, incapacitating the front thigh muscles (quadriceps) since the knee-cap is essentially hanging loose off the bottom of the muscle. Obviously, the pain is severe and does not permit any weight on the leg.

To treat patellar tendon rupture, use basic first aid and call the doctor immediately. You will need to be seen by an orthopedic surgeon.

Provide support for the leg with an inflatable splint during healing. You will have to have surgery to repair the tendon attachment, and follow the above rehabilitation recommendations for patellar tendon strain.

Patellar Tendon Complications:

Osgood-Schlatter's Disease: Occurring only in adolescents, this condition is a degeneration (osteochrondritis) in the shin bone's growth

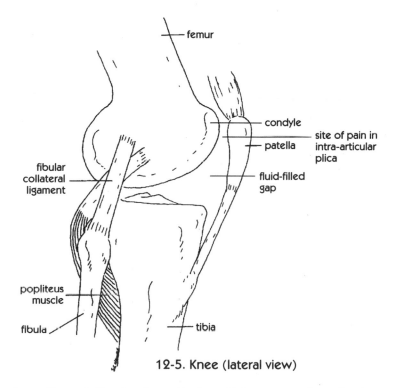

12-5. Knee (lateral view)

plate where the patellar tendon attaches. Pain occurs when the tendon is stressed during activity and when you try to kneel. The condition
is aggravated by excessive pronation (flattening) of the arch, especially with running. Discontinuing aggravating activity can cure this
condition, but it may take as long as six months. Surgery is rarely indicated, yet may be done to clean up parts of the tendon or to help
the disrupted bones to heal. Rehabilitation is the same as for patellar
tendon strain. Most adolescents outgrow this condition. Orthotics,
homeopathics, and knee exercises are most helpful. See Chapter 18
for details.

Pain under the Knee-cap (Intra-articular Plica)

You may think you have degeneration of cartilage (chondromalacia) or
maltracking of the patella if you have pain under the knee-cap. However, tests might show that the cartilage is perfectly normal, and the
knee-cap well-aligned. What you actually have is an inflammation of a
fold of the soft, fatty tissue under the knee-cap (intra-articular plica).
This is fairly common in runners and walkers. See Fig. 12-5.

Two to three pouches may be formed by this soft tissue. With repeated use of the knee, and compression of the knee-cap against the thigh bone (femur), the plica becomes rubbery and hard. You may feel a snapping sensation in the knee-cap; in the late stages, the gristle can actually become firm enough to erode the cartilage.

To treat intra-articular plica, try an orthotic if there is a foot imbalance affecting the knee. An orthopedic surgeon can remove the plica through a small incision with the aid of an arthroscope which has a tiny TV camera on the end of it. Recovery takes about three weeks, and is enhanced by using homeopathic remedies:

Homeopathic injections may also be tried by your physician instead of surgery to dissolve small plica. He or she may try injecting one of the following remedies with Wydase, a natural softening enzyme found in the body:

Ruta Grav if stiff and sore;

Rhus Tox if very, very stiff;

Calcarea Phosphorica if worse any change in weather.

Calcarea Carbonicum if knee pain is worse on rising from a seat and climbing stairs; if there is stiffness and discomfort while sitting.

A cortisone injection may be used, but one injection only.

Pain on the Top of the Knee-cap(Pre-patellar Bursitis)

Anyone who has worked on his or her knees knows that it's not much fun. Carpet-layers, housemaids, plumbers are all likely to suffer from this prosaic pain. Aikidoists *walk* on their knees—Samurai Walk. Excessive pressure on the knee-cap is the main cause of inflammation of the fluid-filled pouch (bursa) which lies between the bone and its covering (Fig. 12-4). A hard blow to the knee-cap, such as falling from a height or being kicked in the knee, will cause the bursa to swell. Sometimes the bursa becomes quite enlarged, but may not be very painful, and you still may be able to walk fairly well. Kneeling or squatting, of course, brings more pain.

For pre-patellar bursitis or mild pain, avoid kneeling on the knee or putting pressure on it. Keep the knee straight whenever possible so you don't stretch out the bursa. Apply ice over the bursa if it feels painful. Wear knee pads if you must work on your knees, but only in *mild* cases of bursitis. Otherwise, you must see your doctor.

Homeopathic injections of *Ruta Grav* are very effective in reducing bursitis, as are oral homeopathic remedies. Take one of the following remedies—four pills four times a day until better:

Ruta Grav; potency of 6, 12, or 30 when it's sore, stiff, and you are apprehensive; the knee feels worse with prolonged motion.

Take *Rhus Tox;* potency of 6, 12, or 30 if very stiff; worse after rest and initial motion; better with heat and continued motion.

Take *Rhododendron;* same potency; when the knee feels worse with an approaching storm.

Take *Benzoic Acid* when the joint cracks with motion, and when there are painful nodules.

Take *Pulsatilla* for wandering joint pain.

Take *Silica* for spongy swelling.

Take *Ledum* if your knee is cool to the touch and feels better with a cold pack; an inflamed knee may also be warm to the touch.

Take *Bryonia* if it's red hot and swollen. worse *any* motion; better cool. After any of these remedies have been taken for a few days, take:

Take *Calcarea Fluorica* which is very good for bursas; take a single 1M dose (only under direction of physician) or 6x without a prescription.

Surgical excision and removal may be necessary in severe bursitis. After surgery, an immobilizing splint is used to rest the knee; after four weeks in the splint, you can start rehabilitation exercises (see Chapter 15).

Acupuncture may be useful for bursitis. Exercises help maintain mobility in mild cases of bursitis. Stretch your front thigh muscles (quadriceps) by pulling your ankle behind you towards your buttocks. Keep your hip forward, and bend the knee as far as you can for ten seconds. Gently release, and repeat about six times twice a day or more (see Chapter 15).

Knee-Cap Dislocation

In a severe knee-cap dislocation, there is no doubt about what has happened! The pain is severe, and the knee-cap is lodged to the outside of your knee and will not slip back into place. Under no circumstances should you try, or let anyone else try, to push the knee back into place. Wrap the knee in an ice towel and go straight to the hospital, keeping your knee absolutely still.

Sometimes the knee-cap slips out of place on a recurring basis. For instance, it may slip out as you run or as you run upstairs. You feel pain and cannot put full weight on the leg. When you straighten the knee, you may feel a click and the joint seems to be all right again. The knee will probably swell up and feel painful over the front of the joint. This is called chronic subluxation of the patella.

To treat a severe knee-cap dislocation, don't push the knee-cap back into place. Wrap the knee in an ice towel and go to an emergency room, keeping the knee absolutely still.

For the first 24 hours, take *Arnica* (any potency) four pills every six hours.

With recurring dislocation where the knee-cap slips in and out of alignment, you may find that one sport or activity seems to bring on this problem. You'll have to decide if it's worth risking surgery and a lengthy rehabilitation period to continue that particular activity.

Various forms of braces can help you with knee-cap problems. Use them with the supervision of your doctor and/or physical therapist. They include elastic bandages, Neopreme braces with a hole cut out for the knee-cap, and straps which are applied over the knee-cap and tend to stop it from wobbling.

Pain on the Outside of the Knee
Pain Along the Outer Side (Lateral) of the Thigh (Iliotibial Band Syndrome)

This pain almost always indicates an overuse injury, stemming from repetitive knee movements. It often follows a mileage increase in runners or cross-country skiers. It worsens walking down stairs or bending the knee. See Fig. 12-6.

The iliotibial band is a strong tract that connects the lateral thigh muscle (tensor fascia lata) to the outer part of the knee. It is working when you extend your hip backwards and/or straighten your knee.

There is a fluid-filled sac (bursa) between the iliotibial band and the bone. When you change your normal movement patterns, the friction creates inflammation, perhaps even bursitis. You can feel the tender spot when you flex your knee past 35 degrees. In severe cases a "snapping" of the band occurs around the outer knee (lateral femoral condyle).

The pain may come on suddenly or gradually. Generally, it starts up each time you are playing your sport or running. You may feel a clicking sensation where the tendon rubs over the end of the thigh bone (femoral condyle) at the knee. There can be sharp pain along with tightness and soreness at your hip joint.

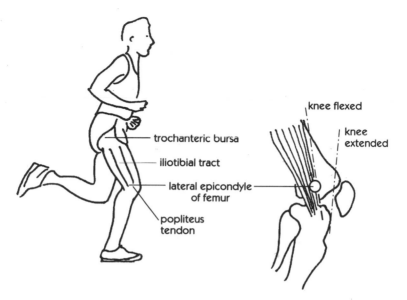

12-6. Sites of Pain in Iliotibial Band Friction Syndrome

Another possible cause of the pain is a direct blow such as playing football where another player falls onto the outer side of your leg.

To treat iliotibial band syndrome, check with your doctor to rule out a medical cause for your pain. Determine what you are doing that caused the stress. For example, are you running too many miles? Are your legs working symmetrically? Does the wear pattern on your shoes indicate a biomechanical foot abnormality?

For pain, apply ice over the inflamed area. Electro-galvanic stimulation or Ultrasound can also help reduce pain and enhance healing.

Substitute race walking for running. Cycle with your seat raised high to help you keep the knee straight. Make sure your shoes are providing proper cushioning and adequate foot control. If shoes are too worn down on the outside, this could be causing the problem. Have a podiatrist check your shoes and any orthotic you might be using which might be over-correcting or over-controlling.

Strengthen the knee by doing two bent-leg and two straight-leg exercises twice a day (see Chapter 15). Stretch the outer thigh. Do ten straight leg raises to the side twice a day.

Your physician can inject under the iliotibial band 1cc of *Ruta Grav* or *Rhus Tox* with 1cc of Xylocaine with ½cc of the softening enzyme, Wydase. If that doesn't work, he or she may inject a long and short-acting cortisone. Be aware that cortisone can cause a white mark under the skin at the injection point.

Take *Rhus Tox* if the knee is stiff and worse on initial motion, but gets better with continued motion. Take 30c four times a day until pain is gone, or;

Take *Ruta Grav* if the knee is better with motion, but gets worse after prolonged movement. Same dose—30c four times a day.

If the pain does not clear up, perhaps indicating a bursa or overly tight iliotibial band, you may need surgery to release part of the tight band and remove any inflamed bursa. Recovery is rapid—within three to four weeks.

Pain on the Outside of the Knee after a Twist or Fall (Lateral-Collateral Ligament Strain)

This injury happens commonly after a fall when you are skiing, running or even walking fast. See Fig. 12-7. Pain on the outside of the knee will hurt more if you sit with the painful knee crossed over your other knee (with the foot of the painful knee resting on top of the opposite knee). This position stretch-es the lateral-collateral (out-side) ligament of the knee.

For lateral-collateral lig-ament strain, use basic first aid.

If you still have pain af-ter a few days, see an ortho-pedist.

You may need a knee-cast or brace followed by physical therapy.

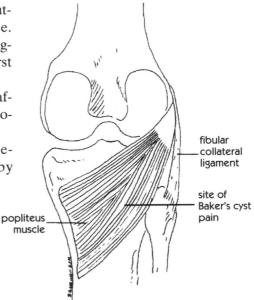

fibular
collateral
ligament

site of
Baker's cyst
pain

popliteus
muscle

12-7. Site of Ligament Injury after a Fall during Skiing, Running or Walking Fast (right knee, back view)

Pain on the Outside of the Back of the Knee (Tendinitis of Biceps Femoris)

Straining these tendons happens with excessive sprinting or long-time overuse from running on banked roads. Pain is felt on the outside of the knee, right above the outside knee bone (the head of the fibula). See Fig. 12-3. Pain is worse going up or down stairs or running and jumping.

To treat tendinitis of biceps femoris, use basic first aid. Rest the knee, and avoid excessive bending or flexing. Walking is all right, but don't bike or run for four to six weeks as you allow the tendon to heal. Gently stretch the hamstrings with exercises. Stay off hills. Avoid any fast running for four to six weeks. You may run slowly with your legs not flexing too much. Avoid jumping, squatting or biking. If anything hurts, don't do it!

If not better within a couple of weeks, see a sports doctor. Injections of homeopathic *Rhus Tox* and *Ruta Grav* may be helpful.

Pain on the Inner Side (Medial) of the Knee Joint

Medial Ligament Strain

Sudden pain on the inner side of the knee usually is the result of a twist to the joint. You may have slipped while running forward, or been tackled in football as you were kicking. Falling sideways with your foot in a ski boot could also cause a strain to the inner ligament. If swelling is visible over the entire joint, you have probably damaged internal structures as well as the ligament on the side of the joint. The torn ligament feels sore and the knee may feel loose on the inner side. See Fig. 12-2c.

There are three levels of damage that may have been done: You may have torn the medial ligament, strained it at its attachments, or pulled away a flake of bone. Gradual pain which gets worse with repeated activity indicates an accumulation of stress. Eventually, the knee hurts on the inside even when you walk or sit down.

To treat medial ligament strain, rest from all painful activity, and apply an ice pack wrapped three or four times a day which usually reduces the pain and swelling. However, if ice increases the pain, then try a heating pad (set to *low,* never high). In this case, your homeopathic remedy would be *Bellis* instead of *Arnica*. Or, alternate hot and cold applications (contrast baths).

Elevate your leg on a pillow or soft chair. To minimize swelling, don't sit or stand with your knee bent. Keep the leg on pillows even in bed if you can sleep that way.

Do not force the knee to bend if this causes pain. Keep your leg straight. To minimize muscle weakening—which inevitably follows this injury—begin quadriceps contractions immediately after the injury. Extend the leg, keeping the knee as straight as possible, and contract the thigh muscles. Try to hold for a count of twenty; do twenty sets two or three times a day.

If the strain is severe, see the doctor immediately, or go to the emergency room of a hospital. You may need a cast or surgical repair.

For the shock of injury take *Arnica*. For pain, bruising and swelling take one of the following (see details under Runner's Knee section): *Arnica, Bellis, Sulphuric Acid, Bryonia, Ledum, Lymphomyosot,* or *Traumeel*.

Once the doctor has diagnosed the exact nature of the injury, you may benefit by injections of one of the following homeopathics in combination with the natural softening enzyme Wydase:

Ruta Grav if stiff; persistent soreness.

Rhus Tox if stiff, restless; worse with initial motion, better with continuous motion; worse when cold and wet, better when warm.

Zeel if the joint is involved.

Traumeel for traumatic injury; for pain, swelling, stiffness.

Unless your doctor advises you not to exercise at all for some specific reason, continue your straight-leg exercises. When the initial pain and swelling have gone away, begin to do gentle, bending exercises. You may swim the crawl and do pool exercises that do not bring pain. Check with your doctor as to when to start weight-bearing knee bends, and light running. Progress very slowly to kicking, squatting, hopping, or running and turning.

If there is continuing pain after treatment, there may be calcified flakes where the ligament was torn away from the bone attachment. You may need an injection of *Traumeel, Rhus Tox* or *Ruta Grav*.

Pes Anserinus Bursitis

This is a pain on the inside of the knee from too much running with a foot or leg imbalance. A fluid-filled sac has become inflamed. Treatment is usually an injection of *Rhus Tox* or *Ruta Grav* with Xylocaine and Wydase. This problem is often mistaken for more serious conditions such as a torn or degenerated medial meniscus or a damaged medial ligament. A simple diagnostic test is to inject the bursa with local anesthetic and a homeopathic remedy. If the pain goes away, even temporarily, then one can assume there is no problem in any other structure within the joint or with the ligament.

Pes Anserinus Tendinitis

This is an overuse injury in the inner knee tendon caused by excessive hill running or excessive speed with biomechanical abnormalities in the leg and foot. This is sometimes confused with medial meniscus tear, so be sure your doctor differentiates the two. Following the treatment steps below should bring a rapid recovery.

For pes anserinus tendinitis or bursitis, basic first aid measures bring relief. Rest from painful activity, use ice packs or a heating pad, keep your leg elevated as much as possible and wrap with an ace bandage. Keep knee straight (extended).

Strengthen the muscles associated with the medial tendon by squeezing a basketball between your thighs. Substitute non impact aerobic activity such as swimming the crawl. Avoid excessive bending or flexing (i.e., no biking, jumping, or fast running). Walking is usually tolerated. Correct biomechanical abnormalities with foot orthoses prescribed by your podiatrist or sports medicine specialist. During recovery try heat, cold or contrast baths and gentle massage.

Take *Arnica* for acute pain in the early phase of the injury (one to two days). Then select either *Rhus Tox* if your legs are restless or *Ruta Grav* if you get tired with continuing motion. After two or three weeks, take *Calc Phos* to finish healing (take for four to six weeks).

Pain and Swelling behind the Knee

Pain and swelling behind the knee can follow tendinitis, tendon strain or a Baker's cyst. Pain in the back of the knee occurs from straining the muscles which insert there, usually the calf muscles (soleus or gastrocnemius). See Fig. 12-7. Or, the hamstrings could be strained from taking too long a stride, running down hill, running too fast, or too much jumping (i.e, too much aerobics). Unaccustomed kicking could also cause strain.

Treatment consists of decreasing flexion (bending), gentle stretching of the calf and hamstrings, massage, physical therapy, and homeopathic remedies for tendinitis. Tendinitis problems usually heal within six to eight weeks. If healing seems to be slow and there is still a lot of pain, a homeopathic injection by a physician may speed up healing and bring relief.

Tendinitis of the Hamstrings, Gastrocnemius, Soleus, or Popliteal

This pain in the back of the knee is caused by excessive running, or by a strain in tennis, basketball or baseball, or even trauma as in football.

For tendinitis in the back of the knee, rest and reduce your bending and flexing activities for awhile. Stretch out your calf muscles in the back of the leg. Try hot, cold or contrast baths.

Select one of the following homeopathic oral remedies:

Rhus Tox for stiffness; worse sitting; for restlessness in legs; if knee feels better after moving around; if worse with initial motion; much worse cold; better heat; problem may come after becoming overheated and cooling off too suddenly.

Ruta Grav for soreness and stiffness.

Causticum if not relieved by motion (try if *Rhus Tox* doesn't work); better with warm bed; if much worse in cold air, but all right with damp weather.

Acupuncture can be very helpful. Structural integration work such as Rolfing, Hellerwork may be done after the pain has gone. Consider a movement practice such as T'ai Chi. Therapeutic yoga is excellent for increasing flexibility in the back of the leg as well as the whole body. Rosen work or Trager work could help loosen tightness as well as uncover unconscious rigid emotional attitudes.

Baker's Cyst

Runners and tennis players may develop this pain where the upper leg meets the lower leg in back. A knee injury such as torn cartilage in the knee joint (meniscus) will cause a swelling at the back of the knee which is called a Baker's cyst (Fig. 12-7).

To treat Baker's cyst apply an ice towel to alleviate the pain.

Rest from painful activity, and elevate the leg often during the day. Call the doctor, as you will need assistance in curing this condition. Treatment usually consists of injections (try *Ruta Grav* with or without cortisone and draining by an orthopedist; if necessary, you may have a surgical removal of the cyst. Take *Ruta Grav.* For rehabilitative exercises for the knee, see Chapter 15.

Pain within the Knee Joint

Posterior Tear of the Medial Meniscus

Running can cause a tear in the inner fibro-cartilage (menisci) between the end of the thigh bone (femur) and the end of the shin bone (tibia). See Fig. 12-2 a, and b. Damage is more common following a severe twisting injury or spain.

With this injury, you may feel instant pain, and will not even be able to move the knee or bear weight on it. Swelling may start either immediately or a few hours later. The knee may look very bloated or just slightly swollen. One sign of a torn cartilage is the feeling that the knee is "locked"; if you shake it gently, it seems to release with a click. Because of the pain, you might not feel the locking sensation until you've recovered enough to move it a little. The locking feeling means that a torn part of the cartilage is jammed between the shin bone and the thigh bone. The knee may periodically lock, then release. A manipulation may unlock it; if, however, it keeps locking, see an orthopedist. You may have to have the torn portion of the meniscus removed with arthroscopy.

Tearing of the medial meniscus occurs when your leg is bearing your full weight when, at the same time, an abnormal sideways movement twists the bones and cartilage inside your knee joint. It is not uncommon in football, where you may have been running forward and been pushed sideways by a tackle. Or, your foot might have been trapped inside a ski-boot as you fell forward. Over-lunging in fencing is another possibility. In all cases, the injury happens when sudden stress occurs with the knee bent. A cartilage tear can also occur when the leg is straight, such as when you miss a drop kick in football.

To treat cartilage tears in the knee, use basic first aid. Keep the knee extended and stretch; avoid excessive bending. Use an ace wrap and a neoprene brace; crutches if you need them. Go immediately to a sports medicine specialist. If the knee is not cured with rest, and at home measures don't work, you may need surgery to repair the degenerated portion of the cartilage. In the meantime take:

Stage One remedies (first 24 hours). Select one. Take two to four pills (any potency) for up to six hours. See details under Runner's Knee section.

> For shock take *Arnica.*
> For pain, bruising and swelling select one:
> *Ruta Grav, Arnica, Bellis, Sulphuric Acid, Bryonia, Ledum, Traumeel,* or
> *Lymphomyosot.*

If surgery is indicated, the arthroscopic method can often be done with local anesthetic. You may return to running or sports probably within one to two months. WARNING: Since you may have relatively little pain after surgery, don't be tempted to resume activity too quickly. Be sure to check with your doctor about your activity program.

Tear of the Cruciate Ligaments

The thick, strong stabilizing ligaments that criss-cross within the knee (cruciate ligaments) can also be torn as a result of the same conditions described above—traumatic injury in a weight-bearing bent knee undergoing abnormal twisting. When the cruciates are torn, the knee is swollen and feels loose and "lax." The leg feels as if it is "shifting" under the knee. When you are seated, someone can easily pull your knee forward with little resistance.

To treat cruciate ligament tear, follow basic first aid. Go to a sports medicine specialist immediately. Take *Arnica* or *Traumeel* for shock. After the first twenty-four hours, select another homeopathic remedy as recommended in the previous section.

The cruciate ligament tear creates a very unstable knee. You may need a brace and medically supervised physical therapy or surgery, depending on the degree of injury.

The most important aspect of non-surgical treatment is rehabilitative exercise to strengthen hamstrings. The doctor will advise you to build up the hamstrings for four to six weeks. Following the hamstrings routine, go on to quadriceps strengthening (with a semi-flexed knee).

For rehabilitation and prevention, you may need orthoses to correct biomechanical imbalances as diagnosed by your doctor.

Use anti-inflammatory medicines as needed for pain—Advil, Motrin, or Feldene. Avoid using them if you are allergic to aspirin. Do not take any pain-killing drugs so that you can continue walking, running or playing sports.

Surgery is indicated if the ligament is torn, as it will not heal or mend on its own. Incidentally, homeopathic *Aethusa Cynapium* is good to take before surgery if you have extreme fear of general anesthesia. If you don't have extreme fear, but, still are very anxious prior to surgery, take *Aconite*. After the removal of the torn pieces of cartilage, new tissue will form from the remaining cells, although the new cartilage will not be as sturdy as the original. The ligaments may have to be augmented with artificial material.

What to do after surgery:

Select one of the following homeopathic remedies (see details under Runner's Knee section:

> *Arnica, Sulphuric Acid, Bryonia, Ruta Grav, Rhus Tox.* In two weeks, following *Ruta Grav* take *Calcarea Phosphorica* if it's worse cold, damp or worse with a change in the weather. Two weeks following *Rhus Tox,* take *Calcarea Carb* if it's worse after rising; worse when climbing stairs.

As swelling goes down, your doctor will recommend non-weight-bearing knee bending exercises, along with daily quadriceps contractions. Gradually, you proceed to half-squats with no twisting, then a variety of movements to rebuild strength and flexibility. Full recovery time depends on the severity of the injury and complexity of the surgery. You may resume normal functioning anywhere from six weeks to six months.

Any sudden increase in swelling or pain is a sign that you are overdoing exercise. Your knee, even if not very painful, is still recovering from a severe trauma. Be very careful not to risk re-injury.

Knee Pain from a Medical Condition

Two medical conditions that affect the knee joint are osteoarthritis (wear-and-tear degeneration with aging) and rheumatism (spontaneous inflammatory arthritis). If you have a pre-disposition for gout, increased activity may precipitate a flare-up. In addition to osteoarthritis and rheumatism, another medical (i.e., non-injury) condition of the knee joint could be referred pain stemming from problems in the back, hip, or thigh.

Knee-Cap Pain (Chondromalacia)

Sometimes general knee-cap pain is called chondromalacia. Actually, this pain is very seldom found in runners or walkers since vigorous exercise keeps the joints healthy. Chondromalacia is a late stage of degenerative arthritis between the knee-cap and the thigh bone. Once degeneration begins, the progression from a mild softening of the cartilage to a substantial wearing away of tissue is rather rapid.

To treat chondromalacia, if pain is severe, anti-inflammatory medications can be used such as Advil, Motrin, and Feldene. Do not take any of these drugs if you are allergic to aspirin or have ulcers, and take them only to relieve pain during the day or night. Select one of the following homeopathic remedies. For specific characteristics of remedies, see the Runner's Knee section.

> *Arnica, Rhus Tox, Ruta Grav, Rhododendron, Calcarea Phosphorica, Calcarea Fluorica, Calcarea Carbonicum.*

Electrical stimulation in conjunction with muscle exercises will enhance healing. Quad sets are very important. See Chapter 15.

Orthoses. If aggravation of the knee-cap is linked to faulty foot mechanics, a foot orthotic can be made by your podiatrist.

Cleaning out the joint and smoothing cartilage (arthroscopic surgery) may be very helpful. If the patella is out of alignment, surgery may be indicated.

Chapter **13**

 # HIP, PELVIS, AND GROIN INJURIES

God requires a faithful fulfillment of the merest trifle given us to do,
rather than the most ardent aspiration to things to which we are not
called.

—Saint Francis de Sales

A Personal Story

My awareness of hip problems in runners came into full bloom many
years ago when I was an admittedly addicted, hard-core, marathoner. I tell this story both to illustrate a common hip problem for zealous
runners, and to demonstrate how easy it is to get out of balance with
one's sport.

I had been invited to give a talk at the Aerobic Center in Dallas by
Dr. Ken Cooper, the founder and popularizer of aerobics here in the
United States. The day before the talk, I was also going to participate
in the Dallas-White Rock Marathon. I was excited because my speaking and running companion would be my old friend George Sheehan,
an M.D. who is a great authority on running.

In those days, I thought I was indestructible. To prove this, after
Dallas, I was scheduled to go on to Hawaii one week later to give another talk for the American Medical Jogger's Association, and then
run in the Honolulu Marathon. I thought I was in good enough shape
for these back-to-back marathons as I was then logging in about seventy
miles per week with a twenty-mile run on weekends. No problem.

Running two marathons a week apart violates all common sense as
well as the rules of exercise physiology. Somehow, I felt the rules didn't
apply to me. I was to find that I, too, was mortal.

There was a high degree of electrical excitement at the starting
line in Dallas the day of the marathon. I started the race at a brisk

pace, enjoying the beautiful course, running with a group of women who were running, frankly, faster than I had planned to. My friend, George ambled up beside me, remarking that if I could keep up this pace, I might set a personal record. Well, that fueled my ego a bit, and I began imagining myself as running a sub-three-hour marathon.

Nina Kussack, the former Olympian marathoner, was out of the race because of an injury. She had promised to give George and me fluids every 3 to 5 miles. Our fluid that day was beer. We were testing a new theory of George's that it would be okay to consume carbohydrates while on the run. Well, I soon realized that beer was not going to be a good idea, so I switched to water. George began feeling weak and had a mild case of heat prostration. He dropped back. I was somewhat concerned for him, but even more concerned about my personal record that day. I managed about a 3:09 race, and I was pleased. George loped in 5 or 10 minutes later and fell to the ground, feeling dizzy and weak. We gave him lots of water, and that ended our experiment with beer as a fluid replacement.

That day was also the beginning of one of my more serious running injuries. During the banquet and talks that evening I noticed a tightening over my right hip. I also had a "snapping" sensation with pain over the outside of my right knee. Despite the pain, I told Harry Cordellos, the celebrated blind marathoner, that I would run ten miles with him the following day in preparation for the Honolulu Marathon. What was I thinking of?

The next morning I was quite stiff, tired, and worn out. Common sense said I shouldn't go running with Harry. Lacking that virtue at that stage of my life (being a Phase Three runner!), I ran with Harry. My hip was sore and stiff, and the knee was giving me problems. After 2 miles, it warmed up, and I did all right. The next morning, however, I had a serious problem—difficulty in simply walking! Every time I bent my knee, there was pain on the outside of the joint. My hip hurt with every step I took. The pain was right over my hip bone—in the area of the greater trochanter.

To give you the medical diagnosis, I had a greater trochanter bursitis with an iliotibial band friction rub (Fig. 13-1). A very small, skinny muscle, the tensor fascia lata, which balances the thigh muscle (quadriceps), had fatigued and tightened up (Fig. 13-1). It started snapping over the knob on the outside of the hip bone. The iliotibial band that runs down the outside of the thigh to the knee was also snapping over the outside of the knee due to tightness. The fluid-filled sac be-

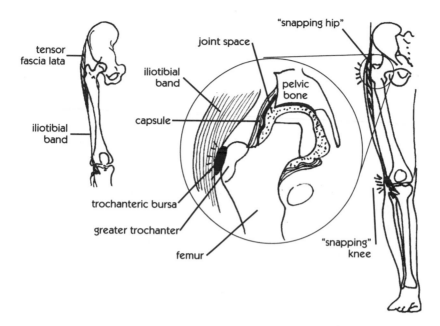

13-1. Greater Trochanter Bursitis and Iliotibial Band Friction Rub

tween the tensor fascia lata muscle and my hip bone had gotten inflamed (bursitis). I also had bursitis in the knee and under the iliotibial band.

Well, even though I was having trouble walking downstairs and walking down hills—even though my leg was snapping and painful—I wouldn't give up the idea of running another marathon in five days. I had a colleague give me an injection in the knee and hip to alleviate pain in the bursas, and began to prepare for the race. In those days, I didn't know about homeopathic remedies, and I would certainly have used them knowing what I know now.

I did run the marathon in Hawaii, in a great deal of pain, and didn't enjoy it at all. The lesson I learned about giving the body time to recover has been permanently ingrained in my somewhat dense mind.

Hip Structure and Function

The hip flexor muscles are the main muscles which pull the thigh bone forward when you walk. All forward kicking movements involve them, as does the movement of lifting the legs up while in a lying position. Hip flexor muscles also pull your lower back forward when you sit up from a lying position. When you sit in a chair, the muscles hold the posture. If you have shortened or tight hip flexors, you will tend to have a sway back. Problems with hip flexors relate directly to back problems, and can be the cause or result of spinal problems, especially if your hips are not symmetrical. Of course, asymmetry leads to overstrain and overuse injury.

The two most important of these muscles are iliacus and psoas major. Because they are so closely associated, we call them by one name—iliopsoas. Attached to the lower vertebrae (lumbar) of your spine, psoas major extends down across the front of your hip joint to fix onto a small bump of bone on the inside of the top of the thigh bone, called the lesser trochanter. Iliacus spreads right over the inside of your hip bone (ilium) down to the inner edge of the front of your sacrum and is fixed to the inner edge of the thigh bone along with the psoas. These two muscles are buried well below other muscles and are crossed by a main artery and a nerve.

Pain in the Hip Flexors

You may feel pain in the hip flexors while walking forward, especially up stairs, or when you press your leg against resistance. A sudden severe strain stops you from being able to draw your leg back at the hip, and it's very difficult to walk. This pain is caused by excessive hill-running, jumping, aerobics, or running on slippery surfaces such as ice or snow.

To treat hip flexor pain apply ice or heat, whichever feels better.

Use *Arnica* for initial trauma and for initial bruising and pain. Use *Bellis* for deep bruising and pain if heat makes it feel better and cold cannot be tolerated. Use *Rhus Tox* if you are much stiffer after resting, and you feel restless trying to get comfortable with your pain; if worse with initial movement or better with continued motion.

Use *Ruta Grav* if the hip is better with rest; if tired and cranky after too much activity or movement; if stiff, sore, bruised and achy; if you feel moody, fretful and despairing about the injury; if pressure feels better; if your hip feels worse lying down; if it tends to be a more prolonged problem as compared to *Rhus Tox*.

In general, avoid painful activities of any kind. Using crutches will not be advisable because holding your leg forward at the hip to walk with crutches makes your condition worse. As soon as you can, start stretching the muscles to minimize their tendency to shorten. At first, it's enough just to straighten your leg at the hip while you are standing. As the pain lessens, slowly begin to pull the leg behind you, holding for a few seconds. As you progress, you should be able to stretch the leg fully behind you, supported by your other bent leg. Don't push to do activity through any pain. Substitute swimming to keep in shape.

In the next few days, for pain, bruising and swelling take 2 to 4 pills every four hours of one of the following:

Arnica if there is a bruised feeling on initial trauma;

Bellis if a heating pad feels better than a cold pack;

Sulphuric Acid if *Arnica* hasn't helped; *Bryonia* if you cannot move easily or bear to be touched; if the hip feels better with pressure or better with a cold pack; *Ledum* if your skin feels cool to the touch and feels better with a cold pack; *Lymphomyosot* if there's a lot of swelling. Take ten drops twice a day; *Traumeel* for initial pain and trauma after straining hip.

If you wish, you can also take Advil, Motrin, Feldene, or Naprosyn with or without homeopathic remedies. Be sure to check with your doctor, and be aware that these drugs may exacerbate stomach problems, ulcers or kidney problems.

A mild injury to the hip flexors may heal in a few days if you discontinue painful activities and gently stretch the muscles immediately.

If the pain keeps coming, even when you're not moving, see your doctor for x-rays to rule out stress fracture. Physical therapy may be very helpful. Ask your physician about homeopathic injections of:

Rhus Tox if stiff with initial motion; restless or sore.

Ruta Grav if very stiff and you're cranky; if pressure feels better; if hip is worse lying down; use *Causticum* if very stiff; worse with cold dry weather; not better with continued motion. Take *Calc Phos* after using one of the previous three remedies if the hip feels worse with changes of weather or worse when cold and damp.

After your injury has healed, body work is excellent for gaining more ease and flexibility. Read the section describing Heller work, Trager, Feldenkrais, Rosen work, and Rolfing. Therapeutic yoga and T'ai Chi are extremely beneficial for restoring balance and general flexibility. In addition, you may want to learn the breathing and movement techniques of Chi Gong for gaining flexibility, strength and increased energy flow.

Snapping Hip
(Bursitis in the Greater Trochanter)

This injury is definitely caused by overuse of the hip muscles, creating friction around the fluid-filled sacs (bursas) in the hip. See Fig. 13-1. The bursas become thick and impede the tendon that slides over them, causing a snapping sound. Race walkers get greater trochanteric bursitis due to the excessive rotation and swinging of the leg at the hip. Beginning runners who cross their legs over when running may get this pain. Women with a wide pelvis may be susceptible to this malady when they begin a running program with no correction for their biomechanical imbalance.

Other people who are at risk are cyclists, players of contact sports, and swimmers who get bursitis from doing the whip kick.

For a "snapping" hip with no pain, you probably don't have to worry about the snapping sensation. If you do have pain, ice the area or apply heat, whichever feels better. Discontinue pain-causing activities immediately. Take homeopathic remedy *Arnica* for pain and swelling if it feels sore and bruised. For other oral homeopathic remedies, see the list in the preceding section.

Injections of homeopathic remedies are very useful for this condition. Three or four injections should reduce the problem in combination with rest from painful activities. Your physician can combine 1cc of one of the remedies below with ½cc of the natural enzyme Wydase:

> *Arnica* for pain and swelling; *Ruta Grav* for stiffness and weariness; *Traumeel* for an exhausted, unsteady feeling.

Orthoses to correct biomechanical imbalances will provide a long-term solution. Strengthening and stretching thigh muscles is very important. See Chapter 15.

Anti-inflammatory drugs such as Advil, Motrin, Feldene, or Naprosyn may be helpful for pain relief, but should not be taken before running. This will mask pain and further damage your leg. Check with your doctor before taking these drugs. Take them with food to avoid damaging the lining of the stomach. Do not take these drugs if you have ulcers or kidney problems.

Since a snapping hip is a preventable overuse injury, I would definitely recommend some form of body work to help you stretch out tight structures. Rolfing, Feldenkrais, Trager, Rosen work, Heller work, yoga, and Alexander technique, to name a few, can offer increased vitality and flexibility.

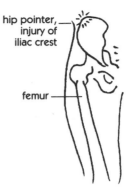

Hip Pointer

An injury known as a hip pointer is a bruise (contusion) on the rim of the pelvic bone (iliac crest). See Fig. 13-2. The iliac crest is the place you put your hands when you stand with your hands on your hips. A bruise in this area may come from a blow, for instance, from a football helmet. A hip pointer can also be caused by muscle

13-2. Site of Hip Pointer Injury.

pulls from track and road racing as well as with other sports. A severe pull could cause some detachment of muscle fibers from the pelvic rim. The abdominal and oblique muscles attach to the inner margin of the iliac crest, and the muscles of the thigh attach to the outer margin. Therefore, if you have tight over-used muscles in the abdomen or in the groin, there can be pain. The injured area may become discolored.

To treat hip pointer injury use basic first aid in Chapter 7. Use ice or heat or a combination of both to reduce pain and swelling. See your doctor for treatment and x-rays to rule out three other possibilities: 1) fracture of the iliac crest; 2) a pulling off of the muscle or tendon (avulsion fracture); or 3) inflammation of the growth plate (apophysitis) (Fig. 13-3).

An elastic wrap can be worn to apply pressure to the hip. Take *Arnica* (any dose) for the first twenty-four hours.

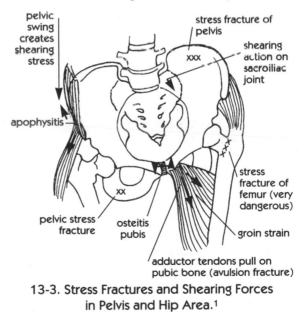

13-3. Stress Fractures and Shearing Forces in Pelvis and Hip Area.[1]

During recovery take either *Rhus Tox* or *Ruta Grav* (see hip flex-or section for characteristics) orally for four to five days, followed by a single 1M dose of *Calc Phos* or a lower dose twice a day for two weeks. Following *Rhus Tox* or *Ruta Grav* take *Symphytum* if there is a stress fracture of the iliac crest. With these more serious conditions, recovery will take two to four months or longer to heal.

For rehabilitation, strengthen abdominal muscles with bent-knee situps, and do lateral thigh raises (out to the side).

If you are involved in contact sports, wear padding and protective gear as recommended by your sports physician or trainer. Foot orthotics can be helpful for hip and abdominal strains when they are associated with poor running form, such as occurs with excessive pronation (flat feet).

In addition to oral remedies, your physician may administer homeopathic injections of:

Rhus Tox if stiff with initial motion; if restless or sore.

Ruta Grav if very stiff; if you feel cranky; if pressure feels better on the injury; if worse when lying down.

Causticum if very stiff; if worse in cold dry weather; when not better with continued motion.

Arnica for sore, bruised, achy feeling.

Traumeel, a combinational remedy, for pain, bruising and swelling.

Take *Calc Phos* after using one of the above remedies if worse with changes of weather; if worse in cold and damp. I don't recommend using cortisone in the hip area. Acupuncture may be helpful for this condition.

Stress Fractures of the Hip

When training is suddenly increased to a new goal, or even slightly raised from an already massive total—say, from forty to sixty miles per week—accumulated microtrauma may lead to a fatigue-stress fracture of the hip or pelvis. Rarely is a stress fracture of the hip caused by an acute blow or trauma.

This injury is becoming more frequent as ordinary people take up running marathons, ultramarathons, and triathlons. Training for and running these Herculean ordeals is no longer only done by a handful of elite athletes aiming for the Olympics. Sometimes, in special circumstances, an older person may even get a stress fracture in the hip from walking.

A stress fracture in the hip feels like a pain deep in the groin. The pain may interrupt your sleep as well as your running. Even taking large amounts of aspirin doesn't help. The only sure confirmation of a stress fracture is a bone scan.

If you suspect you have a stress fracture in the hip, stop running. Immediately make an appointment with a sports orthopedist. Substitute swimming or biking until your diagnosis is made. Continuing to run will only aggravate the fracture, and will delay your recovery.

During your recovery, which will take a minimum of four to six weeks, forego even exercise walking in favor of swimming and cycling. First-rate treatment for a stress fracture of the hip joint should involve an orthopedist for general care, a podiatrist to design a foot orthotic if one is needed, and a physical therapist for rehabilitation.

Homeopathic remedies that will enhance healing are:

Symphytum in the first two weeks to initiate "boneset."

Calcarea Phosphoricum (a single 1M dose) if the injured part is worse with any change in the weather or *Calcarea Fluorica* (a single 1M dose).

Acupuncture can reduce pain and swelling and return energy to the damaged tissue. Massage is always beneficial, but wait until the stress fracture has healed (four to six weeks). Therapeutic yoga is very beneficial after healing. Body work such as Alexander technique, Rosen work, Heller work, Trager work, or Feldenkrais offers increased vitality and freedom of movement after healing. Breathing methods in yoga or Chi Gung will help re-vitalize the body following stress fractures.

Hip Problems Other Than Injuries

Arthritis within the hip joint

Correct any biomechanical imbalances with exercises and/or foot orthotics. A constitutional homeopathic remedy (one that treats your whole body) may help strengthen your entire immune system and help you cope better with this disease. Refer to Chapter 17, Arthritis, for details.

Legg-Perthe's Disease

This is a hip-joint problem with children, usually affecting boys under twelve. See Chapter 18 on Childhood and Adolescence.

Slipped Femoral Capital Epiphysis
This hip-joint problem is more common in the overweight, endomorphic child, especially if he or she takes up running. See Chapter 18 on Childhood and Adolescence.

The Pelvis
Structure and Function
The pelvis is the heart-shaped basin which holds and protects the abdominal organs and and is the first cradle of human life. The pelvis sits at the juncture of the upper part of the body, which is involved with transformative and creative processes, and the lower part of the body which provides mobility.

The two big, flat hip bones (ilia) form the sides of the pelvis, and the shield-shaped bone (sacrum) connects both sides in the back. This connection of hip bone and sacrum is the sacro-iliac joint. The tail bone (coccyx) at the bottom of the sacrum can be felt in the cleft of your buttocks (Fig. 13-4).

In front, two peninsulas of bone come forward forming the symphysis pubis joint; the most pointed parts of the bones are the ischial tuberosities which are your seat bones.

Your pelvis is affected by the way you stand, hold your legs, drop your shoulder, or by the way you habitually carry things. High-heels tilt the pelvis forward, and should especially be avoided in growing girls who may form a permanent curve from this abnormal tilt. Too much weight in the stomach pulls the pelvis forward.

It's important to maintain a good natural curve in the small of the back. Arching and relaxing your back (watch your cat who's a master at this) periodically helps loosen tension in the lower (lumbar) curve. If you have to drive

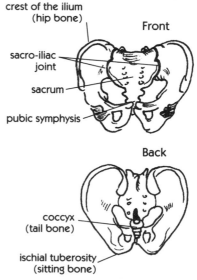

crest of the ilium
(hip bone)

Front

sacro-iliac
joint

sacrum

pubic symphysis

Back

coccyx
(tail bone)

ischial tuberosity
(sitting bone)

13-4. Pelvis

long distances, put a rolled-up towel in the small of the back and see what a difference it makes in your over-all fatigue level at the end of the day.

You should not square your shoulders excessively (soldier's back) nor slump. When lifting weights, you must bend the knees, coordinating the arms and legs in a way that maintains a straight, rigid back. Do not lift and twist at the same time. Alternate arms and hands when carrying packages.

Pain in the Groin

Any pain in the groin should be thoroughly checked out by your doctor since there are a multitude of possible causes. These range from internal problems with organs, such as the bladder or prostate gland, and other inflammatory conditions which must be differentiated from pain caused by sports injuries. Be sure to tell your doctor the background of how your pain began and how long you have been having it.

Injuries in the groin area are sometimes a result of slipping when running on icy roads, straining tendons and muscles as you try to keep your balance. Similarly, you may also pull a muscle when cross-country skiing.

Another possibility for cause of pain in the groin is excessive running on hard surfaces with poorly cushioned shoes—a likely cause of a stress fracture in one of the pubic bones. Repetitive stress in running or cycling can also cause inflammation of the front of the pubis (osteitis pubis) which occurs more commonly in male athletes aged thirty to forty; this condition is described more fully in the section below.

Unless you have very weak bones from osteoporosis, however, it is unlikely that you would get a groin strain from exercise walking. An inguinal hernia is one other possibility with groin pain, but this would also be accompanied by a bulge in the lower abdomen.

Inflammation of the Pubic Bone (Osteitis Pubis)

Repetitive stress from running and cycling can cause pain at the juncture of the two pubic bones in your groin. When the pelvis rotates and shifts in a see-saw motion from running or pedalling, the joint is slightly separated and the cartilage can become inflamed and roughened (Fig. 13-3). Football players are at risk for osteitis pubis because of the accumulated stresses of kicking the football. Sometimes the joint is damaged in a sudden fall with the legs stretched wide apart at the same time pressure is applied—as in a tackle.

Pain from osteitis pubis may come on gradually, starting as an ache. Race walkers are particularly prone to this injury because of the repetitive leg movements. Runners who overstride may also pull this joint. A severe case of over-training usually happens only with high-caliber athletes with a long history of running and racing. Osteitis pubis may sideline them from competition from one to two years.

With a severe trauma, such as falling off a motorcycle, the pain can be quite severe. Sit-ups would aggravate this condition, as would any abdominal strain or violent hip movement. The pain tends to radiate out into the hip, and there may be some swelling. To treat osteitis pubis, begin with ice or heat to relieve pain, whichever feels better. See your doctor as soon as possible so you can begin treatment. Have x-rays to rule out arthritis, rheumatism or gout. Abstain from activities that cause pain. If sex causes pain, don't do it. Gentle massage will stimulate healing in the area.

For pain, bruising and swelling, take one of the homeopathic remedies below in doses of two to four pills (6x-30c) every four hours for twenty-four hours.

> *Arnica* if there is a sore, bruised achy feeling; a cold pack may help numb the pain; *Bellis* if a heating pad feels better than a cold pack; *Sulphuric Acid* if *Arnica* doesn't work within six hours; *Bryonia* if you cannot bear to have the pubis touched, but pressure makes it feel better; *Ledum* if pubic area feels cool to the touch and feels better with a cold pack; injured area may also feel warm; *Lymphomyosot* if very swollen. Take ten drops twice a day.

During recovery take one of the following remedies in potencies of 6, 12, 30 or 200c once a day for three to four days:

> *Rhus Tox*—if you are very stiff and sore first thing in the morning or after sitting or lying down; if you feel better with continued movement or better with light massage; if your pain is worse with a cold pack, and better with warmth; if you feel restless, continually moving around to get comfortable. Take *Ruta Grav*—if you feel better with rest; if you feel stiff, sore, bruised and achy; if your groin feels better with heat; if you feel moody and fretful about the injury; if you are weak, tired and cranky after lots of activity or movement; if there are torn ligaments.

You may also benefit from hydrotherapy and contrast baths. Mild yoga stretching exercises will be very helpful after healing has been established for a couple of weeks.

Anti-inflammatory drugs such as Advil, Motrin, Feldene, or Naprosyn, can be taken for pain relief with or without homeopathics. Check first with your doctor, take with meals, and be aware of possible side effects of nausea, vomiting, or stomach irritation. These drugs can also cause blood in the stools or increase your bleeding time if you have an injury. Don't take them if you have ulcers or kidney problems.

Swimming and stationary cycling may be all right to help maintain aerobic fitness. Avoid running and walking fast.

Groin Strain

A groin strain is different than osteitis pubis because the damage involves muscles, ligaments and tendons, instead of cartilage (Fig. 13-3). The groin can be strained from a severe over-stretching in a single sudden injury, or from an accumulation of stress. You may have been running on wet and slippery ground or slipped on a patch of ice and forcibly contracted your groin muscles to stop yourself from falling. Athletes who play soccer and football or who compete in track and field events can pull a groin muscle. Sprinters, as well as marathoners, also are at risk for groin strain.

A groin strain injury causes large or small tears to the fibers of the muscles or tendons, as well as stress to the bony tissue of the pelvic ring and pubis symphysis. The pain may be sharp or dull, localized or diffuse. It may radiate into the hip and back.

For immediate relief of the pain of groin strain, apply ice packs or heating pad, whichever feels better. Stop doing any activities that cause pain. See your doctor to rule out stress fracture or arthritis.

For the shock of injury, take *Arnica*—two to four pills for up to six hours. For pain, bruising and swelling, take the same homeopathic remedies listed above in the section on osteitis pubis. For stiffness, take *Rhus Tox* or *Ruta Grav;* refer to osteitis pubis for details on these remedies.

Use ice whirlpool together with electro-galvanic stimulation or Ultrasound therapy for physical therapy.

Anti-inflammatory medicines should be used sparingly, and should not be used to mask pain in order to continue painful activities.

Have a podiatrist or sports medicine specialist check you for biomechanical abnormalities in the legs and feet. Start exercising only on the advice of your doctor.

Inguinal Hernia

With this condition, a part of your intestine is bulging out through a small defect in the supportive tissue (fascia) under the skin and fat of the groin. The inguinal ligament is a band which goes across the top of your leg where the leg bends at the hip. Too much pressure in your abdomen can force other tissues down through the gaps in this tissue, creating a hernia. Walking and running are usually not the cause of hernias, as the problem stems from heavy pressure, such as weight-lifting, forcing the tissue through the fascia. However, a hernia, obviously, will affect your walking and running. If you think you have a hernia, go to a doctor. There's nothing you can do in terms of self-help or homeopathic remedies.

Pelvis Fracture

Pelvis fractures can happen to athletes who fall from a height, such as falling off a horse or falling off a running trail. I recall such an incident myself when I was running a race on a hilly trail east of Oakland, California. It was a cold, rather dark day. One portion of the run was downhill, winding, somewhat slippery and treacherous. At one point there was a hairpin turn, and several runners were going so fast they lost control and actually ran off or fell off the trail. One runner broke his pelvis when he slipped and fell down the hill.

In cases of automobile accidents or other traumatic events, there are often more serious life-threatening problems, and a pelvic fracture may be initially overlooked. If left untreated for too long, a possibly significant deformity may result.

To treat a pelvic fracture at the time of trauma, go immediately to an emergency room. Have an x-ray done. The doctor should check the bladder and internal organs for damage.

Take homeopathic *Arnica* every hour for the first twenty-four hours. Choose either *Rhus Tox* or *Ruta Grav* in potencies of 6, 12, 30 or 200c once a day for three to four days or until better. Refer to the section on osteitis pubis for details of remedies.

Four to five days after diagnosis, take *Symphytum*, oral, 200c or 1M for two weeks to enhance healing. Two weeks after taking the *Symphytum*, take a single 1M dose of one of the *Calcarea Salts* (see page 223 for details or consult a *Materia Medica*):

   Calc Fluor, Calc Phos, or *Calc Carb*

For physiotherapy try a bone stimulator or electrical stimulation. Begin swimming when the fracture is stable, and cycling during the later stages of healing. Exercises during recovery should be recommended by your doctor. Don't try to do anything on your own. Recovery will take a minimum of four to six weeks and could take as long as four to six months.

Pain in the Buttocks (Ischial Bursitis)

Well, the proverbial pain in the backside has a name—ischial bursitis! This troublesome, difficult-to-treat problem occurs in runners (often in adolescents doing speed work) who are over- training and increasing their weekly mileage to levels beyond physiological tolerance.

The ischial bursa is a soft sac that lubricates and cushions the space between the tendon and the sitting bone (ischium). Rest is difficult because the injury is aggravated by sitting (see Fig. 13-5). To treat ischial bursitis, see a doctor and have an x-ray to rule out stress fracture or roughening of cartilage in the joint (osteitis pubis). For temporary relief, apply ice or heat to the painful area. Gentle massage will improve circulation.

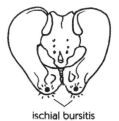

ischial bursitis

13-5. Pelvis
(back view)

Strengthen the hamstrings and gluteal muscles with stair climbing and reverse curls (see Chapter 15). Stretch all the thigh and buttocks muscles.

For pain, bruising and swelling, choose one of the following homeopathic remedies: (take doses of two to four pills per hour for 24 hours)

Arnica if sore, bruised and achy; *Bellis* if heating pad feels better than a cold pack; *Sulphuric Acid* if *Arnica* doesn't work within two hours; *Bryonia* if you cannot bear to be touched in the painful area; *Ledum* if the area is cool to the touch and feels better with a cold pack; (it may also feel warm); *Lymphomyosot* if very swollen. Take ten drops twice a day.

Four to five days after diagnosis, choose one of the Stage Two homeopathic remedies below. Take potencies of 6, 12, 15 or 30 or 200 once a day for three to four days:

Rhus Tox—if you are very stiff and sore first thing in the morning or after sitting or lying down; if you feel better with continued gentle movement or light massage; if your pain is worse with a cold pack and better with warmth; if you feel restless, continually moving around to get comfortable.

Take *Ruta Grav* if injury feels better with rest; if you feel stiff, sore, bruised and achy; if pain reduces with heating pad; if you feel moody and fretful about the injury; if you are weak, tired and cranky after lots of activity or movement; if there are torn ligaments.

An injection of homeopathic remedies into acupuncture points, joints, and ligaments enhance and speed up healing. Your doctor may select one of the injection medicines below, combining with ½cc of Wydase, a natural softening enzyme:

Traumeel for trauma; *Zeel* for joint problems; *Rhus Tox* for stiffness all the time; *Ruta Grav* for stiffness which gets better after movement; *Lymphomyosot* for swelling.

Injections of insoluble *cortisone* are not advised as they can cause degeneration of tissue. I don't recommend injections for young patients. If you are in your forties, injections may be suitable.

Ischial bursitis can be quite bothersome, and may take one to two years to heal.

Footnote:

1. Fig. 13-3. Stress Fractures and Shearing Forces in the Pelvis and Hip Area was adapted from a drawing by F. Netter, M.D.

Chapter 14

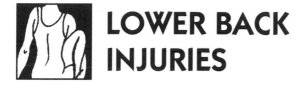

LOWER BACK
INJURIES

Ha! Men throwing their strength to the sky. Walking and bending
and lifting—waves of muscle rocking steaming skin. Throwing our
strength to the sky.
> —Peter Strudwick, footless runner loading a hay wagon,
> from *Come Run With Me*

Structure and Function

Our dreams, aspirations, and accomplishments hang on the spine just as
surely as do our muscles, nerves and ligaments. Built of five bony vertebrae, the lower spine (lumbar) is the lowest part of the back; it stands
ready to perform a vast variety of functions—among them walking,
lifting, twisting, jumping, throwing, dancing, or bowing. The spine and
lower back offer us power, mobility, shock-absorbing resilience and
protection for the spinal cord—the flexible backbone which permits
us to transform our thoughts into actions. The back grants us dignity, hu-
mility, productivity, and the joy of surpassing limitation.

The important parts of the lumbar spine are the five vertebrae bones
with their soft-tissue discs, the ligaments, and the muscles. Sheathed by
the protective canal of vertebrae is the spinal cord (see Fig. 14-1).

The lowest vertebrae, L5, lies on top of the back bone (sacrum),
and establishes the natural curve of the lower spine. A very strong ligament (anterior longitudinal ligament) running from the base of the
skull to the sacrum is attached to the front of the vertebrae. Another
ligament binds the spine in the back, from the sacrum to the second
vertebrae in the neck. There are many other smaller ligaments that
lend strength and flexibility to the structure.

The discs in the spine fit neatly into the flat surfaces between the
vertebrae, and are thicker in the lower back area than in the top por-

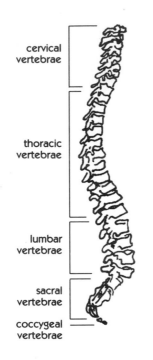

cervical vertebrae

thoracic vertebrae

lumbar vertebrae

sacral vertebrae

coccygeal vertebrae

14-1. Spine (side view)

tion of the back. A major function of the discs is to absorb shock when you land on your feet from a height. The abdominal muscles exert a forward pull on the spine; the extensor muscles running down the back pull the spine backwards. Small rotator muscles in the back work with diagonal stomach muscles when you twist. In the lumbar spine you have the greatest freedom to bend backwards or sideways; forward bending is more limited, and twisting is very restricted. The flexibility of the lower back is tested to the maximum when you dive with a twist.

Your spine is affected by the effects of gravity, your posture, your habitual movement patterns, and by the way you lift or carry weight.

The spinal cord extends from your brain to the level of the second lumbar vertebra. At each vertebra, tiny nerves branch out from the cord. A major injury to the spine, which comprises a big part of the central nervous system, causes paralysis and is usually permanent. The peripheral nerves from the lumbar spine extend to your legs. If the peripheral nerves are injured, the damage is most likely reversible with proper treatment. Pain in the lumbar area can radiate down the legs following the path of the peripheral nerves.

Back Pain

Besides sudden (acute) injury or over-use (chronic) injury, pain in the back can be caused by diseases such as arthritis, tuberculosis, or medical conditions in the lower organs. Be sure to see your doctor and report any symptoms such as difficulty urinating, gynecological problems or intestinal problems.

NOTE: Getting a second opinion is always good medical practice in cases involving serious illness or injury. This is particularly true in the case of back pain. If your doctor recommends surgery for lower back pain, be sure to consult with a second doctor before going ahead with surgery. In addition, if your doctor is recommending *rest* for lower back pain, I would suggest a second opinion as well. For some back problems rest is absolutely necessary, and with others it's not indicated.

The most helpful doctors for back pain are: an orthopedist, a chiropractor, a neurologist, a podiatrist and a neurosurgeon; or, if you can find one, an osteopath. An osteopath, a physician who also does physical manipulation of the body, combines the best of both worlds. If you don't seem to be healing as quickly as you should, or if you are not satisfied with the advice of your doctor, go to another one. Back and spine centers where all specialists work together is an excellent option. Don't have back surgery without a second opinion, because it may be unnecessary.

Low Back Injuries and Sciatica

Low back strain is often associated with biomechanical imbalances of the feet and legs. Short leg syndrome can create problems in the back as can feet that have unequal arches. A short leg absorbs more stress when running and accentuates distresses in the low back and hip. Using the Rule of Three discussed in Chapter 2 on biomechanics, a ⅛ inch limb length discrepancy is, during running, comparable in effect to a ⅜ inch actual deformity at rest. The increased strain is transmitted to the low back.

Sciatica means that the sciatic nerve is inflamed. This large nerve originates in the low back, exits the spinal column, travels down the inner part of the thigh and leg, finally ending at the tips of the toes. When there is an injury to the low back, pain follows the path of this nerve. There may be numbness or pain in the heel or big toe.

Tight buttocks muscles can cause sciatic compression syndrome, again with radiating pain being the key signal. The major culprit in sciatica in athletes and older people is weakness of abdominals. Remember, the abdomen is the front of the back. Since the problem of back pain can be difficult to treat, I recommend a team approach with a podiatrist to handle biomechanical solutions, an orthopedist for diagnosis, a chiropractor for spinal manipulations, and a physical therapist for building up weak muscles to support the spinal cord. Again, if you can find an osteopath, he or she can be very helpful with back problems. If surgery is indicated, an orthopedist or neurosurgeon is consulted. Acupuncture can often help in reducing pain as can homeopathy.

Case History of Sciatica Pain: Evin Schroeder

Evin Schroeder, a thirty-two-year-old attorney, showed up at my office complaining of a nagging, aching pain in his lower back on the right side. The pain, he said, was worse when he was doing downhill running as part of his fitness training.

Common sense made him switch to level ground, but the pain did not go away. Even so, he had persisted in increasing his training mileage, and now the pain was sharp, radiating under the right buttocks and down the leg. He shortened his stride because the leg hurt more when it was straight.

Diagnosis was easy in his case, because the radiating pain down the leg was a sure sign of sciatica. I found that he not only had one short leg, but that he turned both his feet inward when running (excessive pronation). The right foot was even more pronated than the left.

In addition, testing showed that his abdominal muscles were weak. In Evin's case, I had the orthopedist in my office confirm the diagnosis and treatment, and I had our sports chiropractor work on the right sacroiliac joint where there was some "catching" or fixation. I designed foot orthotics for Evin, gave him heel lifts, and recommended bent-knee situps for strengthening the abdominals. I prescribed Advil for the pain and inflammation in addition to homeopathic *Hypericum* for the nerve pain. I advised him to reduce his mileage. He improved in about four weeks, and I didn't see him for another two years.

When he came back after two years of using the orthoses, I had our physical therapist test his musculature with the computerized muscle strength machine (Cybex). We found residual weakness on the entire right side—low back, thigh and right leg. Exercises were outlined for him, and I fine-tuned his orthoses. In addition, I gave him *Calc Phos,* an excellent homeopathic remedy for strengthening the legs and vitalizing the immune system. He has been running fine since this last treatment.

For immediate relief of low back pain and sciatica, apply ice packs or heating pad, whichever feels best. Most importantly, get a correct diagnosis before you do anything else. First, try to find an osteopath for diagnosis and treatment. Or, see an orthopedist to make sure there is nothing mechanically or medically wrong. If you don't have a serious medical problem, then consult a chiropractor for treatment and manipulation. Physical therapists are very helpful too and will be recommended by an orthopedist. A podiatrist can evaluate you for any

biomechanical problems, such as short leg syndrome, excessive pronation, or an imbalance in the back itself. Biomechanical problems account for about 80 percent of chronic low back problems. Evaluation
will also rule out disc degeneration or slippage of vertebrae.

There are several choices of homeopathic remedies for low back
pain. Take doses 6-30, generally two to four pills four times a day until better. Select one:

Arnica if bruising pain; if better with heat, but cold pack may
numb injury and lessen pain and swelling; very sensitive to
touch—it even hurts when lying on a firm mattress; worse with
motion; *Zinc* for restless back pain with shooting pains along
the nerves; if you feel worse being over-heated; *Bryonia* for back
pain that gets worse as you move around; if you feel better with
rest and back brace; if you tend to be very irritable; if better with
a cool pack.

Take *Hypericum* for tail-bone pain or radiating nerve pain;
if you feel very sore, and ice or cold makes pain worse;

Magnesium Phosphoricum for back pains which come and go
suddenly; if pressure feels worse; if there is cramping; if you feel
worse with an uncovered back and leg. Take *Ruta Grav* if you are
stiff and bruised; if you feel worse when sitting and have a burning-
type pain. Take *Kali Carb* or other *Kali Salts* for a stitching pain
predominantly on the left side (may also be on right side), or
knife-like pain; if you must turn to the side in bed to help you
rise. Take *Rhus Tox* if you feel worse with initial motion, but better with continued motion; for right-sided back pain with a burning or aching pain; if you are restless, stiff, and feel worse in the
cold or with an ice pack; much better with heat. Take *Pulsatilla*
for migrating back pain which is changeable; if you feel worse in a
warm room, better with a cool breeze; if your back is better walking slowly, and worse with heavy exertion; *Calc Salts* for over-
work strain of low back; for lumbago with or without sciatica; if
your back feels worse in cold, wet weather; *Ledum* when your
back feels worse with heat, but better with a cold pack.

Don't run. Avoid impact sports. Follow the advice of your doctor
after a proper diagnosis. Once you have your diagnosis, gentle massage
may help to relax you and stimulate healing.

Acupuncture may help after a medical diagnosis has been made.

Physiotherapy will be helpful in educating yourself about back
problems. Your doctor will recommend a physiotherapist.

Hot tubs may help for muscle spasms. Back injuries can be great-ly helped by many body work disciplines. Look into Alexander tech-nique, Rolfing, Heller and Trager work, Rosen work, Feldenkrais, and other systems of energy healing. The important thing to remember is that you must get a standard medical diagnosis before going to any of the alternative treatments. You must know what you are dealing with before treating pain.

I have found that structural integration work, such as Rolfing, while often very beneficial, may not last without accompanying or-thotics. Be sure to discuss any of the alternative treatments you choose with your orthopedist, podiatrist, chiropractor, or osteopath.

Hill running creates substantial problems for sensitive low backs. Going up hill tightens the buttocks (gluteal) muscles; going down hill produces overstriding and increased shock. A daily program of yoga or T'ai Chi could be one of the best possible solutions for back pain and continued health and vigor.

Lumbosacral Strain

Any type of low back pain is going to effect your walking and run-ning program. Lumbosacral strain is a catch-all term for any back con-dition that has no readily identifiable cause. This is certainly not a glamorous injury generating a lot of sympathy! Pain in the lower back can be a result of spending long hours sitting at a desk, behind the wheel of a car, or hunched over a book. Wearing high heels, another cause of low back pain, increases strain to the small of the back espe-cially if your stomach muscles are weak.

Low back injuries are common in football players, especially young players. Once an injury to the back occurs it can follow you into mid-dle-age. The pain is due to extreme muscle spasm and tightness. Many of my patients have had improvement of low back pain with walking and running. Muscles warm up and the rhythmic activity eases ten-sion and relaxes the back. Of course, too much of a good thing can aggravate the back.

To treat lumbosacral strain, avoid any activity that brings on pain. Ice may be applied for temporary relief of pain, alternating with a heating pad (set to *low,* never high) wrapped in a towel.

See a doctor and get a clear diagnosis of what kind of low back pain you have before you do any treatment on your own. See an os-teopath, chiropractor, podiatrist, orthopedist, or a good family practi-tioner. Biomechanical foot imbalances should be checked by a podiatrist. Eighty-percent of low back problems have a foot imbalance as the cause. One way to determine if the foot is the main problem is to have your podiatrist give you temporary foot orthotics, and if the back gets better, then have permanent ones made. Imbalances in the back should be checked by an orthopedist, chiropractor, or osteopath.

You may need a better chair for your desk—one with low back support. Your doctor may give you a soft corset to hold the back area more firmly. However, a corset should be used only as a temporary measure for pain relief, as muscles tend to atrophy if not used and strengthened. When you are no longer in pain, have your doctor recommend back-strengthening exercises.

When standing, don't allow the back to sag or slouch. When driving, support your low back with a pillow or rolled towel if you drive long distances. When sleeping, you may also need a firm board under your mattress for better support while you sleep. A futon is a healthy mattress for low-back pain.

Homeopathic remedies for low back pain are listed below. Select one in doses of 6-30; take two to four pills four times a day until better:

Rhus Tox is a good back remedy if you feel worse in cold, wet weather; if you are stiff, restless, but feel better if you keep moving. After two weeks follow with *Calc Carb*. Take *Kali Carb* if your key symptom is that you feel better sitting; for a stitching pain on the left side, or knife-like pain; if you must turn to the side in bed to help you rise; if you're better sitting, not moving around; if you love sweets, and are set in your ways! Take *Sulphur* if your key symptom is that you feel better sitting and worse standing; if you are a philosophical type person; if you are overweight and feel worse with heat. *Pulsatilla* for migrating, changeable pain in the back; if you feel worse in a warm room, better with a cool breeze; if your back is better walking slowly, and worse with heavy exertion. Take *Arnica* for soreness; if your back feels "beaten up"; worse when touched; worse with motion; lame; for initial treatment; usually better heat. Take *Bryonia* if you cannot move very well or bear to have your back touched, but pressure makes it feel better; if better with a cold pack.

Ledum if foot feels cool to the touch and feels better with cold pack. *Hypericum* for tail-bone pain or radiating nerve pain; if you feel very sore, and ice or cold makes pain worse. *Calc Salts* are the main remedies for chronic low back pain; choose between

Calc Carb, Calc Phos, and *Calc Fluor.* See page 223 for details or consult a Materia Medica for characteristics.

Note on comparing remedies: If your key symptom is that you feel better sitting, select either *Kali Carb* or *Sulphur.* If your key symptom is that you feel worse when you sit, take *Rhus Tox, Pulsatilla, Zinc* or the *Calc Salts.*

If your key symptom is that you feel worse stooping, *Kali Carb, Rhus Tox* or *Sulphur.* If your key symptom is that you feel worse standing, take *Sulphur, Ruta Grav Calc Salts* or *Bryonia.* If your key symptom is that you feel better after walking, take *Rhus Tox* or *Pulsatilla.*

If your low back pain is very bad, then see a doctor. Otherwise you can begin to follow the regimen of treatment and exercise below:

- Exercise for strengthening the back and abdominal muscles are a must as soon as your pain decreases. See Chapter 15 for back exercises. However, any exercise that causes pain should be avoided for the time being.
- Anti-spasmodic medications such as Flexeril relieve muscles spasms; anti-inflammatory medicines such as Advil, Motrin, Feldene, or Naprosyn may be taken, provided you are not allergic to aspirin or have an ulcer. These medicines should be taken with food to avoid irritating the lining of the stomach.
- Deep tissue massage is very helpful in reducing tension in the painful muscles, as is chiropractic manipulation. Rolfing, a form of deep manipulation of the body's holding tissue (fascia), can be very helpful for back problems, but should be done only after a standard medical diagnosis has been made.
- If you have chronic low back problems with no serious medical cause, you owe it to yourself to investigate the various forms of body work now available: Heller work, Trager, Feldenkrais, Rosen, Rolfing, Alexander technique, and others. Check the referral list in Chapter 20 for body workers in your area.
- Participating in any kind of movement practice such as T'ai Chi is very helpful; yoga is an age-old method of retaining youthful flexibility.
- Back pain often responds well to acupuncture treatments. Try acupuncture after serious medical conditions have been ruled out by medical diagnosis.

Herniated Disc

Intervertebral discs, those
elastic bundles of tissue between the vertebrae, are subject to constant stress and
the possibility of degenerative tears as well as dehydration (see Fig. 14-2). The
most vulnerable discs lie between the fourth and fifth
lumbar vertebrae, deep in

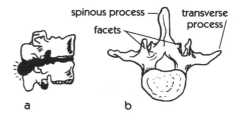

14-2. Lumbar Vertebrae
a) Herniated disc
pressure causes disc to bulge out.
b) Structure of a vertebrae.

the lumbar curve. A sudden blow or twist can generate as much as
1,000 to 1,500 pounds of force when a hundred pound weight is lifted.

In a herniated disc injury, pressure forces a disc to bulge out (her-
niate) beyond the bony borders of the vertebrae. The tissue is then
pressing on the spinal cord or spinal nerves. Like tiny neon lights, the
painful, excited nerves show up on computed tomography (CT) scans,
revealing the precise extent of the problem. MRI is also commonly
used to evaluate disc and nerve tissue. Thermography helps pinpoint areas of inflammation in the back.

In the acute phase of this injury, avoid any painful activity. Apply
ice packs and/or heating pad, whichever feels better.

Select one of the following homeopathic remedies for the first twenty-four hours. Take in doses of 6 30 four times a day until better.

> *Arnica* if very sore bruising pain; better warm, but cold pack
> may numb injury and lessen pain and swelling; very sensitive to
> touch; worse lying on a hard mattress; worse with motion; *Bellis*
> if very deep bruising; soreness; if heating pad feels better than a
> cold pack; *Bryonia* if your onset of pain was slow, and if twisting
> and turning makes the pain worse; if you can't stand to be
> touched; *Rhus Tox* if movements such as twisting and turning
> makes it feel better; much worse cold, damp; much worse cool-
> ing off after overheating; *Ledum* if back feels cool to the touch
> (may also be warm) and feels better with cold pack; *Hypericum*
> if there is sharp, intense nerve-like pain; *Zinc* if there is a bad
> pain at the tail-bone, and you feel worse with sitting. Take *Caus-
> ticum* if the pain is worse rising from a seat; much worse when
> cold or dry; very stiff and tight like *Rhus Tox,* but is not better
> from continued movement; *Pulsatilla* if you have migrating back

289

pains; if you feel worse in the heat, and prefer a breeze or lots of air; *Calc Carb* good for herniated disc pain as well as *Calc Phos* and *Calc Fluor* (choose according to type of constitution (see page 223); *Nat Mur* if you are withdrawn, need solitude, and keep your feelings in; if you eat salty food and *must* lie on something hard when your back hurts.

For pain relief take anti-inflammatory medicines like Advil and Motrin, Feldene, or Naprosyn if you do not have a history of aspirin allergy or ulcers.

Mild to moderate disc protrusion is treated successfully by a physical therapist, chiropractor or osteopathic physician. Get a second medical opinion first, however. Also, you may do well to visit a comprehensive spine center. Severe disc protrusion and herniated disc often needs surgery by an orthopedist or neurosurgeon.

Select one of these two homeopathic remedies following surgery:

Arnica for shock, pain, swelling, general recovery.

Hypericum for nerve irritation and sharp pain.

Following recovery from surgery, it's important to do a lot of walking and a minimal amount of sitting.

Facet Syndrome

Facets are joints between vertebrae (Fig. 14-2b). They can become inflamed, and must be distinguished from disc disease because the treatment is very different. The pain, however, is similar to disc disease, and onset can be gradual or sudden in the low back. It may be caused by poor posture, twisting, or bending. It feels like something is out of place. There is a dull, nagging feeling in the back, and the muscles may be tense or in spasm. It can be quite uncomfortable.

Unfortunately well-intentioned family physicians often confuse a facet syndrome with disc disease and prescribe rest, which is helpful for some low back pain, but is wrong for facet syndrome.

They may even go so far as to put you in traction in the hospital, which is an extreme measure for this injury, and could possibly even contribute to more weakness and stiffness in the back. If you are told you need hospitalization or traction, get a second opinion from a good chiropractor, osteopath, orthopedist, or physical therapist. Be sure the doctor you consult has considerable experience with athletes and physical medicine.

To treat facet syndrome, it's important to get a correct diagnosis. Distinguish whether you have facet syndrome or a herniated disc or

---

Fat Wallet Syndrome

Andy Lawrence was a middle-aged runner who came to me with progressive pain underneath his left buttocks. He was sure that this was running-related. My examination, however, revealed that he had good form and no biomechanical weak links. There was no sciatica or arthritis.

I was stumped until I asked about his daily activities. Since he was a travelling salesman, I asked him to show me how he sat. I noticed that he had his wallet in his left rear pocket which was also where the pain was! He said he always carried the wallet there. I suggested he move it to a coat pocket; from then on—no more pain. A short time later, I read an article in an orthopedic journal called "The Fat Wallet Syndrome" and have since seen at least a dozen other patients with a similar problem.

---

other problems. X-rays or MRI may be needed.

For an adjustment, go to a chiropractor, osteopath, or physical therapist who can gently move the vertebrae, realigning the bones. This movement is called mobilization. Mobilization returns the facets to their correct position, releasing the tension created by pain and muscle spasms. Manipulation is a more forcible adjustment than mobilization.

Orthoses and heel lifts can help this condition. Check for limb length discrepancy (one leg shorter than the other). You may need a foot orthotic inside your shoe or a heel lift.

It is essential to start rehabilitative back exercises to strengthen muscles to prevent future misalignment. Get professional advice from a physical therapist. *Gentle* massage may help the painful area.

Choose one of these oral homeopathic remedies (take two or three pills of any potency four times a day):

Hypericum for nerve pain; *Ruta Grav* if sore and stiff; *Rhus Tox* for stiffness.

If there are spasms along the spine, you may need trigger point injections in the painful spots which often correspond to acupuncture points. Have your physician inject with the above remedies. After two weeks of healing take *Calc Phos.*

After the acute phase of pain is over, Rolfing or other body work may be very helpful. Acupuncture also can be helpful after the acute phase of pain is over.

Non-steroidal anti-inflammatory drugs (NSAIDs) such as Advil, Motrin and others may be taken with or without homeopathic remedies. Do not take NSAIDs if you are allergic to aspirin or have ulcers.

Other Back Problems
Arthritis of the Back

This condition may be caused from old injuries or bone spurs on the spine. The discomfort progresses slowly with much stiffness which increases in cold, wet weather. Most effective treatment is usually constitutional homeopathy and physical therapy. The best homeopathic remedies are the *Calcarea Salts,* and other constitutional remedies (which a homeopathic practitioner will select based on an analysis of your personal characteristics). For acute problems use either *Rhus Tox* if stiff with initial motion, but better after prolonged movement; tends to be restless type or *Ruta Grav* if very stiff and sore; worse motion; cranky, irritable type. Refer to Chapter 17 on arthritis.

Scoliosis

Scoliosis is an abnormal curvature of the spine (Fig. 14-3b). An osteopath, chiropractor, orthopedist, or podiatrist will evaluate you for biomechanical imbalances such as short leg syndrome or pronation (flattening) of the feet. You will need exercises, physical therapy, and possibly braces. Rolfing—deep structural manipulation of the connective tissue—may be helpful, but check with a medical doctor before starting this treatment. Even with Rolfing, you may need braces.

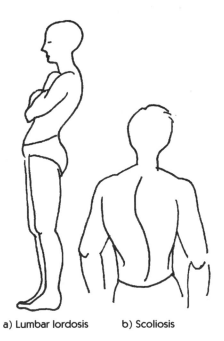

a) Lumbar lordosis   b) Scoliosis

14-3. Spinal Abnormalities

Stress Fracture

If you have prolonged pain and swelling in the back, you may have a stress fracture in the spine. A stress fracture in the vertebrae could occur with hard running or falling. A bone scan will usually show if a stress fracture is present. As with all stress fractures, rest and avoidance of painful activities is essential for four to six weeks. You must be under the care of a doctor for this condition.

Chapter **15**

FITNESS EXERCISES

There is no disease but stagnation. There is no remedy but circulation.
—Ancient Chinese adage

Commonly Asked Questions about Conditioning Exercises and Running

"I don't have time to stretch. Can't I just start off running slowly, and when I feel warm, pick up the pace?"

Yes, you can, as long as the unexpected doesn't happen. If you don't do flexibility exercises you are not going to be prepared for the eventuality of over-stretching. Be aware that the longer you run, the tighter you're going to get, which will limit the range of motion in your joints and ligaments. Your stride will shorten, and your running will be less efficient.

It's much better to take the time—even if it's only three times a week—to really stretch.

"What if I warm up by walking fast or jogging before I start stretching? Wouldn't that be better than stretching with cold muscles? "

Yes. Good idea. You can also warm up on an exercise bike.

"How long should I stretch?"

Stretch at least 20 minutes on the days that you run. The first 10 minutes (before you run) should be easy. After you get back from running, try some of the longer, deeper stretches.

Frequency in Practising Different Types of Exercises

- Stretches may be done every day, 10 minutes before strenuous activity and 10 minutes afterwards.
- Quad sets and other exercises not involving weights may be done every day.
- Muscle strengthening exercises with weights should be done every other day or every third day. Weight training, even with light weights, may cause soreness and you'll need one to three days to recover. Remember: To improve the figure and not build muscle mass, use light weights with more repetitions. To build mass and increase strength, use heavier weights with fewer repetitions.

Everyday Stretches

Fig. 15-1 shows a very good routine to fine-tune the muscles you use in normal activity. Doing these exercises each day allows you to get rid of accumulated tension so that you can use your body with greater ease.

The Warm-Up for Runners, Walkers, and Sportspeople

The purpose of warm-up exercises is to prepare the body for the demands of running or playing a fast-paced sport by raising the temperature and increasing blood flow to the muscles. If you're still tempted to skip this part of your routine, take another look at what a good warm-up provides:

- increased blood flow to muscles
- higher rate of oxygen exchange between blood and muscles
- more oxygen released within muscles
- higher metabolic rate
- faster nerve impulse transmission
- decreased muscle relaxation time following contraction
- increased speed and force of muscle contraction
- increased muscle elasticity
- rehearsal effect (the body practices muscular patterns to be used later)

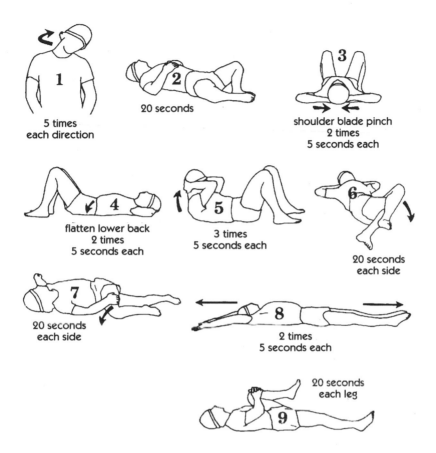

15-1. Everyday Stretches: 10 to 15 minutes.
(adapted from *Stretching*, Anderson)

- reduced risk of abnormal electrocardiogram
- increased flexibility of tendons and ligaments

Pre-warm up
- Pre-warm your muscles and increase breathing by doing one of the following for 3 to 5 minutes:
- running in place
- walking up and down stairs
- free-form dancing
- or do 15 minutes on an exercycle
- Progress to: Fig. 15-2.

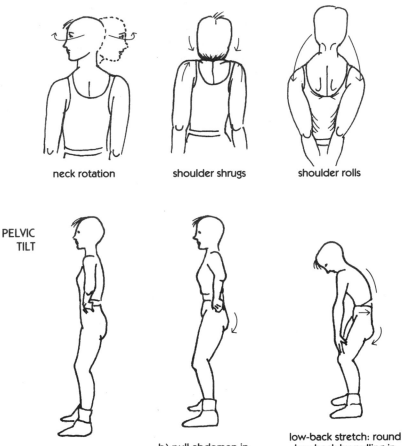

neck rotation   shoulder shrugs   shoulder rolls

PELVIC
TILT

a) knees slightly bent

b) pull abdomen in,
tuck buttocks under

low-back stretch: round
low back by pulling in
abdomen with extreme
posterior pelvic tilt

15-2. Pre-warm-up Routine for Shoulders, Abdomen, Pelvis, and Low-back

- 4 side-to-side neck rotations
- 4 shoulder shrugs
- 4 shoulder rolls
- 4 pelvic tilts
- 4 low-back stretches
- Progress to the 12-step warm-up routine shown in Fig. 15-3.

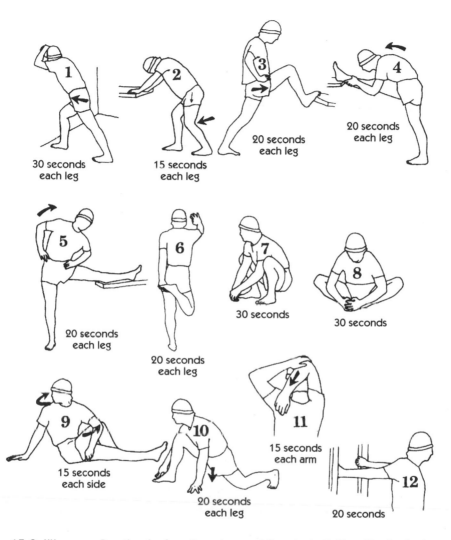

15-3. Warm-up Routine before Running and Sports Activities (9 minutes)
(adapted from *Stretching*, Anderson)

Remember: Back off if you feel a burning sensation in the muscles. The rule of thumb in exercise is that mild discomfort is all right, but there should not be pain. If there is pain, don't do the exercise.
Now you can run!

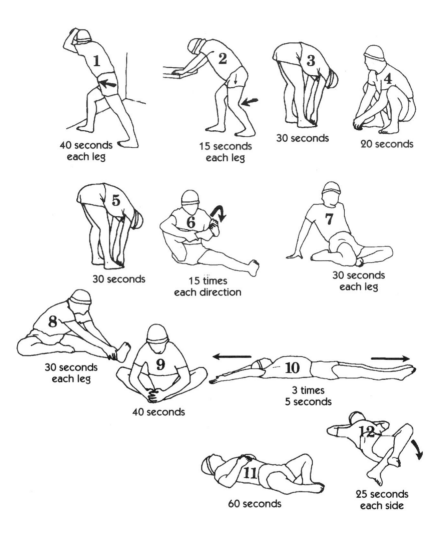

15-4. Cool-down (9 minutes)
(adapted from *Stretching,* Anderson)

Cool-down

Allowing your heartbeat to gradually lower to 120 beats per minute or less helps prevent excessive pooling of blood in the lower extremities, reduces muscle soreness, and promotes faster removal of metabolic wastes such as lactic acid.

Stretching after a strenuous workout is essential for maintaining flexibility, and is even more important than during the warm-up. Remember: All muscles perform better when stretched to 110 percent of their normal length.

• Walk the last block of your run (about 2 to 3 minutes).

Proceed to the 12-step cool down routine shown in Fig. 15-4.

Prevention and Rehabilitation of Injuries in Running

Be prepared for accidental over-stretching

Running tightens—it does not promote flexibility. Over time, muscles become tighter and stiffer with regular running, increasing the risk of accidental over-stretching. When an unexpected movement happens, muscles that are stiff and short cannot accommodate, and something tears and gives. In order to prevent injury, an athlete must be more flexible and stronger than is necessary just for running. The muscles must be able to respond to a stretch beyond what is ordinarily encountered in running, and be able to handle a heavier load than what is needed for running or other sport. You must be prepared for the unexpected. The following story illustrates my point.

Rehabilitating Nathan Schwarz: (Using strengthening exercises, physical therapy, homeopathic remedies, massage, and yoga)

Running into the unexpected

Nathan, a twenty-seven-year-old accountant came to me complaining of a calf pull. He had pulled the attachment of his Achilles tendon to his calf muscle towards the middle of the inside of the right leg. The injury had happened during the hilly 9-mile Woodminster race near Oakland, California. He was going all-out on the finish of this race on a downhill stretch. Coming around a sharp corner, he had landed on the ball of his right foot on a sudden uphill grade. This forced his foot upwards towards the ankle—stretching the back calf muscles much further than they were used to in normal running. He heard a pop as his calf muscle tore. He was unprepared for the unexpected.

"Not enough time for stretching"

Nathan came to see me about seven weeks after the injury. I asked him what kind of training he did, and he said he almost never included stretching in his routine. "I really just like to run and workout. Stretching takes too much time, and it doesn't burn off any calories," he told me. Typical Type-A behavior, I thought to myself.

Pain and stiffness in the morning and after prolonged exercise

Since the injury, Nate had been running, but much more slowly. He was achy and stiff during the first mile. He couldn't run fast or race, and hills were out of the question. About two or three hours after running, his calf muscles stiffened up so much he limped or shuffled. His calf was very painful in the morning when first walking around, but a hot shower helped somewhat. At night the leg was very restless and he kept moving it to try to get comfortable. Massage made the muscle feel better as did leaning against the wall in wall-pushups that stretched the muscles out.

Extent of damage

Nate, luckily, had torn only about one-fifth of the junction of the muscle to the tendon, and he would not need surgery. The tear was healing. The problem was that the gap had healed with thick, inelastic scar tissue which had begun to adhere to surrounding tissue. This was causing the pain when he used the calf muscle.

General inflexibility and weakness

I checked Nate for general flexibility. He could not even touch the tips of his toes. His calf and hamstrings were very tight, and he could barely move his foot to a perpendicular angle at the ankle. Further testing showed he was weak in all the muscles in the front of his legs (quadriceps and shin muscles). To make matters worse, his inner groin muscles were weak, as were the muscles on the outside of his legs.

He was a perfect example of how running only develops the anti-gravity muscles in the back of the leg, while leaving the other three sides (inner, outer, and front) of the legs relatively undeveloped. He was over-specialized for running straight ahead, and was not fit in an overall sense. As we talked about the need for general strengthening and flexibility, I mentioned that his physical condition also reflected his rather rigid, inflexible, goal-oriented mind set. He listened and said nothing.

Breaking up the scar-tissue adhesions

Nate's symptoms fit the homeopathic remedy *Rhus tox.* He had pain and stiffness with initial motion which gradually lessened with gentle activity, but the stiffness returned after excessive activity. He felt better with warmth (hot shower and hot compresses). I injected a combination of a local anesthetic, *Rhus tox,* and Wydase (a natural softening enzyme) to soften the scar tissue.

Passive stretching and active stretching

Nate was put on a strengthening and stretching program. For strengthening the front of the lower leg, I had him sit on a table and raise and lower his leg with a five-pound paint can hooked over his foot (see Fig. 15-5c). When the leg is brought forward to the straight position, the movement is a "concentric" stretch. When the leg is bent back down, the stretch is an "eccentric" one. Eccentric stretching is mostly what happens during running. Concentric stretching occurs when weights are lifted.

I also had him raise and lower his heel while standing on an incline board to stretch out the Achilles tendon area. The incline board is an example of passive stretching: the stretch is attained and held in a relaxed (not straining) manner. He started at 15 degrees and gradually increased the angle to 45 degrees over the next few weeks.

He also did some slow stretches like the one shown in Fig. 15-4 (8 and 9) in which he stretched, let the breath out, and moved slowly forward, stretching the muscle and holding the position.

Yoga and deep-tissue massage

Nate, being the competitive person that he was, wanted to do more. I suggested that he try some deep-tissue massage to work on the scar tissue adhesions, which he did with one of the practitioners in my office. In addition, he started going to weekly Iyengar yoga classes. In three weeks, he told me that he was feeling more flexibility in his stretching, but he was disappointed that he was still only at a first level class.

Physical therapy and ultrasound

Nate was determined to try all methods of regaining a balanced body. He went on a physical therapy program in my office, using ultrasound and electro-galvanic stimulation to continue to soften the scar tissue.

Homeopathic treatment

To soften the scar tissue even further, I gave him an injection of homeopathic medicine and gave him a single 200c oral dose of *Rhus tox*. Following that I put him on two tablets a day of 12c *Rhus tox* to help with the healing. After six weeks, he was about 75 percent improved, although his inflexibility had still not improved beyond level one in the yoga class.

The happy ending

In three weeks Nate returned to see me, very happy that he was about to move to the second level in yoga. His teacher had told him that his muscles had been exceptionally tight and that it had taken a longer-than-usual time to reach the second level. "I realize now," he said, "that the running hadn't really helped me to get fit, other than exercising my cardiovascular system."

At this point he was 100 percent improved. In fact, he said, "You know as I get more physically flexible, I'm feeling a lot more relaxed. I feel different. Do you think there's a connection?" I told him I thought it was highly possible.

Muscle Strengthening

There are three ways to strengthen a muscle:

Isometric. This method contracts the muscle as hard as possible, but there is no movement. For example, holding a basketball between your knees and pushing in is an isometric exercise.

Isotonic. This method contracts a muscle while it is being moved, shortening it while it's moving. An example of an isotonic exercise is when you hold a 5 lb. weight and bring the weight up to your shoulder (bicep curl).

Isokinetic. The reverse of isotonic, this method contracts the muscle while it is lengthening. Isotonic exercise occurs as you extend your arm back down again after holding the weight at the shoulder. In running, many of the muscles contract isokinetically (contracting while lengthening).

It's important to do isometric, isotonic and isokinetic exercises to make sure your muscles are strengthened for the various movements that take place in sports. In fact, resistance training, the use of free weights, weight machines or calisthenics should be done by runners to maintain upper-body strength. New guidelines were published in 1990 by the American College of Sports Medicine after following runners for the past ten years. Those who did not practice upper-body training were found to have an overall loss of muscle mass.

Exercising after Injury

For every day you are away from running or a workout, you lose 3 days of training. This applies not only to those who are performing at high levels of training or competition but also to the everyday runner and walker.

If you have have been laid up with an injury for over two weeks, you must take it very easy when you return to exercising, running or playing sports. While the body adapts to stress rapidly, it also becomes desensitized to stress rapidly. If you are a recovering runner, start with a maximum of 15 minutes a day at slow paces for the first week. Increase workouts by *5 minutes* a day per week. At least one day during the week must be spent resting.

After you can run up to 45–50 minutes a day fairly slowly, then you may begin to speed up the pace and perhaps start some interval work. From then on, you're on your own.

My rule of thumb is: If you begin a run with stiffness and pain and it goes away as you run, then it's okay to keep running. However, if your initial soreness becomes worse or you develop pain while running, then you should stop running. If you are racing and develop serious pains—stop.

Rehabilitative Muscle Strengthening Exercises for Knee Injuries

Warning: Do the following exercises only with the supervision of your doctor.

Strengthening the front of the leg (quadriceps muscles):

Leg lifts (15-5a, b). Use either version of Figs. 15-5a or b which keeps lower back supported while lifting leg. Avoid doing leg lifts lying flat on the floor as this strains the lumbar region. Do three sets of 20 lifts, holding each lift for 1–2 seconds.

Quad exercise with weight (15-5c). Make your own weights with pillow cases or a paint can filled with rocks or sand. Start with no more than 5 pounds on the front of your ankle. Sit on a table and lift leg to straight position. Hold for a count of 20. Do 20 sets 2 or 3 times a day.

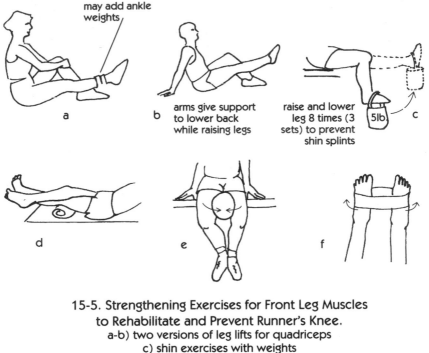

15-5. Strengthening Exercises for Front Leg Muscles
to Rehabilitate and Prevent Runner's Knee.
a-b) two versions of leg lifts for quadriceps
c) shin exercises with weights
d) quad sets—static contractions
e) isometric thigh-squeeze with ball
f) strengthening outer thigh muscles with elastic band

Increase weights 2 pounds a week to a maximum of 40 pounds.

Quad sets (15-5d). Quad sets contract the quadriceps forcefully, especially the inner portion. Sit or lie down and place a rolled towel beneath your knee joint so that the knee is bent about 15 degrees. Then put one leg on top of the other and straighten out the bottom leg, using the upper leg as a weight. Hold this contraction to a count of twenty and do twenty of these twice a day.

Strengthening Inner Thigh Muscles

Ball squeeze (15-5e). Put a basketball between your legs and press your legs together for a count of twenty; relax. Do twenty sets.

Strengthening Outer Side of Thigh

Foot pull (15-5f). Put an old inner tube or elastic band around your feet, and pull apart, trying to separate the legs as much as you can; hold for a count of twenty; relax. Do twenty sets.

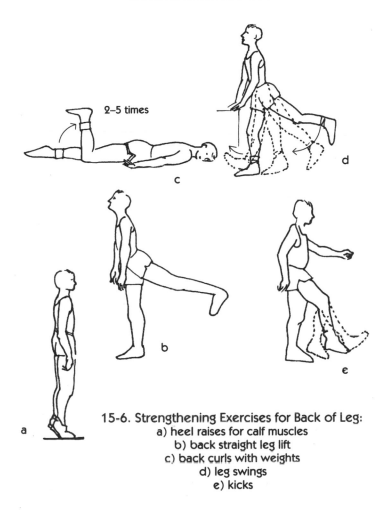

2–5 times

15-6. Strengthening Exercises for Back of Leg:
a) heel raises for calf muscles
b) back straight leg lift
c) back curls with weights
d) leg swings
e) kicks

Strengthening the Calf Muscles

Raise up and down on the balls of your feet (Fig. 15-6a). Do twenty sets.

Strengthening the Back of the Thigh (Hamstrings)

Leg lifts (Fig. 15-6b). Extend the leg straight backward and lift as high as you can, keeping leg straight. Do twenty sets each leg.

Curls (15-6c). Put weights on ankles and curl leg towards buttocks. Start with 5 pounds. Do eights curls each leg, three sets.

Leg swings (15-6d). Stand and swing straight leg forward and back. Do eight swings each leg, three sets.

307

Kicks (15-6e). Stand without supports, and kick as if kicking a ball. Kick until tired, rest a few seconds, continue for three sets each leg.

Stretching Exercises

Standing quad stretch (15-7a). After doing the above strengthening sets, stand and pull back your foot with your hand until the heel touches your buttocks. Then lean forward and pull the foot back, stretching the muscle a little further. Use opposite arm to pull leg towards other side to stretch different muscles in back of leg (Fig. 15-7b).

Yoga stretch for hamstrings (15-7c). Sit on the floor with one leg extended and one leg bent so that your foot is flat against your upper thigh where it joins the groin. Lean forward from the base of your spine, keeping your back straight (not rounded). Extend the arms reaching for your ankle. If you can, hold your big toe, pulling forward so that your torso lies parallel to the extended leg. Breathe into the pose. Stretch out on the exhale, extending only as the muscles permit. Hold for a count of ten, and return slowly to an upright sitting position. Repeat on other side. Then extend both legs and stretch forward, keeping your back straight and holding the ankles or big toes.

Supported hamstrings stretch (15-7d). According to your level of flexibility, use a stool, chair seat, or table to support your leg. With one leg straight and heel on the floor, bring your head toward the knee of the extended leg until it feels uncomfortable, then let up a little bit. Hold for a count of ten. Relax. Repeat for one minute, then do the same exercise with the other leg.

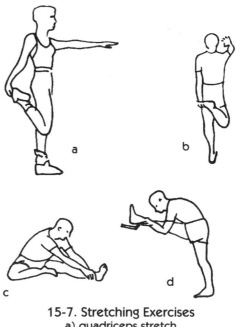

15-7. Stretching Exercises
a) quadriceps stretch
b) quadriceps stretch, alternate arm pull
c) yoga stretch for hamstrings
d) hamstrings stretch with support

Exercises for Hamstrings and Plantar Fascia

Side-to-side stretch (15-8a). With knees slightly bent, move side to side, keeping feet in one place. Stretches and strengthens back of leg and feet. Do eight times, three sets.

Back of leg stretch (15-8b). With knees bent, push against table to strengthen and stretch calves. Do eight times, three sets.

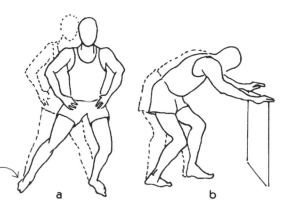

15-8. Muscle Stretches
a) stretch for hamstrings, plantar fasciia
b) back-of-leg stetch

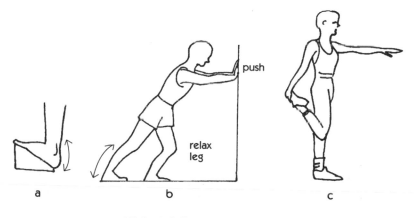

15-9. Achilles Heel Stretches
a) flex-wedge
b) heel cord stretch: hold for count of 20
c) quad stretch lengthens front muscles

Stretching Achilles Tendon

Flex-Wedge (15-9a). Standing at an incline on a Flex-Wedge or edge of stair, stretch out Achilles tendon and calf muscle for 3 minutes.

Wall push (15-9b). With one leg slightly bent, straighten opposite leg back to achieve gentle stretch of lower leg and Achilles tendon. Use wall for support and to push against.

Standing quad stretch (15-9c). This stretch helps to lengthen front muscles which balance the muscles in the back of the leg.

Foot Flexibility Exercises

Describing the alphabet with your toe (15-10a). This exercises all the muscles in the foot to increase range of motion.

Spreading the toes (15-10b). This is a range of motion exercise. Spread toes as far apart as possible, hold 30 seconds. Do five times.

Foot press (15-10c). In this isometric exercise, the bottom foot presses upward and the top foot presses downward to strengthen muscles. Hold for count of ten, three sets.

Walking on tip-toes (15-10d). This increases flexibility in feet and toes. Practice walking on tip-toes 5 or 10 minutes a day.

Picking up towel with toes (15-10e). This exercise strengthens toe and foot muscles and increases range of motion.

describing alphabet with toe

spreading toes

foot press

walking on tip-toes

picking up towel with toes

15-10. Foot Flexibility Exercises

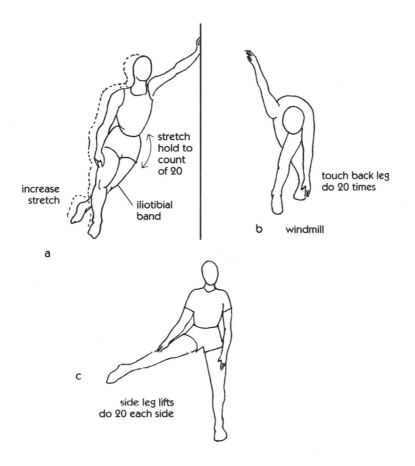

stretch hold to count of 20

increase stretch

iliotibial band

a

touch back leg do 20 times

b   windmill

c

side leg lifts do 20 each side

15-11. Stretches to Relieve Tight Iliotibial Band
(pain on side of leg above knee)

Exercises to Relieve Iliotibial Band Syndrome

(for tightness and "snapping" on upper outside thigh)

Leg stretch (15-11a). Lean against wall at an angle and stretch leg closes to wall behind other leg to stretch side of body and leg.

Windmill (15-11b). With legs crossed, touch back leg twenty times. Do slowly and only if you are flexible. Be careful not to strain lower back.

Lateral leg lifts (15-11c). Raise leg to the side to strengthen muscles on both side of leg. Do eight times, three sets.

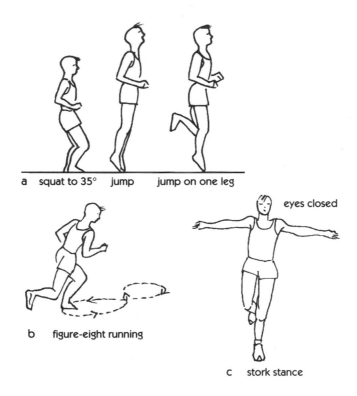

a   squat to 35°   jump   jump on one leg

eyes closed

b   figure-eight running

c   stork stance

15-12. Restoring Balance after Injury

Restoring Balance

Squat and jump (15-12a). Bend knees about 35 degrees and jump. Do twenty sets. Next try squatting and jumping on only one foot.

Figure-eight running (15-12b). Run 5 minutes making figure-eight loops, gradually reducing size of loop.

Stork stand (15-12c). Stand on one foot, eyes closed, arms out-stretched for one minute.

Exercises to Avoid

Straight leg raises from a flat position on the floor (15-13a). In this position, the strain of raising the legs stresses the lower back. A correct leg lift with support for the back is shown in Fig.15-5a, b, p. 306.

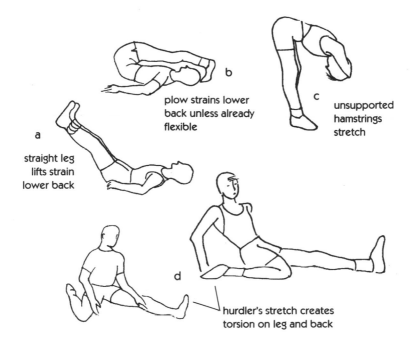

plow strains lower
back unless already
flexible

unsupported
hamstrings
stretch

straight leg
lifts strain
lower back

hurdler's stretch creates
torsion on leg and back

15-13. Exercises to Avoid

The plow (15-13b). This posture is generally unsuitable for most exercisers because it creates too much compression in the neck. Do it only if you are very flexible.

Unsupported hamstrings stretch (15-13c). creates too much tension in the lumbar region. Instead do the supported hamstrings stretch shown in Fig. 15-7d (work hands down leg slowly as you stretch out).

Hurdler's stretch (15-13d). on the floor with one leg bent back produces torsion. Instead stretch the quadriceps with a standing quad stretch as in Fig.1 5-7a, p. 308.

There are pros and cons of running or walking with weights. On the plus side, using hand or ankle weights while running adds to the total mass that must be moved; therefore more energy is used. Using weights also contributes to increased muscle tone and endurance but not strength. No benefit is gained if weights are merely held in the hands when running or walking. Arms must be pumped up and down in harmony with the legs. Walking and pumping the arms with weights is fairly safe and helps to build upper-body strength.

The disadvantage of using hand or ankle weights while running is the increased impact on joints and the lower back.

Using excessive weights may cause imbalances in your posture resulting in strains. All in all, I believe that the disadvantages of running with weights outweigh the advantages. I prefer using rubber-tipped ski-poles for running or walking (exer-striding). See Fig. 3-2 in Chapter 3. If you want to work out with weights, use them in a gym.

Chapter 16

THE SECOND KEY TO HEALTH: NUTRITION

No man ever repented that he arose from the table sober, healthful and with his wits about him.

—Jeremy Taylor (1613-1667)

Food Fit to Eat

"I can't believe you're telling me that a high-protein, low carbohydrate diet is making me lose muscle," exclaimed Phil, a thirty-eight-year-old lawyer who was standing in my office, arms folded, while I was taking his medical history. He had arrived early, mentioning that he was in a hurry. Impatient with my initial inquiries as to his recent emotional states, attitudes, concerns and so forth (all of which are a part of a homeopathic examination), he indicated he didn't have much time for all these preliminary questions. Apparently he felt that even the act of sitting was going to slow down his office visit. He had already interrupted me several times, and was now prepared to argue with me about nutrition. He was the typical Type A personality—competitive in all walks of life. From our brief conversation about running, I knew he fell into the Phase Three category of runners—the obsessive runner.

A professional at probing for answers, he wanted to know more about diet. He had been sure that eating a lot of protein (in his case, about ¾ lb a day) and a minimum of "fattening" carbohydrates was the road to strength, slimness and virility.

Eating for a Whole Life

Looking for a magic diet, a magical supplement, or any other *unbalanced* solution to a problem, is looking for trouble. An attitude of trying to outwit the body for the sake of competition or for other ego reasons may reflect an out-sized concern for control, dominance, or

315

perfection rather than a healthy interest in what's best for the body. If we do things in segments, in parcels, with no sense of wholeness or integration, we also tend to approach recovery and health in terms of "quick fixes." By focusing on protein intake, muscle building, vitamin deficiency, fat-burners, carbohydrate-loading, and other partial approaches to nurturing the body, we lose sight of the whole—joyful health.

Protein and Muscle Mass

Many athletic patients like Phil equate high protein foods with the building of muscle mass. Food alone, whether it's protein or not, does not automatically lead to more muscle. What does build muscle is progressive, high intensity exercise such as weight training *with* enough food to fuel these efforts. If you don't eat enough to match the increased level of energy needed, your body will break down existing muscle. On the other hand, eating massive amounts of protein will not lead to more muscle mass. Excessive protein is stored in the body as fat.

As I explained to Phil, the body uses calories from three sources: protein, fat, and carbohydrates. It will process the foods you eat in different ways depending on your intake and what it needs. For example, both the brain and the brawn (muscles) need glycogen which comes from the glucose in carbohydrates. The most protected part of the body is the brain, and the nutrients for the brain, specifically, glucose, are closely monitored. Under normal circumstances, the brain uses over 60 percent of the glucose in the body. Heavy exercise can use up glycogen stores to the point where the brain experiences a shortage, producing symptoms of dizziness and weakness called hypoglycemia. As supplies start to burn away, the body begins to look for stored glycogen.

That storehouse of brainfood is in your liver—glucose in the form of glycogen. But, this is the savings account for emergencies and your liver, jealously guarding its reserves, would rather convert any available protein to make more glucose than to use the supply stored for a "brainy day." Therefore, as I explained to Phil, because of his low carbohydrate intake and the high demands of his running, even the protein he was eating was being turned into glucose for the brain. The protein that should have been used for normal repair of muscle stress was on its way to the brain instead. Hence, he was losing muscle mass. His diet was almost the equivalent of starvation.

Eating too much protein also stresses the body by giving the liver too much amino acid which is turned into fat. During this process (called deamination) nitrogen is released, turning into ammonia and then into urea. Urea, diluted with water becomes urine. If there is not enough water in the system to dilute the urea, you are becoming toxic; the body will take the water it needs out of your tissues. Your kidneys, by the way, are now working overtime to get rid of the urea. Because of the water loss, you can be fooled into thinking that you are losing weight—which you are—but it's from loss of water not fat. You are dehydrated. Furthermore, excessive protein depletes the body of calcium.

Cholesterol, Fats and Toxins

Alarm systems start blaring—from commercials, advertisements, cereal and milk-cartons—when the word cholesterol comes up. It is a fatty substance manufactured in the body, and therefore is also found in animal foods such as meat, butter or lard. The body uses small amounts of cholesterol for normal functions such as the formation of certain hormones and the production of bile acids in the liver.

Cholesterol deposits are one of the ways excess fat is stored in the body; this fatty "savings account" lines the walls of your arteries. Cholesterol deposits can clog and harden the arteries, which carry blood from the heart, reducing the flow of vital, oxygen-rich blood.

Contrary to the current popularity of fish and fowl as "healthy proteins," eating poultry or fish instead of red meat does not lower cholesterol levels. All muscle foods contain about the same high amount of cholesterol, but meat has higher levels of saturated fat than poultry and fish. Other high cholesterol foods are eggs, lobster, shrimp, crab, and liver. In addition to contributing to higher levels of cholesterol, animal proteins, near the top of the food chain, are usually contaminated with pesticides, herbicides, drugs, and other toxic chemicals found in the farming environment. High level of toxins in the body are obviously undesirable and may contribute to the development of such diseases as arthritis.

Food for Thought

The magical diet that all of us seek to stay youthful, long-lived and slender is no mystery. However, finding what keeps you energized and healthy does take committment—both to educating yourself and to practicing healthy eating. While there are inevitable individual requirements for health, there are also general dietary guidelines that have proven to maintain health and vitality. Many of you will want to read more detailed dietary information. Here are a few suggestions for relevant books:

One of the best books on nutrition is *The McDougall Program— 12 Days to Dynamic Health,* written by John and Mary McDougall, a physician and nutritionist. The McDougalls discuss standard medical practices for diseases from Alzheimer's and arthritis to osteoporosis. They also make dietary recommendations for these diseases. I strongly recommend their book to my patients since it has shopping tips and recipes included to get you started on a low-fat, high-starch diet. They write:

> Meats, fish, eggs, dairy products, lard, vegetable oils, and refined foods all fail as health-supporting foods . . . they are lacking in complex carbohydrates, fibers, many vitamins, and essential minerals . . . these foods contain excessive amounts of the potentially good nutrients and harmful quantities of fundamentally unhealthy non-nutrients. A diet centering around these foods continuously assails us with imbalances and excesses of many kinds, and the body soon reacts with signs of distress that we recognize as diseases.[1]

The McDougall diet eliminates animal foods and almost all fats. They state that 80 percent improvement in health comes from diet alone even without exercise. Of course, exercise is important. For one thing, aerobic exercise burns off fatty deposits in the arteries. Exercise also increases the "good" cholesterol (HDL) and decreases the "bad" cholesterol (LDL). In addition, exercise lowers your fatty acids (triglycerides), and increases the powerhouse cells (mitochondria) in your muscles.

Besides the McDougall's book, I recommend *Food For Sport* by Peter Bruckner and Karen Inge, and *Nancy Clark's Sports Nutrition Guidebook* by Nancy Clark.[2]

Eat and Run

Balanced nutrition through sensible, life-long eating of whole foods is essential for active people. Since many sports place a high priority on being trim, if not thin, getting enough of the right kind of food is even more critical. If not enough important nutrients are taken in, particularly iron, calcium, and zinc, the high energy demands from endurance sports may create serious deficiency states such as anemia and osteoporosis. You may also experience excessive fatigue and be more susceptible to injury. Energy and endurance are the prime factors in peak

Keys to Eating Well

1. Eat to live—don't live to eat. Foods are often eaten because they are fast, fun or festive (or even free), not because they are nourishing.

2. Chew the food. The enzymes in saliva are extremely important for digestion and for maximizing the nutrition of even "not so good" food.

3. Eat produce in season where you live. Local fresh, ripe fruits and vegetable have many advantages over imported, exotic, greenhouse-ripened produce which has been sprayed and waxed with preservatives to prevent spoilage—resulting in higher prices.

4. Eat a variety of foods. Eating different foods each day helps prevent allergic reactions to any one food. The body may develop an intolerance to a food eaten on a regular basis (even one that is nutritious). The most common foods to cause an allergic reaction are: milk, wheat, sugar, coffee, tea and any one kind of meat eaten regularly. These foods are also the ones we usually eat almost every day. Give your body a rest, and protect it from a monotonous diet.

5. Eat nothing that won't spoil—but eat it before it does.

6. Avoid foods with a high toxic content and residue. Animal products contain about 50 percent toxic residue; dairy products (milk, cheese, butter and yogurt) contain 25 percent; vegetables and fruits contain 11 percent; and nuts, seeds and grains contain about 5 percent.

7. Be moderate. Don't burden your body with large quantities of any one food or drink.

8. Don't wash down food with fluids. Too much liquid dilutes the gastric enzymes needed for digestion.

9. Don't cook with aluminum pots and pans as small amounts of aluminum may contaminate your food.[3]

performance. The energy that enables us to exercise is no different from the energy we use to perform our daily functions or to simply rest. However, during exercise, the energy output is about twenty times greater than at rest.

Carbohydrates and Sports

For athletes and non-athletes alike, a diet high in complex carbohydrates (starch) and fresh fruits and vegetables is superior to the typical American diet of high-protein, fatty and sugary processed foods.

There are two kinds of carbohydrates—simple and complex. Complex carbohydrates, beans, lentils, corn, grains, and starches are excellent sources of consistent, dependable energy. Sugar, a simple carbohydrate, has two major drawbacks. First, although it is absorbed quickly, it causes high blood glucose which then triggers increased insulin. The insulin acts to bring down the glucose level—the opposite of what you want when you're burning energy in running or sports. The lowered glucose level is why you feel so tired after the *initial* spurt of energy you feel after eating a candy bar. This up and down energy imbalance is called reactive hypoglycemia. Secondly, sugar adds calories without giving any nutrition.

The most important point to remember about eating carbohydrates is to eat them in their whole, unprocessed form as much as possible in order to derive the most benefit from all their nutrients and fiber. For example, a sugary, processed cereal with wheat germ or bran on top is not a balanced, whole cereal. Grains give you the best nutrients when they are eaten *with* all their parts—the kernel and the outside "bran."

There are many advantages to eating complex carbohydrates. For example, eating whole grains will satisfy your need to chew. Increased chewing and the natural bulk of the food helps you curb a tendency to overeat. Stamina is sustained at a steady level because these foods release energy slowly. In addition, your system will benefit by the roughage which speeds along the digestive process and the elimination of toxins (such as sugar and fat which are absorbed by the roughage). By eating whole grains, along with fresh fruits and vegetable, you receive your vitamins in the proportions that nature has already worked out.

The Sustained Energy Diet

A diet of carbohydrates, fruits and vegetables for athletes results in high-quality, sustained energy. I call this The Sustained Energy Diet.

The Sustained Energy Diet consists of starches, fresh vegetables and fruits. The aim is to reduce fats from animal proteins and even vegetable oils. The small amount of fat that the body needs is found naturally in nuts, seeds, grains and plants. Since our individual bodies may require slightly different foods, I have included a *small* amount of animal protein to be eaten occasionally if desired or needed. Plenty of protein is found in almost all unrefined food, and studies have shown that there is no need to worry about proper "combining" of foods (such as beans and rice) to make a complete protein. Since dairy products may contain fairly high levels of toxic residues and are often implicated in allergies and cholesterol problems, I suggest avoiding dairy on a regular basis.

The Sustained Energy Diet
Complex Carbohydrates

Whole Grains: 2–3 servings daily (about 1 cup each) whole grain bread, brown rice, corn, barley, oats, whole wheat, buckwheat, rye, bulgur, popcorn, kasha, oat groats.

Starches: 2–3 servings weekly of pastas, yams or sweet potatoes.

Protein

Beans: 1–2 servings daily—red, white, kidney, split peas, lentils, chick-peas.

Animal Protein (optional): 0–3 servings weekly of fish, turkey, chicken, low-fat meats, organic eggs (no cured meats or packaged lunch meats with nitrites).

Vitamins and Minerals

Greens, Cooked: 1–2 servings daily of spinach, chard, kale, mustard, collards and turnip tops.

Greens, Raw: 1–2 servings of watercress, lettuce, escarole, parsley.

Vegetables: 1–2 servings daily of broccoli, onions, scallions, leeks, green beans, cauliflower, carrots, zucchini, radishes, butternut squash, celery.

1–2 servings weekly of potatoes, eggplant, tomatoes, peppers if diet includes some calcium.

Sea Vegetables: 2–5 servings weekly of kelp, dulse, irish moss, agar (all calcium-rich).

Fruits: 1–2 servings daily cooked or fresh according to season.

The foods to avoid if possible are:
- All fats, fried food, lard, shortening, nut and peanut butters (small amounts only).

- Steak, commercial eggs, nitrate and nitrite-cured meats and lunch meat.
- Shellfish (limited amounts).
- Cheese, ice cream, sour and heavy cream, yogurt, pasteurized, homogenized vitamin D-fortified milk.
- Iodized salt, commercial soy sauce.
- Coffee, decaffeinated coffee (if taking homeopathic remedies), hot chocolate.
- Fluorinated, chlorinated tap water (except in restaurants), distilled water.
- White flour, white rice (except in ethnic restaurants once in awhile).
- Sugar (white, brown, raw) and honey.
- Canned or frozen foods in quantity (they lack important enzymes and nutrients).

A Word of Advice

If you have read the above and thought "Oh, no. Everything I've been eating is all wrong!" or "Forget it, this is too hard—I'll never be able to give up XYZ," don't despair. Making any changes in your habits requires time and committment. Don't expect yourself to make changes in a week if your diet is very different from the Sustained Energy Diet. Do the best you can. Make choices on a daily basis, and keep your *goal of good health* in mind. Stock up on the right kinds of food, so that good food is always handy. Don't criticize yourself, or make your mealtimes grim and puritanical. Talking about what you "can" or "cannot" eat won't make you the most popular person at the table, nor will commenting on other people's nutritional choices while they're eating. Keep food in perspective along with the other components of your life.

Vitamins and Mineral Supplements

Indiscriminate use of vitamins and mineral supplements often leads to imbalances that are the opposite of what you want to achieve—balanced health. Studies have shown that if your diet is deficient in calcium, iron, zinc, B12, and other nutrients, simply taking supplements does not correct the deficiency.[4] Any nutritional fixing or "tampering" with supplements should be done with the advice of a health practitioner schooled in holistic nutrition. There is no conclusive evidence to suggest that performance will be improved with vitamin—mineral supplements used in excess of the recommended dietary intakes. On the other hand, unless you are only eating fresh, unprocessed foods, chances are your food is deficient in vitamins and trace minerals, so I suggest you take 2 grams of vitamin C and a good multi-vitamin with minerals every day. However, don't expect to compensate for a poor diet with vitamins.

Pre-event Eating

Carbohydrate-Loading

Carbohydrate loading is a week-long regimen that increases levels of glycogen stores through diet and training that has been fashionable in sports for the past few years. I would question it from the point of view that it treats the body as a machine and is not compatible with the holistic view of homeopathic medicine.

Endurance Events

Consider the following eight points in choosing your pre-event meal:

1. Do not eat later than 3 hours before the event.
2. Choose foods high in complex carbohydrates, low in sugars or fats.
3. Eat about 500–1,000 calories.
4. Choose foods with moderate fiber content—nothing heavy.
5. No coffee, tea, soft drinks or beer (all have a dehydrating effect).
6. No new foods that might cause indigestion (remember, pre-event jitters could make your stomach sensitive).
7. No ingestion of sugar or glucose for "instant energy." Eating candy 30 to 60 minutes prior to the event may impair performance as your metabolism will use glyogen stores earlier.
8. Drink as much fluid (preferably water) as you can; drink two glasses of water in the last 30 minutes before you begin.[5]

Watering the Runner and the Walker

You are at least 60 percent water. Dehydration or insufficient fluid intake is stressful and even dangerous to the body. Exercise walkers and runners should drink about a half gallon to three-quarters gallon of water a day, to flush out impurities excreted during exercise.

Research has shown that plain cold water is still the best fluid replacement. Sports drinks which are supposed to replace electrolytes lost through perspiration can actually slow down the absorption of fluid into the body. Plain cold water reaches the cells more quickly than any other type of fluid. Salt tablets are never necessary for exercise, and may be harmful.

Heat Exhaustion

During endurance training or competition, you may lose from 6 percent to 10 percent of your body weight in water. If fluids are not replaced, the body begins to conserve the remaining fluid by switching off the sweating mechanism. Without sweat to cool the body's surface, the core temperature rises. To prevent heat exhaustion, drink water every 3 miles during endurance events.

A medical emergency, heat exhaustion can happen on cool or overcast days as well as hot days. Signs are: muscle cramps in the leg or backside, nausea, vomiting, dizziness, and fainting. Continuing to run with any of these symptoms may lead to a stroke as the body's regulators are no longer able to cope. If core temperature rises more than 2°(C), permanent physical or mental damage can occur. Expert medical help must immediately be given in cases of heat exhaustion or stroke.

First aid for heat exhaustion:
- drink water or fluids immediately
- lie down
- cover with blankets if cold and clammy
- call paramedics or doctor
- take a dose of homeopathic *Arnica* every 15 minutes; or *Glonium* or *Nat Carb*

Smart tips to prevent over-heating
- run in the shade; run early or late when it's cool.
- drink water before, during and after exercise.
- take a 30x dose of homeopathic *Arnica* before event if it's hot outside.
- wear a light-colored hat with ventilation holes.
- wear light-colored, light-weight cotton clothes.
- stop exercising at the first sign of dizziness or headache, faintness or blurred vision.
- be sure to spend time (as much as two weeks) acclimatizing to

weather if competing away from home.
• don't play or run if you're sick or feverish.

Traveler's Diarrhea (*Turista*)

Athletes traveling to competitions in foreign countries need to be particularly prudent about eating food that has been properly cooked and stored. A case of "the runs" can seriously affect performance. Usually diarrhea indicates that the intestinal flora has been disrupted, which sometimes happens merely from being in a different environment, and is not the result of any "germs" that were picked up. Consider the following points when competing in another country.
1. avoid tap water and ice cubes.
2. drink bottled, boiled or carbonated water, soft drinks, and tea (from water boiled 20 minutes).
3. avoid unpasteurized milk products.
4. avoid unpeeled fruit.
5. avoid uncooked vegetables and salads.
6. avoid undercooked beef, chicken or pork.

If you do develop symptoms of diarrhea (loose bowels, nausea, vomiting, fever or cramps):
1. avoid solid food and milk products.
2. drink tea, apple juice, clear soups, bottled water.
3. when symptoms stop, eat light foods such as crackers, boiled white rice or pasta.
4. take homeopathic remedies:

> *Podophyllum* if: Profuse and smelly with much gas passed with stool; early morning about 4:00 am; feels weak and faint afterwards.

> *Arsenicum Alb* if: Simultaneous diarrhea and vomiting; weakness, chilliness, from food poisoning; one of best remedies for *turista*.

> *Veratrum Alb* if: Diarrhea and vomiting, if *Arsenicum Alb* doesn't work.

Special Diet Needs:
Loss of Bone Strength (Osteoporosis)

Since osteoporosis causes about six million bone fractures a year in America, it's important for women to be aware of how it might affect, or be affected by, their exercise programs. Although the effects of this silent disease are seen in old age, bone density can begin to lessen as early as the twenties and thirties. Osteoporosis is the medical term for weak, porous, brittle bones, and is a condition found mostly in white, post-menopausal women. It's found in roughly half of all elderly women and is responsible for shrinking the spinal column and for causing the characteristic unsightly "dowager's hump" or curved back.

Exercising at least three times a week for an hour is one of the best things women can do to prevent osteoporosis, especially when started at an early age. Sustained, weight-bearing activity such as brisk walking, running, tennis, dancing, rope-jumping, basketball, and backpacking encourages the production of bone cells. An activity such as swimming, however, is not a weight-bearing exercise, as the weight of the body is supported by the water. Incidentally, heavier people are less prone to osteoporosis because of the increased weight bearing on the bones. Studies have found that a weight of about 140 pounds lessens your chance of bone loss.

Stretching, yoga and other movement practices stretch the body, increasing circulation and promoting limberness and strength. T'ai Chi, Aikido, and other forms of physical exertion done on a regular basis encourage bone building.

When I see women patients, who in their late forties and fifties have started vigorous exercise (handball and marathon-running) after years of sedentary life, I mention to them that there is a possibility that their bones may already be weakened and brittle. Loss of calcium may have occurred because of the lack of early exercise, especially if their diets were low in calcium or depleted by heavy smoking or drinking. Starting to exercise late in life (or over-train late in life), may put them at higher risk for fractures than, say, a woman who had been exercising from an early age. A fall on the tennis court, for example, might easily break a wrist, arm or shoulder—even a hip.

However, the benefits of brisk walking, light jogging, and other moderate activities usually outweigh the risk of fracture. There is no conclusive evidence yet that osteoporosis can be reversed by exercise once it has occurred.

Besides exercise, a women must be sure not only to eat calcium-rich foods, but avoid substances that hinder retention and absorption of calcium.

Sources of calcium. Getting enough calcium for the post-menopausal women is not as simple as drinking a couple of glasses of milk a day. First of all, the over-all health of the body is usually served best when a variety of foods are eaten so that food allergies don't develop. Obtaining calcium from non-dairy sources is especially important since there is some controversy about using dairy in heavy quantities. For one thing, about 25 percent of the general population lacks the enzyme to digest lactose, a major component of milk.[6]

Another mark against dairy products is evidence that the practice of adding synthetic vitamin D to enrich milk may cause calcium deposits in arteries or kidneys and other soft tissues—not bones.[7] Furthermore, taking the fat out of milk to produce the low-fat products that have become very popular may disrupt the natural balance of elements in the milk so that calcium absorption is lessened.[8] Both the addition of vitamin D and the subtraction of fat change the natural balance of elements in the milk so that it is no longer a whole food. Whenever a food is altered from its "whole" state, the possibility that its nutritive value has been changed is greatly increased. A moderate to high consumption of dairy has, moreover, been linked to skin problems, allergies, and various female reproductive disorders.[9]

Fortunately, there are many calcium-rich foods. I encourage my patients to eat foods such as:
- beans and nuts, sesame seeds, almonds,
- kelp, sardines, canned salmon,
- broccoli, collards, parsley, kale, mustard and turnip tops, watercress and dandelion,
- soups made with bones of fish, fowl or beef (cook with one tablespoon of wine vinegar to draw out calcium into broth.

Outdoor activity, beneficial in so many ways, further helps prevent osteoporosis. In this case, the skin absorbs sunlight and makes vitamin D which is important for calcium absorption.

Calcium depleters. It's not surprising that many of the substances that encourage calcium depletion are also those deemed unhealthy in general. The worst offenders are: tobacco, alcohol, excessive animal protein, caffeine, salt, fats, and vinegar. But other foods which wouldn't seem to be a problem, such as chard (rich in oxalic acid), rhubarb, spinach and chocolate drain away calcium. Furthermore, some researchers have found that foods high in alkaloids such as potatoes, eggplant, peppers and tomatoes also seem to affect calcium balance.[10]

We know that ingesting high amounts of animal proteins cause many problems in the human system. In terms of bone loss, excessive protein causes changes in kidney processes, which, in turn, cause more calcium to be excreted from the body than can be absorbed in the intestines. Therefore, we have one more reason to cut down on meat, poultry and even fish.

Other substances that affect calcium absorption are aluminum (absorbed from food cooked in aluminum pots, from baking soda, and even from the use of some deodorants) and phosphates (in processed foods and sodas).

Drugs such as antacids, antibiotics, anti-depressants, barbituates, cholesterol-reducing drugs, cortico-steroids, diuretics, laxatives, and chemotherapeutic drugs are also known to have an effect on calcium absorption.

Even stomach acid affects how the body uses calcium. It's important to eat slowly, allowing food to absorb acid during chewing; don't wash your food down with fluids.

Calcium supplements have been found to have little or no positive effects on the condition of bones; there is no evidence showing that higher intakes promote greater absorption. Supplements are "add-ons" that may not be in the correct proportion to other elements. In general, it's better to get your calcium from food rather than from supplements since healthy food contains the proper ratio of nutrients to assist absorption. If you have a tendency to develop kidney stones, don't take calcium supplements without checking with your doctor.

When talking about osteoporosis, the subject of hormone (estrogen) replacement therapy inevitably comes up. There is evidence that estrogen helps post-menopausal women maintain healthy bones. However, when hormone replacement is discontinued, calcium excretion is significantly increased. Since hormone replacement therapy may increase the risk of ovarian cancer, there is substantial controversy about whether this is a healthy option for women. This kind of therapy must be discussed in detail with your doctor.

In view of the information we currently know about the loss of calcium from the body, therefore, I recommend that you exercise daily, follow a low-protein diet, and avoid caffeine and phosphate-containing sodas. Osteoporosis *may* be reversible if the calcium loss can be staunched and bones remineralized through good diet. Deformities of the spine or back will not be corrected, however. For more information of this subject, read *McDougall's Medicine—A Challenging Second Opinion.*

Footnotes:

1. John A. McDougall, M.D. and Mary McDougall, *The McDougall Program: Twelve Days to Dynamic Health,* New York, NAL books, 1990.

2. Peter Brukner and Karen Inge, *Food for Sport,* Australia, William Heinemann, 1986; *Nancy Clark's Sports Nutrition Guidebook,* Leisure Press, Champaign, 1990.

3. Correspondence with Alexander A. Wood, D.C., N.D., F.A.N.A., Ontario, Canada.

4. Annemarie Colbin, *Food and Healing,* New York, Ballantine Books, 1986, p. 156.

5. Peter Brukner and Karen Inge, "Sports Nutrition," *Sports Medicine of the Lower Extremity,* ed. by Steven I. Subotnick, D.P.M., M.S., New York, Churchill Livingstone, 1989, pp. 39-64.

6. Colbin, p. 156.

7. *Ibid.,* p. 152.

8. *Ibid.,* p. 155.

9. *Ibid.,* p. 153.

10. *Ibid.,* p. 161.

Chapter 17

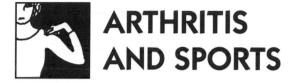
ARTHRITIS AND SPORTS

> Every part of the personality you do not love will become hostile to you.
>
> —Carl Jung

Patients often ask, "Do sports and exercise cause arthritis?" Some people are afraid that too much sports activity may cause excessive wear-and-tear on joints. They want to know how arthritis relates to sports in general. This question prompted me to devote a chapter to this painful, common, and puzzling disease. As an athlete or active person, you should know something about arthritis for two reasons. First, if you already have arthritis, your sport or exercise may be hindered by painful joints. Naturally, you want to know about treatment, diet, and whether or not you should continue to exercise.

Secondly, you may have an injury or painful condition that you think is related to your sports or exercise activity. However, this injury or condition *may* be the signs of early onset of arthritis. There are a variety of factors that could cause arthritis *in combination with increases in sports activity or trauma from sports.* A sports injury may precipitate the disease. It is extremely important that sportspeople be aware of the different types of arthritis, and the possible conditions which may indicate a medical condition rather than an injury.

One of my patients woke up in the middle of the night with a very painful big toe. His first thought was that he had injured his toe in the race he ran that morning. In fact, we found that the race and several other factors had precipitated an arthritic reaction which required medical attention.

"If I have aching in the joints, does that mean I have arthritis?"

Not necessarily. You may have a strain or sprain or bio-mechanical imbalances. You may have an overuse injury, or a localized process that needs attention. However, if any of these conditions are ignored or left untreated, they could progress to arthritis.[1]

"I have a stiff back and a problem with my heel. Is this arthritis or is it related to my running?"

The symptoms that are associated with arthritis are different in every person. They vary in terms of how quickly or slowly they begin and progress; they also vary in the severity of the symptoms. The point for you to remember is that not all "sports injuries" are what they seem to be. Pain, stiffness, inflammation or swelling may indicate the onset of a disease associated with arthritis. Always have a medical doctor rule out or confirm these serious problems by examination, lab tests, or x-ray. Once you know what your condition is, you may look at alternative therapies and seek other opinions.

"What is arthritis?"

Most people think of arthritis as pain in the joints that limit flexibility and motion. It's commonly associated with older people and non-athletic types. Many of us have heard parents or relatives complain about their arthritic joints off and on for years; usually they never seem to get much better, but learn to "live with it." Is arthritis an inevitable part of growing older? Can it be cured? What causes it? Are all types of arthritis the same? Let's take a look at the three types of arthritis:

Rheumatism. Also called rheumatoid arthritis, rheumatism is a systemic inflammatory medical disease known for swelling and pain in the joints. "Systemic" means the disease is present throughout the system, not just present in the joints.

Osteoarthritis. Also called "old-age arthritis," this is a degenerative type in which the cartilage in joints becomes porous and sometimes chips off. Osteoarthritis is a form of "mechanical" deterioration rather than a medical disease.

Arthritis associated with various other diseases. This type of arthritis has other symptoms along with pain in the joints. We'll look at some of the variants of this type.

Rheumatoid Arthritis (Rheumatism)

This is the most common and most crippling type of arthritis. It affects the entire body and destroys the cartilage and tissues in and around the joints. Joints become inflamed, swollen and very painful with motion. The waste products from the inflammatory condition cause the degeneration of joints and cartilage.

Because rheumatoid arthritis exists throughout the entire system, it usually affects both left and right joints (swelling occurs symmetrically). It is a chronic, progressive disease which sometimes goes into remission on its own, and varies individually. For some people, their arthritis develops and worsens quickly. For others, the disease progresses slowly.

Factors causing rheumatoid arthritis

The root cause of rheumatoid arthritis is unknown, but medical research has suggested that arthritis is sometimes linked to:

• Allergic reactions to toxins such as pesticides, fungicides, and other industrial pollutants.

• Drug reactions. Individual reactions to various prescription drugs such as anti-depressants, antibiotics or drugs for high-blood pressure may cause arthritis.

• Allergic reactions to additives, preservatives and yeasts in foods. Gouty arthritis is well-known to be affected by consumption of too much red meat, rich food or alcohol.

• Complications following viral and bacterial infections such as rheumatic fever or Lyme's disease. Some patients are never well following prolonged flu and eventually become arthritic.

• Allergic reaction to the body's own tissue (auto-immune disease). There is growing evidence that for complex reasons the immune system sometimes reacts to the body's own connective tissue (collagen) as if it were a dangerous foreign protein and attacks it. Lupus (systemic eurythmetosis), which affects women in their twenties and thirties, is in this category.

• Heredity seems to play a major role in the development of arthritis. A tendency for rheumatoid arthritis and gout are clearly passed on genetically.

• Other factors such as emotional stress or even cold, damp weather seem to influence arthritis.

• Homeopaths suspect that suppression of symptoms by antibiotics and/or steroid drugs such as cortisone may be linked to the onset of arthritis. In fact, any substance or circumstance that weakens the body's defenses can be linked to rheumatoid arthritis.

Osteoarthritis

Osteoarthritis is caused by mechanical abuse, overuse or simply weak bone mass. Cartilage is worn away in the major weight-bearing joints (e.g., knees and hips), and in frequently-used joints (small joints in the fingers) causing stiffness and pain. In an effort to protect the joints against the degeneration of the cartilage, excessive bone forms at joint margins, causing spurs and decreased motion. If you have bone spurs in your joints, you have osteoarthritis. In rheumatoid arthritis, the joints also deteriorate, but the body doesn't produce extra bone in the form of spurs. Osteoarthritis also differs from rheumatoid arthritis in having less contracture of joints (i.e., bent toes and deformed fingers). In addition, there is not the swelling in symmetrical joints that is found in rheumatoid arthritis. If the degeneration in joint cartilage is severe, use of the joint may be lost.[2]

Causes of osteoarthritis

• Too much local stress on the joints such as with obesity, malposition of joints, or occupational overuse (such as long hours at the computer keyboard).
  • Damage caused by running or playing on hard surfaces.
  • Degeneration of the joint after a fall, sprain or fracture.

Arthritis Associated with Various Diseases

The third type of arthritis is also a systemic disease like rheumatoid arthritis. In this case, arthritis is associated with another medical disease and accurate diagnosis is crucial for proper treatment. These medical diseases may accompany a sports injury, be precipitated through an accidental injury an overuse injury or by increased activity and stress. Most of these conditions can be confirmed by blood tests, x-ray, and other diagnostic procedures.

Since treatment varies according to the type of medical disease present, I have not offered specific treatments for each one. Many of the holistic or homeopathic suggestions, along with conventional treatment, will be appropriate. However, treatment must be done with the advice of your doctor.

Ankylosing Spondylitis

This type of inflammatory arthritis has pain in the back, spine or sacroiliac joints *with* pain in the heel. Therefore, runners should be aware of this condition, characterized by a very stiff back and a very sore bottom or back of the heel or heel bursa (retrocalcaneal bursa). Sometimes a runner who has been running for five or six years suddenly gets a stiff back along with pain in the heel. This is an early sign of the arthritis of ankylosing spondylitis. There is a link to smoking with this disease.

Ankylosing spondylitis is treated medically with drugs, and biomechanically with orthotics; homeopathic constitutional remedies may help. Don't try to treat yourself if you suspect you may have this disease. You must be examined and have a medical diagnosis. Ankylosing spondylitis can be self-limiting and may go away on its own.

Reiter's Syndrome

Reiter's syndrome occurs in young, sexually active men. There is usually pain in the heel or the area around the Achilles tendon. Along with pain in the heel or foot are other medical problems such as inflammation of the eyes, bladder, or urethra. Blood tests will confirm the presence of the disease; there are links to a positive HIV factor.

Lupus

Lupus occurs in young women of childbearing age. Symptoms include fatigue and muscle ache, which, if you are an athlete or very active, might be attributed to overuse injury. However, if you notice a sensitivity to the sun, nausea, brain or kidney problems or have the telltale rash across the cheeks and nose, you may have lupus. The name lupus means wolf and refers to the shape of the rash area which resembles the "wolf face" markings of the animal. The course of this disease is quite variable. Some women may have only a little rash and mild symptoms. Others may get very sick. The disease may progress quickly or slowly or go into remission. Involvement in internal organs can be fatal, and some researchers have tagged energetic Type A women as "lupus types." Active women of childbearing age who experience any of the above symptoms should be checked out with blood tests. It's important to see a good rheumatologist well-versed in this condition. Homeopathy has been used successfully to treat lupus.[3]

Psoriatic Arthritis

Seven percent of those who have psoriasis also have arthritis in three or four different joints. In those who don't have a full-blown case of psoriasis, there may be early signs of the onset of psoriatic arthritis such as small holes or pits in the nails or shiny patches of skin behind the ear. These signs may accompany pain and swelling in the joints. If you are exercising heavily, you may attribute the joint pain to overuse injury and overlook this medical condition. Therefore, pay attention to any concurrent skin disturbances with joint pain.

Gout

Gout is a form of arthritis caused by crystals of uric acid deposited in joints. Joints characteristically become red, hot and inflamed. People with gout either produce too much uric acid or don't excrete enough of what they do produce. It is well-known that an attack of gout may come after consuming too much alcohol (which is dehydrating and impairs kidney functions) and very rich food. Increases in running mileage or sports activity can trigger inflammation and a gouty reaction. The onset of gout may be acute (e.g., occurring suddenly during the night) or chronic (beginning gradually). Gout usually attacks the big toe. If gout occurs after a race or mileage increase, you may think you have an overuse injury or stress fracture because of the pain and inflammation and be tempted to treat it yourself. Be sure to get a medical diagnosis for your condition, particularly *if you have any family history of gout or arthritis.*

Polymyositis or Dermatomyositis

These two conditions refer to arthritis associated with muscle disease—weakness of muscles around hips or shoulders. Dermatomyositis is further complicated by a skin problem in addition to the muscle problem. Both types of diseases associated with arthritis are chronic and progressive.

Scleroderma

With scleroderma, there is scarring of the skin along with arthritis. The skin becomes very tight, especially on the fingers. There may be an allergy to cold which is called Raynaud's phenomenon. Raynaud's disease involves many systems of the body—cardiovascular, digestive tract, skin, joints, and kidneys.

"Can sports or exercise cause rheumatoid arthritis?"

No. Sports activity alone will not cause rheumatoid arthritis which is a systemic medical condition brought on by a variety of factors including additives in the diet, stress, allergies to drugs, yeasts, and toxins. Sensible exercise enhances nutrition in the joints and contributes to flexibility. If you are a runner or sports person and have rheumatoid arthritis, don't exercise to the point of bringing on pain. However, *do* exercise for cardiovascular fitness, immune system enhancement, weight loss, stress reduction and flexibility, all of which will have a positive effect on the disease.

"Do sports cause osteoarthritis?"

Yes and no. If you have healthy joints, keep them that way and don't push beyond your limits. Healthy joints benefit from well-balanced exercise (e.g., running, swimming, yoga).

In a two-year study done on members of the 50-Plus Runners Association, forty-one long-distance runners aged fifty to seventy-two years were compared to forty-one matched controls to find out if repetitive, long-term physical impact (running) caused damage to joints. While female runners had a slightly higher incidence of bone spurs in the spine and the knees, overall results showed no link between running and osteoarthritis. In fact, runners' bones were stronger (had more bone mineral). Another study by Richard S. Panush, MD, at the University of Florida also concluded "that long-duration, high-mileage running need not be associated with premature degenerative joint disease in the lower extremities."[4]

On the other hand, once joints are damaged by overuse or trauma, you risk further degeneration of the cartilage (osteoarthritis) with ill-chosen (high-impact) sports activities.

If you have had trauma to a joint (e.g., hip, knee or ankle) and have some osteoarthritis, find exercises that don't cause pain. If you cannot run without pain, switch to low-impact exercise such as swimming or cycling.

Treatments for Rheumatoid Arthritis and Osteoarthritis

There is no known conventional medical treatment to cure arthritis. Chronic arthritis, unfortunately, worsens over the course of the lifetime, and if it is severe, no known conventional treatment can alter its progression completely. However, arthritis is known to go into remission, making it difficult to determine for sure if a particular treatment may have contributed to the easing of the affliction.

Conventional treatment for rheumatoid arthritis attempts to do three things: decrease inflammation; improve function and flexibility; and repair damaged joints.

• **Decrease or stop the inflammation**. This is done primarily with aspirin or non-steroidal anti-inflammatory drugs (NSAIDs). However, aspirin may be dangerous if you have a heart or kidney problem, if you have asthma, nasal polyps (growths), gout, bleeding tendencies, or stomach ulcers. Aspirin should be discontinued if there is any stomach bleeding, blood in the stools, or ringing in the ears.

Non-steroidal anti-inflammatory drugs (NSAIDs) such as Advil, Naprosyn, Feldene, or Indosin may cause stomach problems and increased fluid retention. Diuretics given to reduce fluid retention may be a contributing factor to the development of gouty arthritis.

A severe inflammatory process must be reduced because the waste products formed eat away the joints and cause unbearable pain. In severe cases cortisone injections (a potent steroid medicine) may be given. Another common form of cortisone, Prednisone, may be given orally. Unfortunately there are severe side effects with cortisone such as degeneration of tissue, fluid retention, swelling of the face, facial hair growth on women, and increased susceptibility to infection.

In very severe arthritic cases, gold salts or methotrexate—a cancer drug—are given to slow down the inflammatory process. Gold salts have a side effect of causing kidney problems. Methotrexate is an immuno-suppressant that reduces the immune system's inflammatory response, and leaves the body more susceptible to infections. Methotrexate also causes blood-marrow and liver toxicity.

• **Improve flexibility and function**. Physical therapy and movement therapy are two methods used to improve function in arthritic joints.

• **Repair damaged joints**. Surgery is another conventional treatment for severe joint deformity. Surgery is done if the deformity is severe and the joints are degenerating. Damaged joints are either cleaned out surgically or fused to prevent further motion. Inflamed joints may be helped by removing the diseased joint capsule, which may also decrease the severity of long-term joint damage.

"What is the standard medical treatment for osteoarthritis?"

Osteoarthritis is a mechanical wearing-down (degeneration) of joints and generally does not have the debilitating inflammatory process of rheumatoid arthritis. Therefore, drugs with more dangerous side effects, such as methotrexate or cortisone, are not used in its treatment.

If joints are badly damaged, avoid high-impact sports such as running, jumping, basketball, and high-impact aerobics to prevent further damage.

Take aspirin or NSAIDs (e.g., Indosin or Naprosyn) for pain and inflammation. Normally, osteoarthritis does not require the use of the strong drugs such as cortisone, gold salts, or methotrexate which are used to control the inflammation of rheumatoid arthritis. Decrease abnormal biomechanical stress on joints with orthotics or braces, and increase the range of motion and flexibility in the joints with physical therapy or surgery. Keeping flexible helps decrease pain. Lose weight if you're more than twenty pounds overweight.

"Can homeopathic remedies help arthritis?"

If treated early before extensive joint damage has occurred, there may be remission or cure with homeopathic remedies. If treated in later stages, homeopathy can slow down the progression of the disease and patients may be able to decrease conventional arthritis medicines, thus avoiding their dangerous side effects. Homeopathic remedies strengthen the immune system and reduce the process of arthritic inflammation. They also help with pain, stiffness and swelling, and may even prevent the disease from getting worse.

In a double-blind, placebo-controlled clinical trial at St. Bartholomew's Hospital, London, researchers found that homeopathy is an effective treatment for a common rheumatic disease, primary fibromyalgia, also known as fibrositis. Thirty patients were given two lots of treatment for one month each. Neither the patients, the doctors, nor the assessors knew which treatment was the real homeopathic remedy, *Rhus Tox* (poison ivy), or the placebo. Statistical analysis of the results showed a highly significant effect from the remedy. The report was published in the *British Medical Journal,* the official publication of the British Medical Association, an organization not generally supportive of homeopathy.

An earlier study published in the *British Journal of Clinical Pharmacology* (1980) also showed that 82 percent of those given a homeopathic remedy experienced relief of the symptoms of rheumatoid arthritis as compared to only 21 percent of those given a placebo.

Homeopathic Remedies for Short-term Joint Pain

If you've had joint pain, swelling and stiffness for a few days or up to two or three weeks, you may want to try a homeopathic remedy for relief. If a homeopathic physician is not available for consultation in your area, you may select one of the remedies listed below. If you don't get better in a few days or so, you may have selected the wrong remedy, in which case you can try another one. If the pain continues beyond a couple of weeks, you should get a conventional medical diagnosis.

For short-term arthritis or joint pain select one of the following remedies. Take two tablets of 6, 12, 15 or 30 (x or c potency) four times a day until better.

Rhus Tox is the primary remedy for arthritis with stiffness. Take if the joints are very stiff with initial motion; if you can barely move getting out of bed, yet feel better after moving around. Other characteristics include feeling worse sitting in a car for long periods; much, much better in warm weather; much worse in cold, damp weather; better after a warm shower; if there is a red triangle on the end of the tongue. Take *Ruta Grav* if you're easily fatigued; although somewhat similar to *Rhus Tox,* the pain is characterized as stiff and achy, worse with cold or wet; better by motion, but not too much motion; better warm, but not as dramatically warm as *Rhus Tox.* Take *Ledum* if the joints tend to feel cool (although they can be hot); if the joint is better cool or better with cold water; if always worse with a warm bed (like *Stellaria)*; if there is weakness, numbness and coolness; for arthritis of the small joints; if pains travel upward; worse with any motion (like *Phytolacca* or *Colchicum)*. Take *Bryonia* if arthritis comes on slowly after 5 to 7 hours or more after injury; hot swollen; much, much worse with any motion; very thirsty; if you feel very irritable; usually used after joints have hurt a few hours or more. Take *Rhododendron* if aching is particularly worse before a storm; if much worse with cold or wet, and melting snow; better after a storm passes. Take *Cimicifuga* for arthritis in the fleshy part of the muscle. Take *Stellarium* if you're not

340

sure the joint is better with or without motion; for psoriatic arthritis; if there is a great deal of stiffness; if worse in the morning; worse when warm; worse with heat in bed; worse with tobacco; better in the evening; better with cool air; for sharp, shifting pain that goes to different part of body (similar to *Pulsatilla;* for pain in the calves and legs; (very good remedy for rear foot and subtalar joint). BHI Arthritis[5] is a a combinational prescription; good for people who are taking multiple conventional medicines. Take one pill three times a day until pain and stiffness decrease. BHI Co-enzyme[5] is a general immune-system-booster that doesn't interfere with other drugs.

Homeopathic Remedies for Chronic (Long-term) Arthritis

I recommend having a professional homeopathic constitutional workup done before trying these remedies for chronic arthritis. You need to be given a homeopathic constitutional, a drug particularly keyed to your portrait type, which will be used in conjunction with the following possible remedies:

Causticum for chronic arthritis with great tightness of muscles and tendons; for joints that are severely contracted, especially in finger and toe joints; if better wet and moist; if worse cold. *Pulsatilla* for chronic arthritis that tends to shift around from joint to joint (similar to *Phytolacca* and *Stellaria)*; patient usually has a soft, mild changeable personality; better with consolation; may be a bit weepy; warm people who are better with a cool breeze; better walking outside; better at twilight; likes walking better than more vigorous activity; better with slow, easy movement.

Take *Benzoic Acid* for chronic rheumatism in small joints; in great toe; for pain at the back of the heel; nodules; may have very strong-smelling urine. Take *Colchicum* for chronic, gouty arthritis (main remedy); if very irritable; very weak; much much worse in evening; much worse any motion. *Calc Phos* for chronic arthritis that is worse with change of weather; also for growing children with Still's disease (juvenile arthritis). *Calc Fluor* for chronic arthritis with symptoms similar to *Rhus Tox* patients.

Calc Carb for chronic arthritis similar to *Rhus Tox.* Take *Phytollacca* for chronic arthritis; if it feels better elevating the feet at the end of the day; arthritis in joints, muscles and fascia; similar to *Rhus Tox,* but better warm, dry and with rest; worse with cold damp; for shifting pain; for attachments to tendons to bones; Achilles tendinitis; for much aching in heels and ankles; sore arthritic feet; worse in the morning and with activity; for electrical-like pain. *Silica* for chronic, hereditary arthritis; if you tend to be very cold, sickly; may have delicate features; if better warm, humid and wet; worse icy cold; if there is smelly sweat; offensive-smelling sore feet; sore insteps. *Meddorinum* for chronic, hereditary-type arthritis; for arthritis with a history of venereal disease; if there is high energy in the evening and feels worse in the morning; better at the sea; tends to sleep on stomach; for very sensitive hot feet that feel better walking on cold floors; if you stick your feet out of the covers at night. *Radium Brom* if similar to *Rhus Tox,* but better cool.

Homeopathic Remedies for Unusual Symptoms in Arthritis

a) If joints feel better with coolness (arthritis usually feels better with heat) try *Pulsatilla, Ledum, Radium Brom,* or *Stellaria.* Read the characteristics of these remedies to see which of them most suits your case.

b) If joints feel worse with motion (arthritis usually feels better with gentle motion), try *Ledum, Bryonia* or *Colchicum.*

c) For shifting, migrating pain try *Pulsatilla, Bryonia, or Colchicum.*

"If I have joint pain and am not sure if it's arthritis, can I still take a homeopathic remedy?"

Yes. If you have had a sports injury and continue to have pains in your joints for a few days or weeks, you may have short-term (acute) arthritis. If you have not had an injury, you may have either acute arthritis or the beginning of a chronic condition. In either case, you may try one of the remedies listed below for acute arthritis if you don't have a homeopath in your area and your joint pains haven't improved significantly with conventional medicines. Note: these acute remedies also work for chronic (long-term) arthritis.

If the pain doesn't improve, you may not have selected the best remedy to match your symptoms, *or* you may have a chronic disease

342

which will keep progressing.

Remedies can be ordered from homeopathic pharmacies (see resource section); sometimes remedies are carried in health food stores or pharmacies.

Case History of a Runner with Reiter's Syndrome

William Patterson, a twenty-six-year-old runner in very good shape, was running about 65 miles a week. In training for tri-athlons and marathons, he also biked and swam. William was an executive and single, with an active social life.

He came to see me very anxious about the swelling on his ankle joint (the subtalar joint). He also had inflammation and swelling on the heel. The swelling had started when he increased his training. I asked if there was a family history of gout, and he said no. I asked if he had had any recent medical problems. "Well, I had a urinary tract infection a few weeks ago," he said, "and about two weeks ago I had an infection in my eye."

I x-rayed his ankle and foot but found no stress fracture; there was, however, a fluffy inflammation on the covering of the bone (periosteum) and the subtalar joint was inflamed. My first thought was that he had a form of arthritis associated with another condition.

When I asked if he'd had any problems with his bowels or stomach, he said no (ruling out inflammatory bowel disease with arthritis). Since he was sexually active, I suggested a urine culture for possible venereal disease; it was negative. The blood tests were, however, positive for arthritis. Since he had no back problem, I ruled out ankylosing spondylitis. After looking at the lab tests, and considering all the other clues, I concluded that he had Reiter's syndrome. The condition may have been set off by the urinary tract infection and exacerbated by the increased mileage and training.

These variant diseases with arthritis tend to go away on their own in one to seven months. I treated him with homeopathic *Bryonia* which matched his symptoms (his foot was red, and hot; worse with any motion, better when cool) and told him to rest from exercise. The *Bryonia* was helpful but the ankle was still painful, so I gave him Indocin (an NSAID for pain and inflammation). He was more comfortable and could walk without crutches.

After two weeks, he was much better but still had stiffness in the heel and in the ankle joint. I gave him *Rhus Tox* since this remedy matched his symptoms of stiffness and pain: worse in the morning;

worse with initial motion, and better with continued motion; much better with heat; much worse with cold. Following *Rhus Tox,* I gave him a long-term constitutional remedy and he has not had any further problems.

Case History of a Runner with Gout

John Tuny, thirty-six-year-old business man and runner called my office one morning and said he had to come in right away. He complained of a terrible pain in his big toe joint. "The pain was so bad," he said, "that it woke me up at 4 a.m. I think I must have hurt my toe during the race I ran yesterday morning." While I was examining his foot, I asked him if he had done well in the race. "Yeah, I did," he smiled broadly for the first time, "I won! We went out and really celebrated last night—you know, a nice French restaurant—the whole bit." Apparently he had celebrated with very rich French food and several bottles of fine French red wine.

I wrote in my notes that he had a red, hot toe joint, and that he said it hurt very much to touch it. He had no temperature (thus no infection), and my diagnosis was that it was probably gout. I gave him a local anesthetic and extracted some fluid out of his joint with a needle. I looked at the fluid under the microscope and saw the characteristic crystals of uric acid—confirming gout.

I injected the joint with *Bryonia* and *Traumeel,* and told him to take *Bryonia* orally every hour for three hours, and then to stop unless he needed to take more. I did lab and urine tests to check for kidney problems associated with gout, and took X-rays. These tests showed the early signs of gout, but no major damage. His uric acid level was high (a sign of gout), and he was dehydrated—probably from all the alcohol the night before and not drinking enough water since the race.

His ankle was put into an ice whirlpool with electric stimulation. He was better the next day, but since he had a family history of gout, I sent him to his internist to see if I'd missed anything. The internist found that he is one of those people who produces too much uric acid. The doctor felt that the gout was not bad enough to prescribe drugs and told him just to watch his diet and avoid alcohol. I put him on a constitutional remedy, and he has had no recurrence in three years.

"Is there a holistic treatment for rheumatoid arthritis?"

Yes. A holistic healing regime can be very helpful for increasing the over-all health and well-being of the arthritis sufferer:

- Avoid foods with additives. Additives may cause an allergic re-action which may trigger a series of allergic responses, stimulat-ing the body's immune system to attack its own tissue.
- Increase natural foods. Decrease processed foods (frozen, canned, or smoked).
- Cleansing the body for one to seven days with a raw food diet and fresh juices.
- Reduce intake of fat.
- Drink plenty of water to keep the system flushed of toxins.
- Take 1-3,000 mgs of vitamin C per day for rheumatoid arthritis; calcium and magnesium tablets may be helpful.
- Take Bromeline, an enzyme, if there is cracking of joints and pain. Take between meals. (If taken with meals, Bromeline is a digestion aid.)
- Use hot packs to relieve pain. If joints are hot as well as swollen, a cold water pack or ice pack may work better. (Don't put an ice pack on the left shoulder because of the proximity to the heart.)
- Apply contrasting compresses (very hot and very cold) to the affected area to aid circulation and ease the stiffness. Soaking the joints or the whole body in a hot Epsom salts bath can also relieve pain.
- Take long hot baths to improve circulation and relax tense mus-cles. Exercise in a warm pool.

"I've heard arthritis may be related to emotional stress. Is that true?"

Arthritis, along with other forms of physical disease, does seem to be linked to emotional stress. According to one researcher, Dr. George F. Solomon of UC-Los Angeles Medical Center, the brain and the body's immune system are always in communication. "The impli-cation . . . for the practice of medicine is that patient attitudes and re-lationships with the physician may be as critical as the specific treatments themselves," he said.

Solomon's work suggests that personality factors may predispose a person to autoimmune diseases such as rheumatoid arthritis. Women with a compliant, subservient personality who deny feelings of anger or hostility are particularly prone to autoimmune disease. Interestingly, the suppression of the emotional level parallels the suppression of the physical response (immune system).

If you are the type of person who keeps your feelings in and have arthritis or a family history of rheumatoid arthritis, psychotherapy

345

may be helpful in treating or preventing the disease. Hypnotherapy, in particular, can help identify hidden feelings, allowing them to be released in a healthy way.

"What about some of the folk remedies I have heard about for arthritis?"

There are indigenous herbal medicines and treatments (folk medicine) that have long been used for the relief of arthritis pain. I have not tried all of these, but have listed some of them for your information.

- Wrap painful joints in heated flannel which have been sprinkled with powdered sulphur.
- Honey and cider vinegar. A tablespoon of cider vinegar mixed in a glass of hot water with a teaspoon of honey, taken twice a day as a cleansing remedy.
- Copper bracelets worn on the wrist for arthritis pain. This is an old remedy that has helped many of my patients.
- Camphor (8 parts) and cayenne pepper (1 part) mixed with olive oil (4 parts.) Massage into painful joints. However, don't use anything with camphor in it if you are taking a homeopathic remedy as camphor may antidote the effect of the remedy.
- Cod liver oil (1 tablespoon) and fresh orange juice (2 tablespoons) mixed together well. Take before breakfast or just before bed.
- Dandelion roots (boil 2 or 3 roots) in 2 pints of water for 1 hour. Drink a glass of the tea before each meal. Roots are best picked in the spring.

"What do you recommend as exercise for people with rheumatoid or osteoarthritis?"

Regular low-impact exercise, yoga, and any other form of movement therapy. T'ai chi and yoga can be a great help in preventing both rheumatoid and osteoarthritis as it gently stimulates the entire body, including the joints. Rotation of shoulders, hands, wrists, ankles and pelvis all help relieve stiffness. Another benefit of practicing yoga is that it relieves stress in general.

"What sports should I avoid so I won't get arthritis?"

Sports involving possible heavy impact and injury to joints, such as football, basketball or hockey may lead to joint damage and arthritis following a bad injury.

"If either of my parents had arthritis, will I get it?"

It depends. Heredity plays a part in all disease. If your parents had arthritis, and you are exposed to the same influences they were exposed to (e.g., bad diet, excessive drugs, toxins, or viral disease), you have a greater risk of getting the disease than someone who is exposed to the same influences, but doesn't have the hereditary factor. If you had parents who bottled up their emotions and feelings, and you're the same type of person, you might develop arthritis, too. Heredity plays a big part in the various types of systemic arthritis like gout.

With a family history, you need to take precautionary measures. Your diet should be low in red meat and additives, low in sugar, fats and processed foods, and high in complex carbohydrates. You need to drink plenty of water. You need regular low-impact aerobic exercise, and up to twenty miles of running or walking a week. Reduce the stresses in your life by meditating, participating in fulfilling activities, and staying happy.

"Do children get arthritis?"

Yes. Still's disease is a serious form of juvenile arthritis with high fever and rash (similar to Lyme's disease). I sometimes recommend to families with a history of arthritis that children have a homeopathic workup. However, it's still too early to know if this type of preventive medicine will actually avert the disease later on.

I remember one young patient, Nancy Bollinger, who was referred to me by an osteopathic physician. Nancy was a personable fourteen-year-old girl who had developed arthritis in the knees and ankles about eight months before. She also had terrible plantar fasciitis (pain on the bottom of the foot). She had gone to Stanford medical center in Palo Alto, California, and it was thought she might have either Still's disease (juvenile arthritis) or Lyme's disease (because the arthritis had developed after a flu-like infection with a red rash). No one was quite sure how to treat her.

She told me that her pains shifted from the left ankle and foot to the right. She said even though she was stiff and sore, she always felt better after a gentle walk. She also felt better with the windows open and when there was a cool breeze.

I examined her for biomechanical abnormalities. To help her walk better, I treated her fasciitis and ankle problems by injecting *Rhus Tox* and *Traumeel*. I also made orthotics for her shoes. She had a rather dramatic improvement with the plantar fasciitis and ankle symptoms, but was still sore.

I next did a homeopathic constitutional workup and found she fitted the remedy *Pulsatilla.* The characteristics which matched those of the remedy were: migrating pains; better with a cool breeze; thirstless; compliant personality; young female; and fair-skinned. I took her off *Rhus Tox* and gave her a single 1M dose of *Pulsatilla.*

After two months all her symptoms went away. The limp disappeared, and she started walking normally (with orthotics). What happened next was very interesting.

About six months later, she developed a sore throat—possibly strep throat. She went to her family doctor who gave her an antibiotic. All her old symptoms came back! The antibiotics had antidoted the *Pulsatilla.* She took another dose of *Pulsatilla* and the arthritis and plantar fasciitis disappeared again.

"What about massage, chiropractic, or acupuncture work for arthritis?"

Many arthritic symptoms are improved (but not cured) by gentle forms of mobilization, motion, and massage. A chiropractic treatment may relieve pain if *gentle,* non-forceful, adjustments are done. It's very important to treat the neck gently.

Acupuncture, ayurvedic medicine, shiatsu, applied kinesiology, yoga, and many other forms of healing may help depending on the type of arthritis. Get a proper medical diagnosis and talk to several practitioners about possible treatment.

Summary of Arthritis Treatment

There is a myth that running may cause arthritis over time. In fact, findings have shown that bone mass is greater in people who run long-distance and that healthy joints do not suffer damage. Arthritis stems from either a medical disease or a local injury (the accumulation of stresses to the joints). Normal, biomechanically balanced running does not cause arthritis. In fact, joints require stimulation from weight-bearing exercise in order to remain healthy. "What you don't use, you lose."

Moderate running (under 25 miles a week) decreases the symptoms of mild arthritis and may prevent its occurrence. On the other hand, sometimes very high mileage, especially if done with uncorrected biomechanical problems, can cause osteoarthritis.

If you are a walker or a runner with arthritis, find out what kind you have. Is it one or two joints (osteoarthritis) or many joints (rheumatoid arthritis)? Walking and moderate, low-impact sport is not harmful if you have mild arthritis; in fact, it will make your joints feel better. However, if the pounding on the joints from running gives you pain, don't run. Walk instead, or do yoga, low-impact sports or swimming.

Arthritis symptoms can be controlled and suppressed, but not cured by various western medicines such as aspirin, NSAIDs and cortisone. My advice is to get all the conventional lab work done first so you know what kind of arthritis you're dealing with. Find out what the orthodox diagnosis is and what treatment your doctor recommends. Find out the pros and cons, and ask about alternatives.

With systemic arthritis (rheumatoid arthritis or arthritis associated with other medical diseases) it's important to look at all the physical and emotional factors in your life such as diet, exercise, personal satisfaction and overall lifestyle. Holistic treatment recommends good diet, water therapy, gentle exercise and reduction of stress—all of which are beneficial for chronic arthritis sufferers.

Homeopathic remedies can help with the pain and swelling of arthritis if detected early. Some forms of arthritis *may* be slowed down or even cured by homeopathy. If, however, joints are damaged from overuse, homeopathic remedies probably won't give you back a healthy joint.

Since emotional stress from a bad relationship or a job you don't like may strain and weaken your immune system as much as physical factors, you might consider psychotherapy. A good counselor can provide emotional support to help reduce the pressure of making needed changes.

The treatment options suggested in this chapter are given as an overview, and are not meant to be used without the advice of a physician.

Footnotes:

1. Nancy E. Lane, MD, "Aging, Long-Distance Running, and the Development of Musculoskeletal Disability," The American Journal of Medicine, Vol 82. p. 772.

2. Nancy E. Lane, MD, et.al., "Running, Osteoarthritis, and Bone Density: Initial 2-Year Longitudinal Study," The American Journal of Medicine, May, 1990, Vol. 88, p. 452.

3. For an engrossing story of a patient's view of lupus and her treatment with both prednisone and alternative methods, see Donna Hamil Talman, *Heartsearch: Toward Healing Lupus* (Berkeley, California, North Atlantic Books, 1991).

4. Richard S. Panush, MD, et.al., "Is Running Associated With Degenerative Joint Disease?" JAMA, 1986: 255:1152-1154.

5. BHI-Arthritis and BHI-Co-enzyme are manufactured by Biological Homeopathic Industries, 11600 Cochiti SE, Albuquerque, New Mexico, 87123, 800-621-7644.

Chapter 18

SPORTS INJURIES IN CHILDHOOD AND ADOLESCENCE

> Everytime I climb a tree
> Though climbing may be good
> for ants
> It isn't awfully good
> for pants
> But still it's pretty good
> for me
> Everytime I climb a tree.
> —David McCord

Growing pains are real, be they physical or emotional. Many of the problems associated with running and sports in childhood and adolescence stem from growth spurt complications. Bones grow first, and the muscles and tendons catch up later. While the muscles and tendons grow and expand, the muscles get very tight, achy, and stiff. Children's bodies may become extremely tight. Their muscles ache, and there is inflammation at the attachments of the tendons to bone. Common sites of achiness and stiffness are the front of the knee, the back of the heel, and the bottom of the heel. These areas may appear red and swollen. The pain is aggravated by sports and physical education.

Pain in the Bone Not Near a Joint

The areas where growth takes place in the bones—specifically not near a joint—are called growth plates (apophyses). An injury in a growth area away from a joint is usually of no consequence. Therefore, if an apophysis is inflamed or injured, there may be discomfort, but once healed, there is usually no permanent deformity.

Pain and Swelling at the Knee
(Osgood-Schlatter's Disease)

Osgood-Schlatter's disease (named after the two doctors who studied the problem) involves pain and enlargement around the knee. It occurs beneath the knee joint in the front of the leg. There is a large, often painful bump (see Fig. 18-1). Young people who have this bump usually outgrow the problem in a year or two, but often find it very difficult to run, play basketball, or do jumping sports during a two-year period.

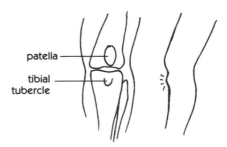

18-1. Osgood-Schlatter's Disease: painful bump on knee in adolescents is usually out-grown in one to two years.

The problem is found more often with children whose feet turn inward too much (excessive pronation).

To treat Osgood-Schlatter's disease, common sense must prevail. Those activities that cause discomfort should be avoided.

See an orthopedist for diagnosis and x-rays.

Select one of the following homeopathic remedies:

Ruta Grav if stiff and sore; if movement makes it better, yet too much activity causes fatigue and pain.

Rhus Tox if it's very sore with initial motion, but gets better with continued motion. Use either one of these remedies for two weeks and then use: *Calcarea Phosphorica* if there is much pain at the tendon attachment; if associated with rapid growth spurt; if the child is the bubbling and outgoing type. Give *Calcarea Fluorica* if there is more bone pain. Both of these *Calcarea Salts* are very good for growing pains associated with bone. I usually give children a 200c dose, and then have them take 12c twice a day for two weeks. These *Calcarea Salts* are very good for children and may even help scoliosis.

Be sure to instruct the child to avoid pain-causing activities such as jumping or squatting. Strengthening and stretching the calf muscles and quadriceps will be necessary. Ask your doctor for appropriate exercises.

Foot orthotics used inside shoes are very important in helping to correct this condition. See a podiatrist. A neoprene knee brace will protect the area and may be useful in very active children. You can buy braces at sporting goods stores. Otherwise, let the child do whatever is comfortable.

Pain in the Growth Plate in the Heel (Heel Apophysitis) or Severe's Disease

This pain occurs most often in children between the ages of ten and fourteen as the growth plate of the heel does not close until late teens. Tension is caused by a too-short, stiff Achilles tendon or a too-short plantar fascia (tendon on the bottom of the foot) pulling on the heel plate. This tension causes pain on the back or on the bottom of the heel. This problem is similar to the adult "pump bump" pain (or heel spur syndrome) described in Chapter 9. See Fig. 18-2.

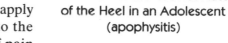

Youngsters who have this pain are often involved in soccer, Little League, cross-country skiing, or track. They complain of swelling and inflammation of the back or bottom of the heel which worsens with activity.

18-2. Pain in the Growth Plate of the Heel in an Adolescent (apophysitis)

To treat heel apophysitis apply an ice pack or heating pad to the heel for immediate relief of pain and swelling. Contrast baths (alternating hot and cold dips) are also helpful.

See a doctor to rule out stress fracture of the growth plate.

Give the child homeopathic *Arnica* for the first 24 hours. Then switch to *Ruta Grav* in potencies of 30x or 12c. Give twice a day for two weeks, then give either:

Calcarea Phosphorica or *Calcarea Fluorica*. Start with a 200c or 1M dose, and then give 12c twice a day for two weeks.

See a podiatrist to determine if the child is toeing-in (supination) or toeing-out (pronation). A simple foot orthotic with a small amount of heel lift and extra padding under the heel will help.

Massage may help, and physiotherapy may be recommended by your doctor.

Case History of Apophysitis

Jerry Garcia, an avid soccer player, was eleven years old when his father, Jose, brought him to see me. Father and son enjoyed running together, and Jerry's team had been doing well so he had been practicing fairly hard. He had started having considerable pain on the bottom of his heel, which was aggravated by wearing soccer cleats and working out on hard surfaces.

I x-rayed Jerry's foot to rule out a stress fracture, and the picture showed that the growth plate on the bottom of the heel had some irregularities which meant he had an apophysitis (growth plate disturbance) and probably a slight stress fracture as well. Since this problem was not near a joint, it presented no great threat other than pain.

Jerry happened to be going through a rapid growth spurt. When teenagers grow and become taller, the bones grow first, putting excessive stretch on the soft tissue. The soft tissue, in turn, pulls hard on the growth plate where it's anchored. This causes an inflammation similar to a heel spur.

Jerry also tended to toe out a bit, and his feet were somewhat pronated (turned inward). I gave him a semi-flexible foot orthotic which was a modification of a ready-made Birkenstock orthotic. It formed a cup for his heel, eliminating excessive pronation, but allowing enough flexibility for him to perform well both in soccer and in running. For more shock absorption, I put in a Viscolas heel on top of the orthosis.

Jerry still had some stiffness and discomfort for two to three weeks while he was healing but was able to play soccer. He was also shown how to stretch his hamstrings, calf muscles, and his Achilles tendon since they were quite tight and might cause another injury. Lastly, I gave him a homeopathic remedy to promote the healing of the growth plate; in this case, the remedy was *Ruta Grav.* About two weeks after the *Ruta Grav,* I gave him one dose of *Calcarea Phosphorica* to help prevent any relapse. His father told me he was fine after that.

Navicular Apophysitis (Kohler's Disease).

This is a serious growth plate problem which requires protection and rest until healing can be established. It generally occurs in younger children aged six to twelve. A cast and crutches are often necessary to prevent further stress to the area.

Bulge in the Arch of the Foot (Os Navicularis)

In this condition, there is usually a big bulge in the arch and the foot is inflamed and painful. Pain is felt with jumping and running fast. A problem of adolescents aged twelve to eighteen, os navicularis happens when two growth plates in the navicular bone pull apart (Fig. 18-3). Because the posterior tibial tendon, which holds the arch up, may be anchored in the part of bone that is pulled away from the main bone, the foot is weaker.

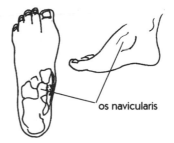

os navicularis

To treat os navicularis, see a doctor for x-rays. This is treated first with *orthotics* (very important), taping and rest. However, sometimes the extra bone has to be removed surgically.

18-3. Bulge in the arch of the foot in teen-agers indicates growth plate problem.

Take *Ruta Grav* followed, after two weeks, by *Calcarea Fluorica.*

Joint Injuries (Epiphyseal Injuries)

Growth plates within a joint are called epiphyses. When an injury happens to this area, damage may be permanent. Fortunately, injuries to the growth plate within the joints are rare, being caused usually by a trauma. The most common place for a epiphyseal fracture to occur is within the ankle joint. Ankle injuries in the growing child must be x-rayed and evaluated to insure appropriate diagnosis and treatment.

If there is a suspected fracture in the ankle joint or foot, take the child to the doctor at once and get x-rays. Give homeopathic *Arnica* immediately to help with shock, pain and bruising. Continue every hour for the first 24 hours. Then choose a remedy below:

Ruta Grav if very painful. *Ledum* if foot feels cool (or warm) to the touch and feels better with cold pack.

Bryonia if inflamed, red, painful; much worse touch and motion (child will not tolerate touching of injured part).

Lymphomyosot if very swollen. Take ten drops twice a day. Symphytum *only after fracture is properly aligned;* use for two weeks. Then go to *Calcarea Fluorica*: take a 200c or 1M dose. The next day begin 12c twice a day for two weeks.

During recovery, depending on the type of fracture, your child will be treated with crutches, a cast, or possibly surgery. Proper treatment of a fracture is essential in a growing child to avoid a permanent growth disturbance.

Do not let the child engage in sports activities for four to six weeks; return to sport must be approved by the doctor. Resumption of activity must be carefully monitored, and under no circumstances should the child resume activity at the same level he or she was doing before the injury. Physiotherapy will be recommended by your doctor after the fracture is healed.

In-toeing and Out-toeing

Young children from one to five years old are very often brought to me by concerned grandparents who worry more about "pigeon-toes" or "knock-knees" than the parent does. Most of the time, there really is no cause for alarm as the children will outgrow these seeming deformities. However, it is a good idea to protect the feet while they are outgrowing these tendencies. A podiatrist can help you find out if the deformity is serious.

A child will compensate for excessive toeing-in by turning the feet out. This is an unconscious reaction on the child's part in order to look like the "other kids." Turning the foot out causes pronation (flattening of the foot), leading to collapse of the arches. It's important to encourage the child to turn out at the hip joint and stretch the hip muscles. I suggest that the child sit cross-legged ("Indian-style"). Foot orthotics are a big help in training the hip to turn out and protecting the feet. Ballet or modern dance lessons are often a help in re-aligning legs and stretching muscles.

Another problem is the young child who is toeing-in or out and who stumbles or trips frequently. This child is always falling down and seems clumsy. He or she should be examined for neurological problems. Sometimes the motor skills have not quite developed, and the parents need to be reassured that there is nothing wrong—that the child will grow at his or her own pace.

Usually a child with flat feet and weak arches will toe-out. Often tightness at the hips causes a duck walk and prevents the legs from naturally rotating inwards.

What Children Can Do For Weak Feet

- Walk on tip-toes.
- Pick up marbles with curled toes.
- Walk on the outside of the foot.
- Balance on a tilt board.
- Bounce on a trampoline.
- Wear a foot orthotic to keep foot straight.
- Roller skate or ice skate.
- Stretch out the heel cord, legs and hips.

For a toeing-in problem, get a diagnosis to check for a hip problem. Once the foot is protected with an appropriate foot orthotic, the child should be encouraged to stretch out the hip muscles, and to walk with the feet straight ahead. Roller skating or ice skating help the feet to point forward.

Once in awhile a child will have very flat, weak feet with looseness in the ligaments. The feet will need protection with foot orthotics; otherwise, the arch will flatten even more.

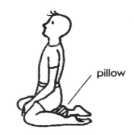

pillow

If one hip turns out, but the other doesn't, x-rays should be taken to rule out a bone or hip problem. If a hip problem is suspected, see an orthopedist. Orthotics will help to correct the misalignment, and stretching exercises for the hips (Fig. 18-4) are necessary. The hip is stretched by sitting on the floor with

18-4. Stretching Exercise to Correct Out-toeing: sit on the floor with legs to side of body or put pillow under buttocks if needed.

the legs bent back with the lower leg bent close to the thighs (along the sides of the body). If the child is not flexible enough to sit with the buttocks on the floor in this position, put a pillow under the seat. If necessary, stretch one leg at a time. Dancing, yoga for children, ballet and gymnastics all stretch and strengthen legs, and help improve alignment.

Limping and Pain at Hip (Legg-Perthe's Disease)

In young, active children, especially boys, pain and limitation of hip movement may indicate a serious hip joint problem called Legg-Perthe's disease after the doctors who studied it. The child with this condition tends to walk with a painful, limping gait and will not want to participate much in sports activities.

There is usually a weakness in the upper thigh due to atrophy (non-use). The child cannot spread the legs very far apart or rotate the leg inward. An x-ray will show that there is a deterioration of the head of the thigh bone (femoral head) where it connects to the hip socket (see Fig. 18-5).

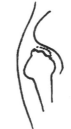

18-5. Legg-Perthe's Disease: head of femur is degenerated within hip joint.

For Legg-Perthe's disease, see an orthopedist—not a chiropractor or any other alternative therapist—for x-rays and treatment. The most common treatment is a brace, worn up to a year, to permit the femoral head to form a new blood supply which will allow the bone to heal. The hips are spread apart about forty-five degrees to prevent the femur from slipping out of the hip joint. The child can still walk and move about.

Surgery, by the way, may be necessary for an adult with this disease, including having a full hip replacement if the degeneration has been severe. Give the child one of the following homeopathic remedies to enhance healing: (check a *Materia Medica* for details of characteristics to help make a selection)

Calcarea Carbonicum, Calcarea Phosphorica, or *Calcarea Fluorica.*

Physiotherapy will be recommended by the doctor. Stretch out muscles and ligaments under the supervision of a physiotherapist.

Hip and Groin Pain with Awkward Gait (Slipped Femoral Capital Epiphysis)

The overweight teen-ager is particularly prone to this injury. Usually, the child first complains of a mild discomfort in the hip, as well as

> **My Advice to Parents of Young Athletes**
>
> If your child has hip pain, take him or her to an orthopedist for both diagnosis and treatment. Stop sports. If there is a foot imbalance or toeing-in or out, see a podiatrist. When in doubt, always check with your pediatrician. For growing pains or growth problems, see a homeopath for a constitutional remedy.

deep groin pain. The pain sometimes radiates down (is referred) to the knee as the condition inside the joint worsens. The child may develop an awkward, wobbling gait, leaning toward the painful side. The affected leg is rotated outward (Fig. 18-6).

The pressure from the child's excessive weight causes slippage of the head of the thigh bone (femoral capital), leading slowly to knock-kneed deformity. On x-rays, the femur looks a little like an ice-cream cone that is melting and tilting off to the side. The tilting of the growth plate interrupts the blood supply, a dangerous situation and may lead to the death of the head of the femur.

Have the child examined and x-rayed as soon as you suspect a problem. Your pediatrician will probably send you to an orthopedist. Treatment in the early stage is centered on preventing further slippage. If there has been a minimal slip, the joint should be stabilized surgically by an orthopedist. Several months are necessary to allow for proper healing. Usually, there will be full recovery.

Rehabilitation by a sports physical therapist, working together with an orthopedist is mandatory. Homeopathic remedies to strengthen the constitution in general are the same as the preceding section.

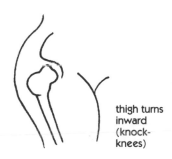

thigh turns inward (knock-knees)

18-6. Hip Pain in an Overweight Child (slipped femoral capital epiphysis)

Chapter 19

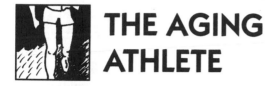 THE AGING ATHLETE

It's better to wear out than to rust out.
—Richard Cumberland, theologian, 1631–1718

Running When You're Older

One question I am asked often is, "What are the long-term results of running? If I run too much when I'm younger, will it cause problems when I'm older?" or "I would like to run forever. What should I do to assure that I will be able to? Just what are the long-term effects of running?"

In order to find out some answers, I decided to write letters to many of the competitive long-distance runners I treated ten to fifteen years ago. I wanted to know if they are still running or if they had suffered injuries which had sidelined them forever. I also wanted to know if they had any advice for younger runners. This is what I found out.

Half of the runners I interviewed are still running strong. Most of them are now in their fifties, sixties, or even seventies. They are running, but they are running less mileage. Instead of the 60 to 70 miles per week run during their competitive years, almost all of them are down to about 30 miles a week now. Some of the older runners, those over fifty or fifty-five years, are running every other day, rather than every day. These people told me that, if they ran every day, they had too many aches and pains to make it worthwhile.

Most of these veterans are swimming, biking, and doing stretching exercises. They all reported that the older they get, the more time they must spend doing warm-up exercises, such as stretching, since their bodies tend to get stiffer and stiffer as the years go on.

Of those who have been "sidelined" (no longer running), most continue to enjoy exercise walking or other sports. Some of these runners had logged as much as 100 miles a week when they were younger. During the last few years, however, some had suffered arthritic changes in joints, and one or two had had hip and pelvis problems.

Of those who were still running, over 70 percent of them told me they expect to be running until their last days on earth. Running is vital to their life. In fact, running is so important to them that they are not willing to compete as much now and risk permanent injury. Interestingly, most of them felt that the high mileage they had done when they were younger was really unnecessary. Many of them now feel that running over 45 or 50 miles a week is venturing into the realm of diminishing returns.

To carry the study a bit further, I interviewed people who were fitness runners, people who had entered the sport during the running revolution in the seventies. Many of them were about thirty-five fifteen years ago. About 60 percent of these athletes are still running. They are running twenty to thirty miles a week, four or five days a week. Occasionally, they might run a 10K race. The other 40 percent have given up running for other sports, and most of them say the reason was because of foot or knee pain. They say that after they got older, their knees or feet hurt more and more when they ran. Even though they had had good shoes and good orthoses, running just wasn't worth it.

Lynne Leahy, however, is one of those exceptional runners who just won't quit despite about five years of recurring stress fractures, hamstring pulls, and frequent ankle sprains. "When I first started running, I had never done any exercise, and my body just wasn't conditioned for the rigors of running," she told me. Lynne is a mere forty-six years old—not really in the ancient runner category yet—but she's been running for fifteen years. "I took it up when I quit smoking and drinking as a diversion from my old wicked ways. I guess I ran about ten miles a week in those days," she said. She still runs a marathon a year but doesn't try to set a record.

She views running as a time for spiritual refreshment and enjoys the dark quiet streets of early morning in her neighborhood.

"I'd have to say I'm obsessed with my running, although about a year and a half ago I relaxed from my 'training mode' and just started running for the pure pleasure of it. I was told many times by doctors that I should stop because of the various injuries. My friends, too, were shocked that I'd want to keep running, but I had to. I just couldn't give it up. I'd change to other exercise while I healed my fractures and sprains, which was good for me. I learned to strengthen myself by swimming, bike-riding, exercise classes, T'ai Chi. I found that it takes about five years to really condition the body for running. I'm keeping my fingers crossed, but I haven't had an injury in three years." Lynne has become a Phase Four runner—sensitive to the needs of her body and committed to running, without striving to set records.

Exceptional Older Athletes

What about the exceptional runners? Bill Rogers and Hal Higdon, both top-flight senior runners, are still going strong. Bill Rogers is looking forward to his current level of competition. Bill Clark, a previous Bay Area great who I remember treating some fifteen years ago, has been sidelined for the past couple of years with a pelvic injury.

Blind marathon runner Harry Cordellos of San Francisco is fifty-three years old this year. He told me, "I just ran my best time in five-and-a-half years—3:17:40—at the Dallas-White Rock Marathon. That was my 117th marathon." When I asked Harry about the training he would recommend to new runners, he was quite vociferous. "Tell them not to worry about setting records. Don't push beyond what's sensible. I've run 39,000 miles so far, and the only injury I ever had was plantar fasciitis."

Harry feels that the attitude about running has changed since the running revolution of the seventies. "I see a real change in running and racing. A lot of the fun has disappeared. People are getting so serious, so sophisticated about training, they're really over-doing their training —and it's ruining their running. People go to some of these hi-tech running camps where there's all this structured interval work and so forth. After awhile they quit running. To me, the main thing is just putting on my shoes, being able to run, and enjoying breathing fresh air."

Like other runners who keep running into their fifties, sixties and seventies, Harry varies his workouts with swimming and using an exercycle. Demonstrating yet again what it means to be exceptional, Harry has just won a place on a disabled water-ski team where he will be doing slalom, tricks, and jumping.

Other runners, such as orthopedic surgeon Stan James of Eugene, Oregon, have given up competitive running in favor of cross-country skiing. He feels that the impact shock of running isn't worth the wear and tear on knees, ankles and feet. On the other hand, Steve Perlman of Slymar, California, is still getting up every morning at 4:30 to run. He averages about 60 miles a week, despite a torn meniscus (knee injury) two years before. He says that now that he's over forty, he has to spend much more time stretching. He also takes two easy days between every long hard run. He avoids races to not push himself into another injury.

One of the most remarkable letters I received was from Walt Stack, the legendary senior runner from San Francisco. Walt is the founder of the Dolphin Club South End Runners, with whom I used to run. He started his letter with his familiar, "Hi, Ole Bean!" It was a handwritten letter in pencil on brown paper. He said he had run 65,000 miles since 1965, as well as the Western States 100 and The Iron Man in Hawaii. He has run in over twenty states, as well as in Athens, Paris, Melbourne, Fiji Islands, Hawaii, Canada, Alaska and even up Pike's Peak. Born in 1907, his current routine includes running five days a week, swimming thirty minutes in San Francisco Bay and biking 6 miles to and from his home. He's an example of how you can run forever if you have the right constitution and body. In typical Walt-style he ended his note with sage advice: "Start off slowly, then gradually taper off!"

Don Lundberg, a seventy-three-year-old runner from Modesto, California, suggests that new runners learn to relax early on, listen to their body, and adjust accordingly. He recommends periodic forced super-deep breathing when running. He runs 6 miles each morning before breakfast except for the day before and after a marathon. Don has run eighteen marathons and doesn't skip running more than two days in a row, even when on vacation. His injuries include a pulled calf muscle and bruised toes from running on rocks. Twice in his running career he has had back problems which prevented him from running—a week each time. He now feels that stretching and calisthenics solved his back problem. He also works out hard every day on his ranch. A college professor by profession, he has run in the World Games in Melbourne and has a record of 3:17:02 at the Napa, California Marathon in 1982.

John Thompson of Glendale, California responded to my inquiry. He's sixty-four and has been running for the past ten years with only two injuries. The first was a heel spur, the second was a painful groin pull. The groin pull sidelined him from running for six months. Since then he's had no problem. "My secret," he wrote, "is to run almost exclusively on horse trails." He used to race two or three times a month and now only races six or eight times a year. "I just enjoy running every day for the pleasure only." His advice to younger runners is to build up mileage slowly and use trails for at least forty to fifty percent of the time. Roads are too hard and eventually lead to injury. He also bikes occasionally for alternate exercise, he said, because he feels it's good to have other recreational activities to fall back on. He has run in eleven marathons, with a time of 3:32 in 1981. "I don't have much speed," he wrote, "but I'm durable."

There are many exceptional athletes who continue to achieve into their later years. Forty-one-year-old Jack Foster stunned the world by running an unprecedented two hours and eleven minutes to finish second in the marathon in the 1974 Commonwealth Games. His progress as a runner did not stop with that race. He went on to establish eight world age class marathon records. This type of achievement is very reassuring for many aging athletes who dream of performing at a world class level.

The world of sports is full of performances of older athletes. Among them are Willie Shoemaker, fifty-six, who continued to win horse races until his retirement in 1989. Carlos Lopez of Portugal, at the age of forty-two, won the Olympic Marathon title in 1984 during the Los Angeles Games despite the searing heat. One year later, he established the current World Marathon Record of 207.12 and also captured the World Cross Country Championship. In 1985, Richard Bass, at the age of fifty-five, became the oldest person to conquer Mt. Everest. At age sixty-five, Ashley Harper became the oldest man to swim the English Channel. Gordie Howe, in 1980, as a fifty-two-year-old grandfather, was named the NHL All-Star for the twenty-second time, an unprecedented feat.

Eighty-seven-year-old Ken Beer of Hillsborough, California, is the holder of fifty-three national senior titles in the United States Tennis Association's octogenarian circuit, which boasts 1,500 members above the age of seventy-five. Quoted recently in a *New York Times* interview, Beer said, "The only way a person stays alive at my age is to take a keen interest in something, and be challenged. For me that's tennis: It gets me outdoors, helps me meet good people. A person without a challenge is on the downhill." Although Beer started playing tennis in his thirties, many of the other senior tournament players came to the game after retirement.

While some people may take any setback as an excuse to slow down, eighty-one-year-old John Lawrence of Hewlett, Long Island, number twenty-three in the national 80's tennis singles ranking, made a speedy comeback to the courts after fracturing his shoulder during a game. He had tripped over some bushes near the edge of the court, breaking his non-playing shoulder in several places. His surgeon told him to expect to be sidelined for six months to a year. However, after spending two months with his arm immobilized, he began working out on the stationary cycle and having physical therapy three times a week. After one and a half months of this routine he was back on the courts, and claims that he's playing even better than before the injury.

To be sure, these individuals are exceptional, but it does give the rest of us hope that we can reach our dreams before we're "too old."

Idleness and Aging

The medical literature strongly suggests that the greatest threat to the health of the aging athlete is not the aging process itself, but rather inactivity. There is less risk in activity than in continuous inactivity . . . it's better to get a good physical examination if you intend to be sedentary to see if you're healthy enough to stand the inactivity. As venerable a physician as Hippocrates said, "Idleness and lack of occupation tend—nay are dragged—towards evil."

It's heartening to hear that regular exercise may be able to retard the physiologic decline associated with old age as much as 50 percent. Taken in this light, regular aerobic exercise really is a fountain of youth. Scientists have shown that life does not begin at forty, but it doesn't have to end there, either. Body systems appear to have been designed to reinforce activity. When there is disuse, a large number of degenerative changes take place.

Obviously, we learn from real life examples and from scientific data that "what you don't use, you lose." Although activity is a must, most of the runners I interviewed mentioned slowing down a bit. They have decreased the total mileage run and regularly give themselves rest days. More time is necessary for stretching and flexibility exercises, and alternative aerobic exercise is helpful to allow the body to recover from those longer runs. Running more than 30 miles a week is usually unnecessary and may be harmful for those runners over forty years of age. As you approach fifty, it may be a good idea to run every other day or run two days, rest one day. It's always good advice to run on natural surfaces rather than on artificial ones. If you do run on roads or concrete, pay the utmost attention to the cushioning ability of your shoes.

Don't compare your running to other peoples' running. If your best friend can run 60 miles a week and never be sore or injured, it doesn't mean you can. High mileage and too much racing increases the risk of injury.

What is Aging?

Aging is a universal, progressively decreasing loss of structural and functional ability with the passage of time . . . from a scientific point of view. However, examples from research studies as well as personal best records of exceptional athletes show there is a vast range of accommodation to the aging process. On any day in your local park you'll see the wiry, panting, grey-haired runner breezing past the dozing senior, cane in hand, on the park bench. Many of the effects of aging are—believe it or not—optional!

Functional and anatomical slow-down (aging) is preceded by attitudinal changes. What you think you become. The physical factors contributing to aging (lifetime habits of smoking, excessive alcohol consumption, a diet of refined foods) combine with the spiritual, mental and emotional factors—loss of interest in life, retirement without a replacement activity, grief and loss. *To decrease the effects of aging, the most important attitude to have is optimism.* Having goals and dreams and an optimistic outlook is even more important than having a "young attitude." Interacting with enough people is important. Run or walk with a friend, if possible.

Getting old, in the western culture, is often equated with failure, and people spend enormous amounts of time and money fighting the process. In other cultures age is equated with wisdom. Elderly people often focus on physical limits, which causes low self-confidence, depression, low motivation. *These* feelings can lead to a vicious cycle of degeneration of the body.

It's a good idea to look at the beliefs you hold around aging, and see if you want to follow along with the majority of society in believing that age is a failure, a loss, and a mistake. You can choose how you enter your latter years. Look for role models of creative, vital older people and start to ask people about how they stay engaged with life.

If you regard your body as a machine, it will disappoint you in the aging process. Instead, value what you have and can do, and if you've focused excessively on physical activity, enlarge your world in other ways. Investigate forms of body work therapy. Travel, to see how older people function in different cultures. Begin writing or painting, and join a community college or adult class.

Although it happens to every body, aging is highly individualized and depends on various factors, such as genetics, lifestyle, and past disease processes. Aging need not be accompanied by disease. It can be a natural process that brings to fruition wisdom and internal growth. Aging implies *losing* vitality, but maturing implies *gaining* wisdom.

How and Where Aging Happens

Different parts of the body may age faster than other parts, depending on stress, lack of exercise or toxins (alcohol, smoke, fat, chemicals) that you ingest. Let's look at the different systems of your body and see how they might be affected by age.

Cardiovascular and Pulmonary System

To run "you gotta have heart" . . . and lungs. Beyond the age of thirty-five, there is an inevitable drop in the maximum amount of oxygen you can hold in your lungs during one breath. Year by year your heart rate slows down with the result that less oxygen is fed to your cells. While inactivity results in lowered aerobic capacity, evidence shows that the cardiovascular system of a person of seventy will respond positively to aerobic endurance training—exercise walking or running. Even though ideally you should be exercising from your twenties, it's never too late to improve your health. The statistics on aerobic capacity for different ages are interesting.

Todd, Taylor and Thaddeus

Let's peek into a cardiologist's office as he does a comparison of three men—Todd and Taylor, both twenty-five-year-old college students, and Thaddeus, an older man of sixty-five. Todd has been working with computers since he was about sixteen. He admits to the doctor that he isn't interested much in sports and doesn't get much physical activity. Taylor, on the other hand, won a track and field scholarship and runs about 60 miles a week. Thaddeus, a retired school teacher, tells the doctor that he has been running 30 miles a week for twenty years.

The doctor tests all three men on their maximum oxygen performance level (VO$_2$ max). Looking over the test results, he says, "Frankly, Todd, I'm not surprised that your VO$_2$ max is only forty because you've never exercised. But you're only twenty-five; you should be much, much higher." Sheepishly, Todd tosses his head slightly and reddens.

"Of course, you, Taylor," says the doctor to the young athlete, "are testing at a very strong VO_2 max of seventy because you're in training and you've got youth on your side." The young man shifts his shoulders back slightly, hands on hips. "But, Thaddeus, you old dog, you did really well for a guy your age. You tested out with a VO_2 of sixty-five—very close to our young athlete, Taylor, here who's less than half your age."

The cardiologist explains that if Todd is to continue to live a life of inactivity, by the time he is Thaddeus's age of sixty-five, his VO_2 max will be thirty to twenty-five. Thaddeus, even at the age of sixty-five, is in far better physical shape, because of his regular aerobic activity of running, than an untrained twenty-five-year-old. In fact, he is only a little bit below a twenty-five-year-old trained athlete.

In testing more than 500 middle-aged men at the Human Performance Laboratory some years ago, Dr. David Costill discovered that one out of ten had oxygen deficiencies because of a poor cardiovascular system. He feels the greatest risk is to people who do not get involved in athletics until middle age:

> The critical years in terms of cardiovascular disease are between 25 and 35. That's the era of a man's life, and a woman's, when the least attention is paid to their physical health. Men and women both are balancing job and family, and don't pay any attention to their endurance ability. Both let themselves deteriorate. Once you build up atherosclerotic deposits in your system, you rarely get rid of them—even by exercise. At best, you can stop the build-up of more deposits, or hope that by being better trained you will have more strength to survive a heart attack should it occur.[1]

Recent research at the American Heart Association on cholesterol, diet and exercise shows that 30 to 40 minutes a day of aerobic exercise and proper diet increase the "good" kind of cholesterol (HDL) which can reverse cholesterol buildup in clogged vessels. In addition, by quitting smoking *and* exercising, you can rebuild your lungs. That means that it's never too late to start!

Berkeley homeopathic educator Dana Ullman once told me, "The best time to start exercising is ten years ago. The second best time is today."

Kidneys and Lungs

Kidney function also decreases with age. Your ability to control fluid volumes decreases, which jeopardizes the function of the cardiovascular system. As you age, you may be at greater risk of experiencing problems associated with overhydration, dehydration, and electrolyte disturbances. In addition, the ability for the lungs to function at their best decreases with the aging process. Older runners may get out of breath more than a younger athlete. An advanced form of lung impairment is called senile emphysema—a term that should get your running shoes on. Exercising regularly and avoiding environmental pollutants and tobacco smoke greatly slows down the aging of the lungs. Regular physical exercise increases gas exchange in the lungs, decreases breathlessness, and strengthens the respiratory-lung musculature.

Vascular System (Arteries and Veins)

It's common knowledge that hardening of the arteries—atherosclerosis—is associated with improper diet and inactivity. Blood vessel walls become inelastic with the aging process unless there has been regular aerobic activity, running or walking. Hard, inelastic blood vessels require more work from the heart to pump the blood through them. This leads to heart disease. Aerobic exercise for at least twenty minutes burns off some of these debilitating deposits.

Central Nervous System

The central nervous system is also adversely affected by the aging process. By the age of eighty, there is a 15 percent decrease in nerve conduction velocity. The ability to coordinate complex motor activities and maintain balance reduces each year after the age of forty. This deterioration is accelerated when there is inactivity. The reaction times of aging athletes slow down, and they must train regularly to preserve a superior skill level.

Muscles and Bones

The greatest problem in the musculo-skeletal system is brittleness of bones due to lack of calcium (osteoporosis). Women are at far greater risk of losing calcium than are men. Men lose bone mass at about 0.4 percent each year after the age of fifty. They don't have a significant bone loss until their eighties. Most women, on the other hand, lose bone mass at the rate of 0.75 percent to one percent each year beginning in the early thirties. This rate may go as high as three times that amount during menopause, and remain high for several years thereafter. At this rate, many women lose more than thirty percent of bone mass before their seventies. This is why senior women may break a wrist or hip from a relatively minor pressure.

Osteoporosis can be a serious consideration for older women who run or play sports, particularly if they started their program at age fifty or older. However, for women who have been regularly active, bone loss is less of a concern. Fitness walking, aerobics and running all decrease the risk of calcium loss. The skeleton needs regular muscular traction and the effects of gravity to keep healthy. (Astronauts become osteoporotic in outer space!) Gravity increases the thickness of bone and the strength of the various dynamic tissues within the bone. Bone and all parts of the skeleton are dynamic and constantly changing according to the stresses applied to them. When there is inactivity, bone loses its strength, and cartilage loses its elasticity. The same is true of muscles, ligaments, and tendons.

Post-menopausal women or those who have had a hysterectomy can help prevent osteoporosis, not only by exercising, but by reducing consumption of animal protein which contributes to calcium loss. It's also important to increase intake of vitamin C and complex carbohydrates. Avoid additives in foods which can cause metabolic changes leading to arthritis as well as osteoporosis.

Connective Tissue (Muscles, Ligaments and Tendons)

We previously assumed that connective tissue was inert. We were wrong. Muscles, ligaments and tendons are just as subject to change as all the other parts of the body. Activity promotes their strength and flexibility, whereas inactivity leads to weakness and stiffness. It's no mystery why you feel stiffer as you get older—it's the inelasticity of connective tissue. Therefore, it's important to spend time stretching and warming up. If you're an older runner and you injure a tendon or ligament, it will take longer to heal. Severely damaged ligaments may never return to their original length. Injury will permanently disturb their normal stress-strain characteristics and will cause irreversible damage or failure.

A real problem is the Achilles tendon, which begins losing its blood supply after the age of thirty or thirty-five. It becomes stiffer and less resistant to stress. Tendo-Achilles ruptures in the master athlete create a serious problem and weekend warriors are also prone to this injury. Older women should not wear high heels, and should keep stretching the Achilles heel tendon.

Running and Arthritic Joints

A question that patients always ask me is, "Will running produce arthritic changes in my joints? Will my knees become arthritic if I continue to run?" The answer to this, emphatically, is "No." If, however, you train, race and run when there is pain in your knee joint, pain in your ankle joint, or pain in your foot, this could lead to arthritis. Arthritis is especially likely if there is inflammation with pain. The inflammatory processes within a joint can damage the cartilage, causing it to soften. Once cartilage becomes inflamed, arthritis can be the end result. So, be sure to check out a pain with your doctor rather than "toughing it out."

Articular cartilage, that Teflon-type material within the joints, requires regular mechanical stress and loading to remain healthy. Too much or too little stress causes weakening of the cartilage and eventually may lead to arthritis and stiffness of the joints.

I frequently see cartilage that has become weakened in people who fractured their ankle and were put in a cast for several weeks. Although the fractures heal, the cartilage of the immobilized leg gets thinner because there has been no stimulation to provide nutrients to the area. This leads to early degeneration and arthritis or stiffness in the joint. The skeleton must be kept active to facilitate adequate blood supply. *Cartilage deterioration comes not from the aging process but from inactivity.*

At times, a doctor presupposes that older athletes with a knee problem have arthritis and tells them to decrease their training. By assuming that all joint pain is arthritis, based on the age of the patient, the doctor will not look further for possible injury. However, a master athlete who has been training may have torn the cartilage within the knee joints. A torn cartilage, as distinct from arthritis, needs immediate diagnosis and treatment such as removal of the torn portion. Without appropriate treatment, these master athletes are at greater risk of developing degenerative knee changes. For more information on arthritis see Chapter 17.

Skeletal Muscles

As far as muscles go, there is little evidence of any major changes in muscular structure before the age of seventy, although there is some increase in stiffness and decrease in elasticity. Muscle strength decreases beyond the age of fifty. By age sixty-five, you still have 75 to 80 percent of your peak strength. Stretching and aerobic activity will keep your muscles strong and supple.

The Active Elder

Age and disease are not synonymous. Disease is caused by inactivity on all levels—spiritual, mental, emotional and physical. Senior athletes such as Walt Stack and thousands of others prove everyday that activity and enthusiasm for life leads to more life—not degeneration. People who stay active and have hobbies do well and live longer than those who give up and sit down. Whatever you do—do something, and do it with zest and regularity. Celebrate your age. Remember what author Henri-Frederic Amiel said in 1883 in his *Journal Intime:*[2]

> To know how to grow old is the masterwork of wisdom, and one of the most difficult chapters in the great art of living.

Footnote:

1. D. Costill: "Physiologic basis for training," Track & Field News Publications, Palo Alto, CA. 1979.

2. Henri, Frederick Amiel, *Journal Intime,* Edmond Scherer, 1883.

Chapter 20

TREATMENT RESOURCE GUIDE

How to Find a Homeopath in Your Area

To find a homeopath in your area, check the yellow pages of your telephone directory under Physicians, Homeopathy. If you do not find a listing for a homeopath, call one of the homeopathic organizations listed below for information.

All of the pharmacies and homeopathic businesses listed here offer mail-order services. In addition to the companies listed, many health food stores and conventional pharmacies also carry homeopathic remedies.

I recommend that you purchase a home remedy kit in order to be prepared for common ailments and injuries. Also, it is more economical to buy a kit than to buy remedies individually.

Sources of Homeopathic Medicines

Ainsworth's Homoeopathic Pharmacy
38 New Cavendish Street
London, W1M 7LH, England

BHI-Heel (Biological Homeopathic Industries)
11600 Cochiti SE
Albuquerque, New Mexico 87123
800-621-7644
Note: BHI carries injectable homeopathic medicines for intra-articular, intra-fascial or soft tissue injections for health practitioners. They have combinational medicines (oral, topical, and injectable) as well as single remedies; they manufacture Traumeel (often used in sports injuries), Lymphomosot, BHI-Arthritis and BHI-Coenzyme.

Boericke and Tafel, Inc.
2381 Circadian Way
Santa Rosa, CA 95407
707-571-8202 or 800-876-9505

Boiron-Bornemann, Inc.
1208 Amosland Road
Norwood, PA 19074
215-532-2035 or 800-258-8823

Dolisos America
3014 Rigel Avenue
Las Vegas, NV 89103
702-871-7153 or 800-824-8455

**Hahnemann Homeopathic
Pharmacy**
1918 Bonita Avenue
Berkeley, CA 94704
510-548-5015

Helios Homoeopathic Pharmacy
92 Camden Road
Tunbridge Wells, Kent TNI
2QP, England

**Homeopathic Educational
Services***
2124 Kittredge Street
Berkeley, CA 94704
510-649-0294
800-359-9051 (for orders only)

Luyties Pharmacal Company
4200 Laclede Avenue
St. Louis, MO 63108
314-533-9600 or 800-325-8080

A. Nelson & Co. Ltd.
5 Endeavour Way
Wimbledon SW19 9U1T
England

Standard Homeopathy
210 W. 131st Street
Los Angeles, CA 90061
213-321-4284 or 800-624-9659

**D.L. Thompson
Homoeopathic Supplies**
844 Yonge Street
Toronto 5, Ontario, Canada
M4W 2H1

*Homeopathic Educational
Services is the largest seller of
homeopathic books, tapes, and
software. Contact them for their
complete catalog.

Homeopathic Organizations

**National Center
for Homeopathy**
801 N. Fairfax #306
Alexandria, VA 22314
703-548-7790

**American Institute
of Homeopathy**
1585 Glencoe
Denver, CO 80220
800-848-5477

376

**International Foundation
for Homeopathy**
    2366 Eastlake Avenue E.
    Suite 301
    Seattle, Washington 98101
    206-324-8230

**California State Homeopathic
Medical Society**
    Richard Hiltner, M.D.,
    President
    169 East El Roblar
    Ojai, CA 93023
    805-646-1495

**Pacific Academy
of Homeopathic Medicine**
    1678 Shattuck Avenue #42
    Berkeley, CA 94709
    510-549-3475

**British Homoeopathic
Association**
    27A Devonshire Street
    London, WIN IRJ, England

Society of Homoeopaths
    2 Astrian Road
    Northampton NN14HU,
    England

Holistic Health Resources

Individual practitioners can be found in local newspapers
distributed free in health food stores in most areas.

American Holistic Medical Association
    6932 Little River Turnpike
    Annandale VA 22003
    703-642-5880

Natural Medicine

**National College of
Naturopathic Medicine**
    11231 SE Market Street
    Portland OR 97216
    503-255-4860

**Ontario College of
Naturopathic Medicine**
    60 Berl Street
    Toronto, Ontatio, M8Y 3C7
    Canada

**John Bastyr College of
Naturopathic Medicine**
    144 54th Street
    Seattle, WA 98105
    206-523-9585

Herbal Medicine

Herbal Studies Course
219 Carl Street
San Francisco CA 94117

Herb Research Foundation
1007 Pearl Street, #200
Boulder, CO 80302

Manipulative Therapies

For Sports Massage:

The American Massage Therapy Association
Department of Information
1130 West North Shore
Avenue, Chicago, IL 60626
312-761-2682.

American Osteopathic Association
212 East Ohio Street
Chicago IL 60611
312-280-5800

American Healing Academy
(for craniosacral therapy)
PO Box 4175
San Francisco, CA 94101
415-753-2615

For Physiatrists:

The American Academy of Physical Medicine and Rehabilitation
122 South Michigan Avenue,
Suite 1300
Chicago, IL 60603-6107
312-922-9366

The Association of Academic Physiatrists
8000 Five Mile Road,
Suite 340
Cincinnati, OH 45230
513-232-8833

The National Chronic Pain Outreach Association
4922 Hampden Lane
Bethesda, MD 20814
301-652-4948

American Chiropractic Association
1916 Wilson Blvd. Suite 300
Arlington VA 22201
703-276-8800

Palmer College of Chiropractic
1000 Grady Street
Davenport IA 52803
319-324-1611

Body Work Therapies

Body Therapy Center
368 California Ave.
Palo Alto, CA 94306
415-328-9400

Rolf Institute
PO Box 1868
Boulder CO 80302
303-449-5903

Hellerwork
415 Mt. Shasta Blvd. #4
Mt. Shasta, CA 96067
916-926-2500

**The American Center
for the Alexander Technique**
142 West End Avenue
New York NY 10023
212-799-0468

Lomi Bodywork School
222 Grahn Drive
Santa Rosa, CA 95404

For Therapeutic Touch:

**Nurse Healers and Professional
Associates Cooperative, Inc.**
175 Fifth Avenue
Suite 3399
New York, NY 10010.

**Reiki—
Trinity Metaphysical Center**
227 Highland Terrace
Woodside, CA 94062

**Trager Institute
for Psychophysical Integration
and Mentastics**
300 Poplar Avenue
Mill Valley CA 94941
415-388-2688

Feldenkrais Guild
PO Box 11145
San Francisco CA 94101
415-550-8708

**International Institute
of Reflexology**
Box 12462
St Petersburg FL 33733
813-343-4811

The Rosen Institute
2315 Prince Street
Berkeley, CA 94705
510-845-6606

Touch For Health Foundation
1174 North Lake Avenue
Pasadena CA 91104
213-794-1181

Asian Therapies

Center for Chinese Medicine
2303 S. Garfield Avenue,
Suite 202
Montcrey Park, CA 91754
213-573-4141

American College of Traditional Chinese Medicine
455 Arkansas
San Francisco, CA 94107

Academy of Chinese Culture
420 14th Street
Oakland, CA 94612
510-763-7787

Acupressure Institute
1533 Shattuck Avenue
Berkeley, CA 94709
510-845-1059

Emperor's College of Traditional Oriental Medicine
2515 Wilshire Blvd
Santa Monica, CA 90403
213-453-8833

Five Branches Institute
College and Clinic of
Traditional Chinese
Medicine
200 Seventh Avenue
Santa Cruz, CA 95062
408-476-9424

Movement Therapies

Integral Yoga Institute
227 West 13th Street
New York, NY 10011
212-929-0586

American Dance Therapy Association
2000 Century Plaza, Suite 230
Columbia, MD 21044
301-997-4040

Siddha Foundation
PO Box 600
South Fallsburg, NY 12729
914-434-2000

Internal Spiritual Martial Arts

Almost every urban area in the United States has Aikido dojos and T'ai Chi schools. See local free newspapers for schools near you.

U.S. Aikido Federation and New York Aikikai
142 West 18th Street
New York, NY 10011
212-242-6246

Aikido Today Magazine
Arete Press
480 West Sixth Street
Claremont, CA 91711

(contains listings of schools and articles about aikido)

Cheng Hsin School of Internal Martial Arts (T'ai Chi)
Peter Ralston, Director
6601 Telegraph Ave.
Oakland, Ca 94609
(510) 658-0802

Psychotherapy

American Psychological Association
1200 17th Street NW
Washington, DC 20036
202-833-7600

American Society of Clinical Hypnosis
2250 East Devon, Suite 336
Des Plaines, IL 60018
312-297-3317

Bodynamic Institute
959 Kains
Albany, CA 94706
510-526-6201

Alchemical Hypnotherapy Institute
2310 Warwick Drive
Santa Rosa, CA 95405
800-950-4984

Academy for Guided Imagery
PO Box 2070
Mill Valley, CA 94942
415-389-9324

California Institute of Integral Studies
Box CG, 765 Ashbury Street
San Francisco, CA 94117
415-753-6100

Silva Mind Control
6 East 39th Street
New York, NY 10016
212-684-6477

Biofeedback Society of America
4301 Owens Street
Wheatridge, CO 80033
303-420-2889

Paranormal Therapies

Healing Light Center
  204 East Wilson
  Glendale CA 91206
  213-244-8607

World Research Foundation
  15300 Ventura, Suite 405
  Sherman Oaks, CA 91403
  818-907-5483

The Radionic Association
  16a North Bar
  Oxfordshire OX16OTF
  England
  0295-3183

Homeopathic Remedies

Remedies mentioned in this book are listed alphabetically by their Latin names which are used worldwide, followed by their commonly used short name. The original substance from which they are derived is listed parenthetically.

Remedies are available in non-prescription potencies of 6, 12, 30x or c. (Lower case "x" indicates that there is one part homeopathic substance to nine parts alcohol/water solution. Lower case "c" indicates that there is one part homeopathic substance to ninety-nine parts alcohol/water solution). The more dilute the solution, the more potent. Potencies of M (one part homeopathic substance to 1,000 parts of solution) are available by prescription.

Aconitum Napellus, Aconite—(Monkshood)
Aethusa Cynapium, Aethusa—(Fool's Parsley)
Antimonium Crudum—(Black Sulphide of Antimony)
Apis Mellifica, Apis—(The Honey Bee)
Arnica—(Leopard's Bane)
Arsenicum Album—(Arsenious Acid)—Arsenic Trioxide
Baryta Carb—(Carbonate of Baryta)
Belladonna—(Deadly Nightshade)
Bellis Perennis, Bellis—(Daisy)
Benzoicum Acidum—(Benzoic Acid)
Bryonia—(Wild Hops)
Calcarea Arsenica—(Arsenite of Lime)
Calcarea Carbonica—Ostrearum, Calc Carb—(Carbonate of Lime)
Calcarea Fluorica—Fluor Spar, Calc Fluor—(Fluoride of Lime)
Calcarea Phosphorica, Calc Phos—(Phosphate of Lime)
Calcarea Silicata, Calc Sil—(Silicate of Lime)
Calcarea Sulphurica, Calc Sulph—(Sulphate of Lime-Plaster of Paris)
Calendula Officinalis, Calendula—(Marigold)
Cantharis—(Spanish Fly)
Causticum—(Hahnemann's Tinctura acris sine Kali)
Cimicifuga Racemosa, Cimicifuga—(Black Snake-root)

Cocculus—(Indian Cockle)
Colchicum—(Meadow Saffron)
Colocynthis—(Bitter Cucumber)
Cuprum Metallicum—(Copper)
Gelsemium—(Yellow Jasmine)
Glonoine—(Nitro-glycerine)
Graphites—(Black Lead)
Hamamelis Virginica—(Witch-hazel)
Hekla Lava—(Lava Scoriae from Mt. Hecla)
Hepar Sulphuris Calcareum, Hepar Sulph—(Hahnemann's Calcium Sulphide)
Hypericum—(St. John's-wort)
Ignatia—(St. Ignatius Bean)
Kali Bichromicum—(Bichromate of Potash)
Kali Carbonicum—(Carbonate of Potassium)
Ledum—(Marsh-Tea)
Lycopodium—(Club Moss)
Magnesia Phosphorica, Mag Phos—(Phosphate of Magnesia)
Natrum Carbonicum, Nat Carb—(Carbonate of Sodium)
Natrum Muriaticum, Nat Mur—(Chloride of Sodium)
Paeonia—(Peony)
Phytolacca—(Poke-root)
Pulsatilla—(Wind Flower)
Radium—(Radium Bromide)
Rhododendron P—(Snow Rose)
Rhus Toxicodendron, Rhus Tox—(Poison-ivy)
Ruta Graveolens, Ruta Grav—(Ruc-bitterwort)
Sabadilla—(Cevadilla Seed)
Sanguinaria—(Blood Root)
Staphysagria—(Stavesacre)
Stellaria Media—(Chickweed)
Symphytum—(Comfrey-Knitbone)
Thuja Occidentalis, Thuja—(Arbor vitae)
Urtica Urens—(Stinging-nettle)
Veratrum Album—(White Hellebore)

Index

References to figures are in **bold** type. Foreword and footnotes are not indexed.